Simple TOC

T0195465

MUSCULOSKELETAL ANATOMY COLORING BOOK

Fourth Edition

Joseph E. Muscolino, DC

Owner, The Art and Science of Kinesiology and Learnmuscles.com
Stamford, Connecticut

ELSEVIER

Elsevier
3251 Riverport Lane
St. Louis, Missouri 63043

MUSCULOSKELETAL ANATOMY COLORING BOOK, FOURTH EDITION ISBN: 978-0-323-87816-6
Copyright © 2024 by Elsevier Inc. All rights reserved.

Notice

Practitioners and researchers must always rely on their own experience and knowledge in evaluating and using any information, methods, compounds or experiments described herein. Because of rapid advances in the medical sciences, in particular, independent verification of diagnoses and drug dosages should be made. To the fullest extent of the law, no responsibility is assumed by Elsevier, authors, editors or contributors for any injury and/or damage to persons or property as a matter of products liability, negligence or otherwise, or from any use or operation of any methods, products, instructions, or ideas contained in the material herein.

Previous editions copyrighted 2018, 2010, and 2004.

Content Strategist: Melissa Rawe
Director, Content Development: Ellen Wurm-Cutter
Publishing Services Manager: Julie Eddy
Senior Project Manager: Cindy Thoms
Design Direction: Maggie Reid

Printed in India

Last digit is the print number: 9 8 7 6 5 4 3 2 1

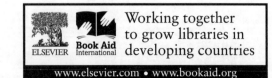

www.elsevier.com • www.bookaid.org

Introduction

Sciences have long been taught in a classroom format in which an instructor lectures to students and the students have textbooks to read at home. Unfortunately, lecture format and textbook reading do not cater to the kinesthetic element of learning that is present in all of us. Toward that end, coloring books of anatomy and physiology are useful tools for approaching and learning class material in a manner that is not possible via lecture and textbook format alone. However, I do not believe that coloring books should replace quality classroom instruction and quality textbooks; rather I believe that coloring books of anatomy and physiology are valuable adjunctive learning tools that should be used in conjunction with classroom learning and textbook reading.

For this reason, I recommend the *Musculoskeletal Anatomy Coloring Book* to aid you as you endeavor to learn the structure and function of the musculoskeletal system, as well as the other major systems of the human body. With regard to an adjunct textbook for learning muscles and how the musculoskeletal system functions, I recommend *The Muscular System Manual: The Skeletal Muscles of the Human Body, 5th edition* (Elsevier, 2024) and *Kinesiology: The Skeletal System and Muscle Function, 4th edition* (Elsevier, 2024). For learning the kinesthetic skill of muscle and bone palpation, I recommend *The Muscle and Bone Palpation Manual, 3rd edition* (Elsevier, 2023). Also, for quizzing muscle attachments and actions, I recommend the *Musculoskeletal Anatomy Flash Cards* available on the accompanying Evolve site.

Beyond being simply a coloring book, this book is also designed to help the reader learn the information in a number of ways. First, regarding muscles, the two hurdles for the new student are learning the attachments (origins and insertions) and actions of the muscles. In the part on muscles (Part 3), the text information of the attachments is written next to the locations on the illustration where the actual muscle attachments are located. As you color the muscles from attachment to attachment, I recommend that you integrate this written information by saying the attachments out loud. To help learn the actions of the muscles, arrows that visually demonstrate the line(s) of pull of the muscle have been placed within the muscle. As you color in these arrows, note the actions that are caused by the line of pull demonstrated by the arrows. Putting the attachment and action information together with the illustration, and kinesthetically coloring at the same time, allows for a fuller integration of the information that you need to learn!

This book is also designed to allow the student to quiz himself/herself. Throughout the book, wherever you find blank lead lines pointing to a structure, use that opportunity to quiz yourself on being able to identify the structure. The answer key starts on page 479. There are also quiz questions on muscle attachments and actions that are located at the end of each chapter of Part 3. Further, on each right-hand page of a two-page muscle spread in Part 3, there are illustrations showing the individual muscle being studied within its larger group of muscles. For another opportunity to quiz yourself, write in the directional terms around these illustrations (e.g., anterior, posterior, lateral, etc.). Check your answers by turning to the illustrations at the beginning of each chapter in Part 3.

Although this book covers every major system of the human body, its emphasis is the musculoskeletal system. More specifically, the major emphasis of this book is the muscular system.

This book is organized into four parts with sixteen chapters.

Part 1 is composed of Chapter 1 and contains essential information on kinesiology (essentially muscle structure and function). I strongly recommend reading this entire chapter before continuing with the rest of the book. It will give you a context to better understand all that you will be learning throughout Parts 2 and 3 of this book.

Part 2 is on the skeletal system and comprises Chapter 2, covering the bones of the body.

Part 3 is the core of the book and comprises Chapters 3-13, covering all the major skeletal muscles of the body.

Part 4 comprises Chapters 14-16 and covers the other systems of the body. More specifically, Chapters 14 and 15 cover the nervous system and arterial system, the understanding of which is important toward learning innervation and arterial supply to the skeletal muscles. Chapter 16 covers tissue structure and the other major systems of the human body.

The answer key to the self-testing pages that are included throughout the book is located after Chapter 16.

Regarding the use of colors, of course you may use any that you like to color the various structures. However, there are certain colors standardly used for the anatomical structures of the human body, and I recommend the following to you as guidelines:

- Red is classically used for blood vessels that carry "oxygenated" blood (arteries of the systemic circulation and veins of the pulmonic circulation) and blue is used for all blood vessels that carry "deoxygenated" blood (veins of the systemic circulation and arteries of the pulmonic circulation).
- Red is also used for coloring the muscles of the body. Therefore, to make muscles distinct from blood vessels that have been colored red, perhaps a different shade (I recommend a lighter shade) of red can be used for the muscles.
- The attachments of muscles (tendons and aponeuroses) and other fibrous fascia are usually colored white; given that the page is already white, you may simply leave them uncolored. However, since this is a coloring book and the purpose of this book is to learn kinesthetically by coloring, I recommend that you do color them. A light shade of color would be best.
- Yellow is classically used for nerves.
- As for coloring bones, I recommend the following:
  1. When coloring the bones in Chapter 2, color the entire bone lightly with a light shade of color, different from those used above; a light yellow to beige color is most often used. Then use a darker color to color over the landmarks on the bone that you feel are important to you and you want to learn. This will help these landmarks to stand out visually as well as help root them kinesthetically.
  2. When coloring the bones in Part 3, I recommend that you use a different color for each of the muscle's two bony attachments (if there are more than two different bony attachments for a particular muscle, you may use more colors). Further, I recommend that you color the attachment of the muscle that is usually fixed (i.e., the origin) with a darker color to convey upon it a feeling of being heavier and more stable. Conversely, I recommend that you use a lighter color for the attachment that usually moves (i.e., the insertion) to convey a feeling of being lighter and therefore more mobile.
- Cartilage is always lightly shaded; pale blue is usually used.
- When coloring the many systems of Chapter 16, beyond the conventionally used colors that are mentioned above, please note the following: the liver is usually a fairly dark brown, the gallbladder is usually green, fat is usually yellow, lymph is usually green, and the brain and spinal cord are usually a light brown.
- The purpose of this book is for you to learn by coloring, and hopefully enjoy yourself along the way. If you prefer to use colors different from those recommended above, and it will add to your enjoyment and learning,

please do so. They are only guidelines. Most important is that you enjoy and learn!

Because this is a coloring book and not a textbook, the text in this book has been kept to a minimum. This has been done for two reasons: (1) excessive text tends to clutter the page and obscure visualization of the structures being colored and learned; and (2) the inclusion of text forces the illustrations to be smaller, which also makes visualization and coloring more difficult. Further, I feel that coloring books are best used as adjuncts to textbooks, not as a replacement. Although this coloring book can certainly stand on its own, in many ways it is a companion to *The Muscular System Manual: The Skeletal Muscles of the Human Body, 5th edition* (Elsevier, 2024), which is strongly recommended for students wishing to learn more about the musculoskeletal system. Having said this, a new chapter on muscle function has been added to allow this book to stand better on its own, when needed.

However, since an understanding of what is being colored is crucial, and the handiness of having some of that information accessible in the same book is helpful, the introductory text in Chapters 3 and 16 are included. Chapter 3's introduction is a very practical approach that gives you a method to understand how muscles work; the more you understand, the less you have to memorize! Chapter 16's introduction is a brief overview of each of the major systems of the body. I strongly recommend reading these two introductory sections before diving into the coloring.

ACKNOWLEDGMENTS

I would like to begin by thanking Barry Antoniow in Canada for first giving me the idea to develop a musculoskeletal anatomy coloring book. It has been long needed, and I appreciate Barry's insight. Since so much of the artwork for this coloring book has come from the *Muscular System Manual,* I would like to acknowledge the beautiful, crisp, and clear illustrations drawn by the artists of that book: the principal artist, Jean Luciano; and the additional artists, Rosa Cervoni, Barbara Haeger, and J.C. Muscolino. The quality of these illustrations greatly aids the reader in learning musculoskeletal anatomy. And I thank the entire crew over at Elsevier for their work in creating this book: Melissa Rawe, Content Strategist; Ellen Wurm-Cutter, Director, Content Development; Cindy Thoms, Senior Project Manager; and Maggie Reid, Senior Book Designer.

I must thank my entire family for their unending support as I spent hour after hour at the computer working on this book. Without their unconditional support, none of this would have been possible.

Lastly, I would like to say that studying by using coloring books has to be one of the more creative and fun ways to learn anatomy. For this reason, I would like to dedicate this book to my children, Randi and J.C., who have consistently taught me to try to keep creativity and fun in my approach to life.

Table of Contents

CHAPTER 6 MUSCLES OF THE PELVIS, 183

CHAPTER 7 MUSCLES OF THE THIGH, 213

CHAPTER 8 MUSCLES OF THE LEG, 251

CHAPTER 12 MUSCLES OF THE HAND, 391

CHAPTER 13 OTHER SKELETAL MUSCLES, 413

PART 4 NEUROVASCULAR SYSTEM, TISSUE STRUCTURES, AND OTHER SYSTEMS OF THE BODY

CHAPTER 14 THE NERVOUS SYSTEM, 423

How Muscles Function: The Big Picture

1

OVERVIEW

This chapter has two major thrusts: it explores the "big picture" of how muscles function concentrically (i.e., contracting and shortening) to create joint actions, and it offers easy methods that can be used by the student to learn muscles. Regarding muscle concentric contraction function, this chapter explores the idea of fixed versus mobile attachments of a muscle and introduces the concept of a muscle's reverse action(s). Included in this discussion is an exploration of the lines of the pull of a muscle and how they affect the possible actions of the muscle. Other, more advanced topics such as how a muscle can transfer the force of its contraction to another joint that it does not cross and how a muscle's actions can change with a change in joint position are also explored. Regarding learning muscles, a five-step approach to learning muscles is presented in this chapter. This five-step approach breaks the process of learning the attachments and actions of a muscle into five easy and logical steps. Particularly important is step 3, which shows how to figure out what the actions of a muscle are instead of having to memorize them. Specifically for the rotation actions of a muscle, the *off-axis attachment* method is explained. For kinesthetic learners, a rubber band exercise is given to further facilitate learning muscles. Continuing the process of learning muscles, a functional group approach is then given that greatly decreases the amount of time necessary to learn the actions of muscles.

SECTION 1.1 "BIG PICTURE" OF MUSCLE STRUCTURE AND FUNCTION

- A muscle attaches, via its tendons, from one bone to another bone. In so doing, a muscle crosses the joint that is located between the two bones (Figure 1.1).
- When a muscle contracts, it creates a pulling force on its attachments that attempts to pull them toward each

other. In other words, this pulling force attempts to shorten the muscle toward its center. To understand how a muscle creates a pulling force, it is necessary to understand the sliding filament mechanism.

- If the muscle is successful in shortening toward its center, then one or both of the bones to which it is attached will have to move (Figure 1.2).
- Because the bony attachments of the muscle are within body parts, if the muscle moves a bone, then the body part that the bone is within is moved. In this way, muscles can cause movement of parts of the body.
- When a muscle contracts and shortens as described here, this type of contraction is called a **concentric contraction**, and the muscle that is concentrically contracting is called a **mover**.[1]
- Note: A muscle can contract and not shorten! A muscle contraction that does not result in shortening is called an *eccentric contraction* or *isometric contraction*.[2]
- It is worth noting that whether or not a muscle is successful in shortening toward its center is determined by the strength of the pulling force of the muscle compared with the force necessary to actually move one or both body parts to which the muscle is attached.
- The force necessary to move a body part is usually the force necessary to move the weight of the body part. However, other forces may be involved.

SECTION 1.2 WHAT HAPPENS WHEN A MUSCLE CONTRACTS AND SHORTENS?

- Assuming that a muscle contracts with sufficient strength to shorten toward its center (i.e., concentrically contract), it is helpful to look at the possible scenarios that can occur.
- If we call one of the attachments of the muscle *Bone A* and the other attachment of the muscle *Bone B,* then we see that three possible scenarios exist (Figure 1.3)[3]:
  1. *Bone A* will be pulled toward *Bone B.*

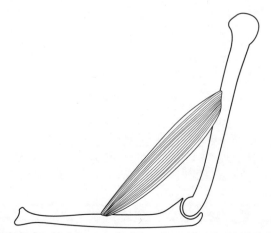

Figure 1.1 A generic muscle is shown; it attaches from one bone to another bone and crosses the joint that is located between them.

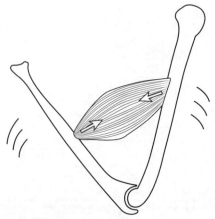

Figure 1.2 Muscle shown contracting and shortening (i.e., a concentric contraction).

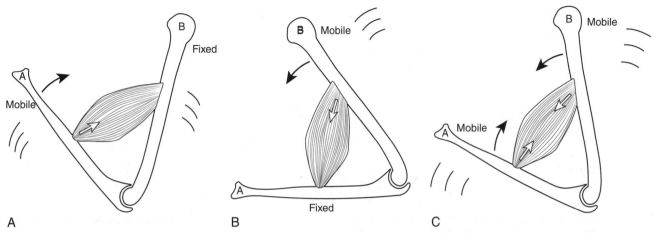

Figure 1.3 The three scenarios of a muscle contracting and shortening. In **A,** bone A moves toward bone B. In **B,** bone B moves toward bone A. In **C,** bone A and bone B both move toward each other.

2. *Bone B* will be pulled toward *Bone A.*
3. Both *Bone A* and *Bone B* will be pulled toward each other.

- Essentially, when a muscle contracts, its freest attachment moves.
- If an attachment of the muscle moves, it is said to be the mobile attachment. If an attachment of the muscle does not move, it is said to be the **fixed attachment** or **stabilized attachment**.[4]
- Note: We usually think of a typical muscle as having two attachments and a typical muscle contraction as having one of its attachments fixed and its other attachment mobile. However, it is possible for a muscle to contract and have both of its attachments mobile, as seen in Figure 1.3C. It is also possible for a muscle to contract and have both of its attachments fixed (as occurs during isometric contractions).
- When a muscle contracts and one of its attachments moves, the muscle creates a joint action. To fully describe this joint action, we must state three things[5]:
  1. The type of motion that has occurred
  2. The name of the body part that has moved
  3. The name of the joint where the movement has occurred

As an example to illustrate these concepts, it is helpful to look at the brachialis muscle. One attachment of the brachialis is onto the humerus of the arm, and the other attachment is onto the ulna of the forearm. In attaching to the arm and the forearm, the brachialis crosses the elbow joint that is located between these two body parts (Figure 1.4).

When the brachialis contracts, it attempts to shorten toward its center by exerting a pulling force on the forearm and the arm.

- Scenario 1: The usual result of the brachialis contracting is that the forearm will be pulled toward the arm.

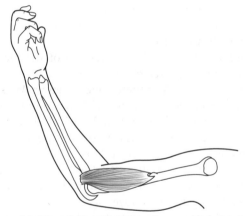

Figure 1.4 The right brachialis muscle at rest (medial view).

This is because the forearm is lighter than the arm and therefore would be more likely to move before the arm would. (In addition, if the arm were to move, the trunk would have to move as well, which makes it even less likely that the arm will be the attachment that moves.) To fully describe this action, we call it *flexion of the forearm at the elbow joint*, because the forearm is the body part that has moved and the elbow joint has flexed (Figure 1.5A). In this scenario, the arm is the attachment that is fixed and the forearm is the attachment that is mobile.

- Scenario 2: However, it is possible for the arm to move toward the forearm. If the forearm were to be fixed in place, perhaps because the hand is holding onto an immovable object, then the arm would have to move instead. This action is called *flexion of the arm at the elbow joint* because the arm is the body part that has moved and the elbow joint has flexed (see Figure 1.5B). In this scenario, the forearm is the attachment that is

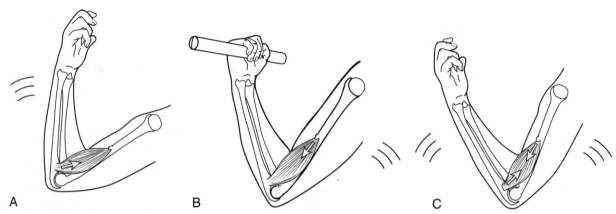

Figure 1.5 The three scenarios that can result from a shortening (i.e., concentric) contraction of the brachialis muscle. **A,** Flexion of the forearm at the elbow joint. **B,** Flexion of the arm at the elbow joint. **C,** Flexion of the forearm and the arm at the elbow joint.

fixed, and the arm is the attachment that is mobile. This scenario can be called a **reverse action**, because the attachment that is usually fixed, the arm, is now mobile, and the attachment that is usually mobile, the forearm, is now fixed.[6]

- Scenario 3: Because the contraction of the brachialis exerts a pulling force on the forearm and the arm, it is possible for both of these bones to move. When this occurs, two actions take place: (1) flexion of the forearm at the elbow joint and (2) flexion of the arm at the elbow joint (see Figure 1.5C). In this case, both bones are mobile and neither one is fixed.
- It is important to realize that the brachialis does not intend or choose which attachment will move or if both attachments will move.
- When a muscle contracts, it merely exerts a pulling force toward its center. Which attachment moves is determined by other factors. The relative weight of the body parts is the most common factor.
- However, another common determinant is when the central nervous system directs another muscle in the body to contract, which may stop or "fix" one of the attachments of the mover muscle. If this occurs, this second muscle that contracts to fix a body part would be called a **fixator** or **stabilizer** muscle.[7]
- It follows that if a muscle does successfully shorten, and one attachment is fixed, then the other attachment must be mobile.

SECTION 1.3 FIVE-STEP APPROACH TO LEARNING MUSCLES

- Essentially, to learn about muscles, two major aspects must be learned: (1) the attachments of the muscle and (2) the actions of the muscle.
- Generally speaking, the attachments of a muscle must be memorized. However, times exist when clues are given about the attachments by the muscle's name.[4]

- For example, the name *coracobrachialis* tells us that this muscle has one attachment on the coracoid process of the scapula and that its other attachment is on the brachium (i.e., the humerus).
- Similarly, the name *zygomaticus major* tells us that this muscle attaches onto the zygomatic bone (and that it is bigger than another muscle called the *zygomaticus minor*).
- Unlike muscle attachments, muscle actions do not have to be memorized. Instead, through an understanding of the simple concept that a muscle pulls at its attachments to move a body part, the action or actions of a muscle can be reasoned out.

Five-Step Approach to Learning Muscles

- When a student is first confronted with having to study and learn about a muscle, the following five-step approach is recommended:
  - Step 1: Look at the name of the muscle to see if it gives you any "free information" that saves you from having to memorize attachments or actions of the muscle.
  - Step 2: Learn the general location of the muscle well enough to be able to visualize the muscle on your body. At this point, you need only know it well enough to know:
    - What joint it crosses
    - Where it crosses the joint
    - How it crosses the joint (i.e., the direction in which its fibers are running)
  - Step 3: Use this general knowledge of the muscle's location (step 2) to figure out its actions.
  - Step 4: Go back and learn (memorize, if necessary) the specific attachments of the muscle.
  - Step 5: Now look at the relationship of this muscle to other muscles (and other soft tissue structures)

of the body. Look at the following: Is this muscle superficial or deep? In addition, what other muscles (and other soft tissue structures) are located near this muscle?

Figuring Out a Muscle's Actions (Step 3 in Detail)

- Once you have a general familiarity with a muscle's location on the body, then it is time to begin the process of reasoning out the actions of the muscle. The most important thing that you must look at is the following:
  - The direction of the muscle fibers relative to the joint that it crosses

  By doing this, you can see the following:
  - The line of pull of the muscle relative to the joint. (When a muscle contracts, it creates a *pulling* force. It is this pulling force that can create motion—in other words, joint actions. Note: Muscles do not push, they *pull*!)
  - This line of pull will determine the actions of the muscle[6] (i.e., how the contraction of the muscle will cause the body parts to move at that joint).
  - The best approach is to ask the following three questions:
  1. What joint does the muscle cross?
  2. Where does the muscle cross the joint?
  3. How does the muscle cross the joint?

Question 1—What Joint Does the Muscle Cross?

- The first question to ask and answer in figuring out the action(s) of a muscle is to simply know what joint it crosses.
- The following rule applies: If a muscle crosses a joint, then it can have an action at that joint.[5] (Note: This, of course, assumes that the joint is healthy and allows movement to occur.)
  - For example, if we look at the coracobrachialis, knowing that it crosses the glenohumeral (GH) joint tells us that it must have an action at the GH joint.
  - We may not know what the exact action of the coracobrachialis is yet, but at least we now know at what joint it has its actions.
  - To figure out exactly what these actions are, we need to look at questions 2 and 3.
- Note: It is worth pointing out that the converse of the rule about a muscle having the ability to create movement (i.e., an action) at a joint that it crosses is also true. In other words, if a muscle does not cross a joint, then it cannot have an action at that joint. However, this rule is not 100% accurate. Sometimes the force of a muscle can be transferred to another joint, even if the muscle does not cross that joint.[5]

Questions 2 and 3—Where Does the Muscle Cross the Joint? How Does the Muscle Cross the Joint?

- Questions 2 and 3 must be looked at together.
- The *where* of a muscle crossing a joint is whether it crosses the joint anteriorly, posteriorly, medially, or laterally.

- It is helpful to place a muscle into one of these broad groups because the following general rules apply: muscles that cross a joint anteriorly will usually flex a body part at that joint, and muscles that cross a joint posteriorly will usually extend a body part at that joint; muscles that cross a joint laterally will usually abduct or laterally flex a body part at that joint, and muscles that cross a joint medially will usually adduct a body part at that joint.[6]
  - Notes: (1) Flexion is nearly always an anterior movement of a body part, and extension is nearly always a posterior movement of a body part. However, from the knee joint and farther distal, flexion is a posterior movement and extension is an anterior movement of the body part. (2) Abduction occurs at joints of the appendicular skeleton; lateral flexion occurs at joints of the axial skeleton.
- The *how* of a muscle crossing a joint is whether it crosses the joint with its fibers running vertically or horizontally. This is also very important.
  - To illustrate this idea, we will look at the pectoralis major muscle. The pectoralis major has two parts: (1) a clavicular head and (2) a sternocostal head. The *where* of these two heads of the pectoralis major crossing the GH joint is the same (i.e., they both cross the GH joint anteriorly). However, the *how* of these two heads crossing the GH joint is very different. The clavicular head crosses the GH joint with its fibers running primarily vertically; therefore, it flexes the arm at the GH joint (because it pulls the arm upward in the sagittal plane, which is termed *flexion*). However, the sternocostal head crosses the GH joint with its fibers running horizontally; therefore, it adducts the arm at the GH joint (because it pulls the arm from lateral to medial in the frontal plane, which is termed *adduction*).[5]
- With a muscle that has a horizontal direction to its fibers, another factor must be considered when looking at *how* this muscle crosses the joint (i.e., whether the muscle attaches to the first place on the bone that it reaches, or whether the muscle wraps around the bone before attaching to it). Muscles that run horizontally (in the transverse plane) and wrap around the bone before attaching to it create a rotation action when they contract and pull on the attachment.[5]
  - For example, the sternocostal head of the pectoralis major does not attach to the first point on the humerus that it reaches. Instead, it continues to wrap around the shaft of the humerus to attach onto the lateral lip of the bicipital groove of the humerus. When the sternocostal head pulls, it medially rotates the arm at the GH joint (in addition to its other actions).

- In essence, by asking the three questions of step 3 of the five-step approach to learning muscles (What joint does a muscle cross? Where does the muscle cross the joint? How does the muscle cross the joint?), we are trying to determine the direction of the muscle fibers relative to the joint. Determining this will give us the line of pull of the muscle relative to the joint, and that will give us the actions of the muscle—saving us the trouble of having to memorize this information!

SECTION 1.4 **RUBBER BAND EXERCISE**

Visual and Kinesthetic Exercise for Learning a Muscle's Actions

Rubber Band Exercise

- An excellent method for learning the actions of a muscle is to place a large colorful rubber band (or large colorful shoelace or string) on your body, or the body of a partner, in the same location that the muscle you are studying is located.
- Hold one end of the rubber band at one of the attachment sites of the muscle, and hold the other end of the rubber band at the other attachment site of the muscle.
- Make sure that you have the rubber band running/oriented in the same direction as the direction of the fibers of the muscle. If it is not uncomfortable, you may even loop or tie the rubber band (or shoelace) around the body parts that are the attachments of the muscle.
- Once you have the rubber band in place, pull one of the ends of the rubber band toward the other attachment of the rubber band to see the action that the rubber band/muscle has on that body part's attachment. Once done, return the attachment of the rubber band to where it began and repeat this exercise for the other end of the rubber band to see the action that the rubber band/muscle has on the other attachment of the muscle.
- By placing the rubber band on your body or your partner's body, you are simulating the direction of the muscle's fibers relative to the joint that it crosses.
- By pulling either end of the rubber band toward the center, you are simulating the line of pull of the muscle relative to the joint that it crosses. The resultant movements that occur are the actions that the muscle would have. This is an excellent exercise both to visually see the actions of a muscle and to kinesthetically experience the actions of a muscle.
- This exercise can be used to learn all muscle actions and can be especially helpful for determining actions that may be a little more difficult to visualize, such as rotation actions.
- Note: The use of a large colorful rubber band is more helpful than a shoelace or string, because when you stretch out a rubber band and place it in the location

that a muscle would be, the natural elasticity of a rubber band creates a pull on the attachment sites that nicely simulates the pull of a muscle on its attachments when it contracts.
- If you can, you should work with a partner to do this exercise. Have your partner hold one of the "attachments" of the rubber band while you hold the other "attachment." This leaves one of your hands free to pull one of the rubber band attachment sites toward the center.
- A further note of caution: If you are using a rubber band, be careful that you do not accidentally let go and have the rubber band hit you or your partner. For this reason, it would be preferable to use a shoelace or string instead of a rubber band when working near the face.

SECTION 1.5 **LINES OF PULL OF A MUSCLE**

- Because the line of pull of a muscle relative to the joint it crosses determines the actions that it has, it is extremely important to fully understand the line or lines of the pull of a muscle.[6]
- It is helpful to examine four scenarios regarding a muscle and its line or lines of pull:
  - Scenario 1: A muscle with one line of pull in a cardinal plane
  - Scenario 2: A muscle with one line of pull in an oblique plane
  - Scenario 3: A muscle that has more than one line of pull
  - Scenario 4: A muscle that crosses more than one joint

Scenario 1—A Muscle With One Line of Pull in a Cardinal Plane

- If a muscle has one line of pull and that line of pull lies perfectly in a cardinal plane, then that muscle will have one action (plus the reverse action of that action).
- A perfect example is the brachialis muscle. The brachialis crosses the elbow joint anteriorly with a vertical direction to its fibers. All of its fibers are essentially running parallel to one another and are oriented in the sagittal plane. Therefore, the brachialis has one action, namely flexion of the forearm at the elbow joint[5] (as well as its reverse action of flexion of the arm at the elbow joint). The brachialis' line of pull is in the sagittal plane; therefore, the action that it creates must be in the sagittal plane, and that action is flexion (Figure 1.6).

Scenario 2—A Muscle With One Line of Pull in an Oblique Plane

- If a muscle has one line of pull, but that line of pull is in an oblique plane, then the muscle will create movement in that oblique plane. However, when this movement is named, no name for oblique-plane movement

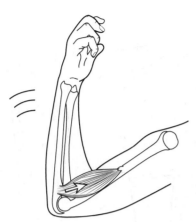

Figure 1.6 The brachialis muscle has one line of pull to its fibers, and that line of pull is located within the sagittal plane; therefore, the brachialis can flex the elbow joint.

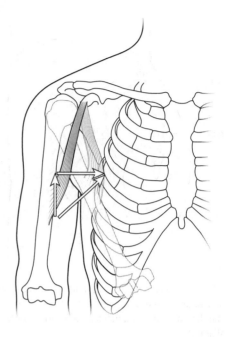

Figure 1.7 Illustration of the motion that is caused when the coracobrachialis contracts (with the scapula fixed and the humerus mobile). This one oblique-plane motion (*yellow arrow*) must be broken down into its two cardinal-plane actions (*green arrows*) when the joint actions of the coracobrachialis are discussed.

exists. Instead, this movement has to be broken up into names for its component cardinal-plane actions.

- An excellent example is the coracobrachialis. The coracobrachialis has a line of pull that is in an oblique plane. That oblique plane is a combination of sagittal and frontal cardinal planes. When the coracobrachialis pulls, it pulls the arm diagonally in a direction that is both anterior and medial at the same time. However, no one name for this oblique-plane motion exists. To name this one motion that would occur, we must break it up into its component cardinal-plane actions of flexion in the sagittal plane and adduction in the frontal plane. Therefore, even though the muscle actually creates only one movement in an oblique plane, we describe it as having two cardinal-plane actions (Figure 1.7).[1]
- For this reason, a muscle that has one line of pull can be said to have more than one cardinal-plane action if that muscle's line of pull is oriented within an oblique plane. Of course, for each of its actions, a reverse action is theoretically possible.

Scenario 3—A Muscle That Has More Than One Line of Pull

- If a muscle has more than one line of pull, then we apply the same logic that was used in scenarios 1 and 2 to this muscle.
- For each line of pull that is oriented perfectly in a cardinal plane, there will be one action possible (along with the corresponding reverse action).
- For each oblique-plane line of pull, the movement that occurs in that oblique plane can be broken up into its separate cardinal-plane components (with their corresponding reverse actions).
  - An example is the gluteus medius. The gluteus medius has posterior fibers, middle fibers, and

anterior fibers, each with a different line of pull on the femur at the hip joint. The posterior fibers pull in an oblique plane; the cardinal-plane components of this oblique plane are extension in the sagittal plane, abduction in the frontal plane, and lateral rotation in the transverse plane. The anterior fibers also pull in an oblique plane; their cardinal-plane components are flexion in the sagittal plane, abduction in the frontal plane, and medial rotation in the transverse plane. However, the middle fibers are oriented perfectly in the frontal plane; therefore, their only action is abduction in the frontal plane.[5] In this example, the posterior and anterior fibers fit scenario 2 (one line of pull in an oblique plane), and the middle fibers fit scenario 1 (one line of pull in a cardinal plane) (Figure 1.8). (Note: The reverse actions of the gluteus medius are movements of the pelvis toward the thigh at the hip joint.)

Scenario 4—A Muscle That Crosses More Than One Joint

- If a muscle crosses only one joint, it is termed a **one-joint muscle**; if a muscle crosses more than one joint, it is termed a **multijoint muscle**.
- If a muscle is a multijoint muscle, then the reasoning that is applied at one joint for each line of pull that

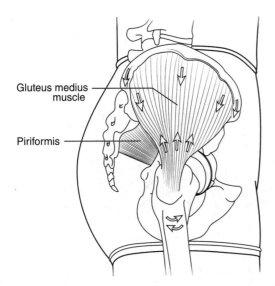

Figure 1.8 Gluteus medius muscle. The gluteus medius has posterior fibers and anterior fibers that are each oriented in an oblique plane. The middle fibers of the gluteus medius are oriented directly in a cardinal plane.

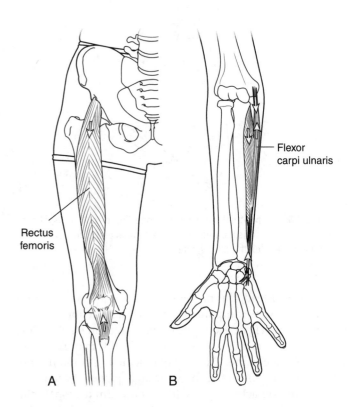

Figure 1.9 Whenever a muscle crosses more than one joint (i.e., is a multijoint muscle), it can create movement at each of the joints that it crosses. **A,** Rectus femoris (of the quadriceps femoris group), which crosses both the hip and knee joints. **B,** Flexor carpi ulnaris, which crosses the elbow joint and also crosses the wrist joint.

the muscle has is applied at each joint that the muscle crosses.

- Many multijoint muscles exist in the human body.
- Examples include the following:
  - The rectus femoris of the quadriceps femoris group crosses the knee and hip joints with one line of pull. Therefore, it can extend the leg at the knee joint in the sagittal plane, and it can flex the thigh at the hip joint in the sagittal plane[5] (as well as create the corresponding reverse actions) (Figure 1.9A).
  - The flexor carpi ulnaris crosses the elbow joint with one line of pull in a cardinal plane and crosses the wrist joint with one line of pull in an oblique plane. Therefore, it can flex the forearm at the elbow joint in the sagittal plane, and it can flex and ulnar deviate (i.e., adduct) the hand at the wrist joint in the sagittal and frontal planes, respectively[5] (as well as create the corresponding reverse actions) (see Figure 1.9B).

Can a Muscle Choose Which of Its Actions Will Occur?

- No. Muscles are simply machines that contract when they are ordered to contract by the nervous system. If a muscle contracts, then whichever motor units are ordered to contract have every muscle fiber within them contract and attempt to shorten.[8] Whatever line of pull these fibers lie within will have a pulling force created that will pull on the attachments of the muscle. When a muscle has only one line of pull, it must attempt to create every action that would occur from that one line

of pull. Only muscles that have more than one line of pull can attempt to create certain actions and not other actions. This occurs when the central nervous system directs to contract motor units that lie within only one line of pull of the muscle (and does not direct to contract motor units that lie within other lines of pull). An example is the trapezius. It has three parts: (1) upper, (2) middle, and (3) lower. Each part has its own line of pull. The upper trapezius can be ordered to contract without the middle or lower parts being ordered to contract. In this manner, a muscle with more than one line of pull can attempt to create some of its actions and not others.[5] Other examples of muscles with more than one line of pull are the deltoid and gluteus medius.

Therefore, we can state the following two rules:
- A muscle with one line of pull attempts to create every one of its actions when it contracts.
- A muscle with more than one line of pull does not necessarily attempt to create every one of its actions when it contracts. It may attempt to create the action(s) of one of its lines of pull without creating the action(s) of another of its lines of pull.

SECTION 1.6 FUNCTIONAL GROUP APPROACH TO LEARNING MUSCLE ACTIONS

- The best method for approaching and learning each action of a new muscle that you first encounter is to use the reasoning of step 3 of the five-step approach. For each aspect of the direction of fibers for a muscle, you apply the questions of *where* and *how* the muscle crosses the joint. This reasoning is solid and will lead you to reason out all actions of the muscle that is being studied.
- However, it can be very repetitive and time-consuming as you apply this method to muscle after muscle after muscle that all cross the same joint in the same manner.
- Therefore, once you are very comfortable with applying the questions of step 3 for learning the actions of each muscle individually, it is recommended that you begin to use your understanding of how muscles function and apply it on a larger scale.
- Instead of looking at each muscle individually and going through all of the questions of step 3 for that muscle, take a step back and look at the broad functional groups of muscles at each joint.
- A muscle belongs to a **functional group** if it shares the same function (e.g., joint action) as the other members of the functional group.[5] The type of functional group that is being referred to in this section is a **functional mover group** (i.e., all the muscles in a group create the same joint action when they concentrically contract). Muscles can also be functionally grouped in roles other than as movers of a joint action.
- For example, instead of individually using the questions of step 3 to learn that the brachialis flexes the forearm at the elbow joint, and then that the biceps brachii flexes the forearm at the elbow joint, and then that the pronator teres flexes the forearm at the elbow joint, and also the flexor carpi radialis, palmaris longus, and so forth, it is a simpler and more elegant approach to look at the functional group of muscles that all flex the elbow joint.
- In other words, the bigger picture is to see that *all muscles* that cross the elbow joint anteriorly flex the forearm at the elbow joint. Looking at the body this way, when you encounter yet another muscle that crosses the elbow joint anteriorly, you can automatically place it into the group of forearm flexors at the elbow joint (Figure 1.10).
- For each joint of the human body, look for the functional groups of movers. In the case of the elbow joint, because it is a pure hinge, uniaxial joint, it is very simple. Only two functional mover groups exist: (1) anterior muscles that flex and (2) posterior muscles that extend.

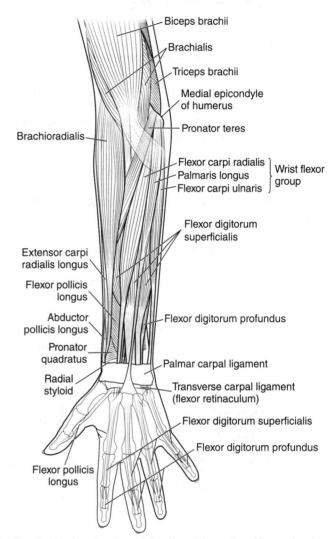

Figure 1.10 Anterior view of the elbow joint region. All muscles that cross the elbow joint anteriorly belong to the functional mover group of elbow joint flexors.

- Triaxial joints such as the shoulder or hip joint will have more functional mover groups[5] (flexors, extensors, abductors, adductors, medial rotators, and lateral rotators), but the concept will always be the same. Once you clearly see this concept, learning the actions of muscles of the body can be greatly simplified and streamlined. (Guidelines to determine the functional group to which a muscle belongs are given in Section 1.7.)

Reminder About Reverse Actions

Remember that the reverse actions of a muscle are always possible,[5] even if they have not been specifically listed in this book! So, each muscle that flexes the forearm at the elbow joint can also flex the arm at the elbow joint.

SECTION 1.7 DETERMINING FUNCTIONAL GROUPS

Understanding the actions of muscles from a functional group approach is the most efficient and elegant method to learn the actions of the muscles of the body.

- The muscles of a functional mover group are grouped together because they all share the same joint action. If their joint action is the same, then their line of pull relative to that joint must be the same. Therefore, it stands to reason that a functional group can also be looked at as a structural group (i.e., the muscles of a functional group are located together).
- Generally, certain guidelines can be stated regarding the location of functional groups of muscles.
  - Note: The general rules presented for learning functional mover groups of muscles are not hard and fast. They are better looked at as guidelines because exceptions to these rules exist. For example, across the ankle joint, frontal-plane functional groups are named as *everters* and *inverters,* not *abductors* and *adductors*. Another example is the saddle joint of the thumb, where flexion and extension occur in the

frontal plane, and abduction and adduction occur in the sagittal plane. Occasional exceptions aside, these general rules or guidelines are extremely valuable!

Sagittal Plane

- All groups of muscles that cross a joint in the sagittal plane can perform either flexion or extension (Figure 1.11).[3]
  - If the muscles cross the joint anteriorly, they perform flexion (except for the knee joint and farther distal).
  - If the muscles cross the joint posteriorly, they perform extension (except for the knee joint and farther distal).

Frontal Plane

- All groups of muscles that cross a joint in the frontal plane can perform either right lateral flexion/left lateral flexion or abduction/adduction (Figure 1.12).[3]
  - If the body part being moved is an axial body part, then the muscles perform lateral flexion to the same side (i.e., muscles on the right side of the body

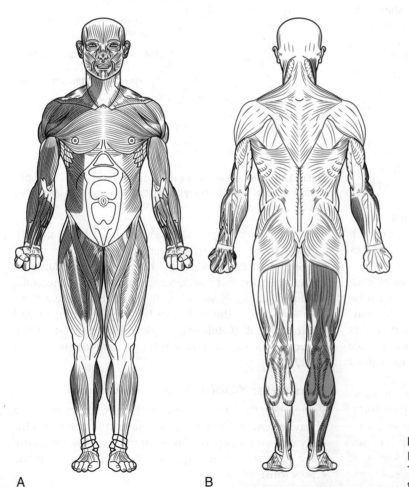

A   B

Figure 1.11 A, Anterior view of the musculature of the body. **B,** Posterior view of the musculature of the body. The flexor functional mover groups are colored red on the right side of the body.

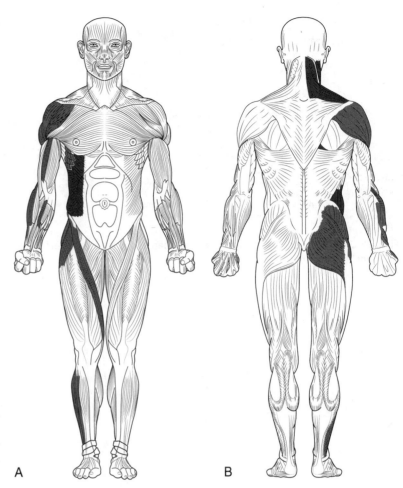

Figure 1.12 A, Anterior view of the musculature of the body. **B,** Posterior view of the musculature of the body. The muscles of the lateral flexor functional mover groups (for axial body joints) are colored red, and the muscles of the abductor functional mover groups (for appendicular body joints) are colored green on the right side of the body.

A   B

perform right lateral flexion; muscles on the left side of the body perform left lateral flexion).

- If the body part being moved is an appendicular body part, then the muscles perform abduction if they cross on the lateral side of the joint, and the muscles perform adduction if they cross on the medial side of the joint.

Transverse Plane

- Transverse plane actions are slightly more difficult to determine because the muscles of a transverse-plane functional mover group are not necessarily located together in one structural group (as are the muscles of the sagittal and frontal-plane functional mover groups).
  - For example, the right splenius capitis and the left sternocleidomastoid both perform right rotation of the neck (and head) at the spinal joints. However, even though these two muscles share the same joint action and are therefore in the same functional group, they are not located together. The right splenius capitis is in the right side of the neck, and the left sternocleidomastoid is in the left side of the neck; furthermore, the splenius capitis is located

posteriorly, and the sternocleidomastoid is located primarily anteriorly.

- Functional groups of the transverse plane perform rotation.[3]
  - If the body part being moved is an axial body part, then the muscles perform right rotation or left rotation.
  - If the body part being moved is an appendicular body part, then the muscles perform lateral rotation or medial rotation.
- An easy method to determine the transverse-plane rotation action of a muscle to place it into its functional mover group is to look at the manner in which the muscle *wraps around* the body part to which it attaches. (Another method to determine rotation actions that is technically more exacting is called the *off-axis attachment* method,[9] presented in Section 1.8.)
  - For example, the right splenius capitis and the left sternocleidomastoid both have the same action of right rotation because they both wrap around the neck region in the same manner (Figure 1.13A).
  - The right pectoralis major and the right latissimus dorsi have the same action of the medial rotation of

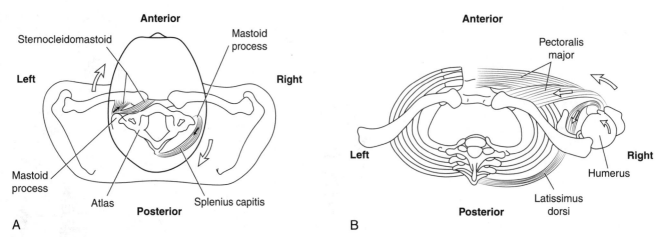

Figure 1.13 A, Superior view of the right splenius capitis and left sternocleidomastoid muscles. **B,** Superior view of the right pectoralis major and right latissimus dorsi.

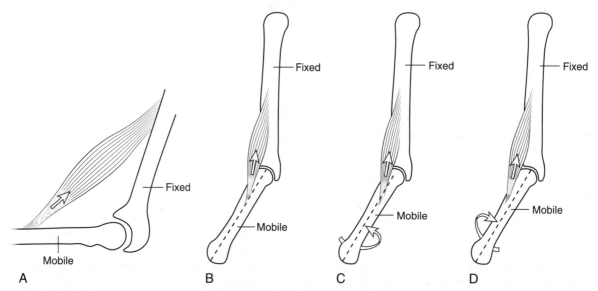

Figure 1.14 A, Side view of a muscle that attaches from one bone to another. **B** to **D,** Oblique views of muscles that cross from the same fixed bone to the same mobile bone. (Note: In all cases, a dashed line indicates the long axis of the mobile bone.) (Note: The muscles, bones, and joint illustrated in **A** to **D** are hypothetical; they are not meant to represent any specific structures of the body.)

the right arm at the glenohumeral joint because they both wrap around the humerus in the same manner (see Figure 1.13B).

- When trying to see the manner in which a muscle wraps, it is usually best to visualize the muscle from a superior (or proximal) perspective, as in Figures 1.13A and B.

SECTION 1.8 OFF-AXIS ATTACHMENT METHOD FOR DETERMINING ROTATION ACTIONS

- Seeing how the direction of a muscle's fibers *wrap* around the bone to which it attaches is a convenient visual method for determining the transverse-plane rotation action of a muscle.[9]

- However, another method can be used to determine rotation actions that might be a little more challenging to visualize at first; but once the rotation is visualized and understood, this method is a more accurate and elegant method to use. This method is called the **off-axis attachment method.**

- Figure 1.14A illustrates a side view of a muscle that crosses from one bone (labeled *fixed*) to another bone (labeled *mobile*). It is fairly intuitive to see that this muscle will move the mobile bone toward the fixed bone. However, to determine whether this muscle can create a rotation motion requires that we see exactly where the muscle attaches onto this mobile bone; more specifically, we need to see whether the muscle attaches *on-axis* or *off-axis*.

- Figure 1.14B is an oblique view that illustrates a hypothetical muscle that attaches onto the mobile bone **on-axis** (i.e., directly over the long axis of the mobile bone represented by the dashed line). When this muscle contracts and shortens, even though the mobile bone will be moved toward the fixed bone, no rotation of the mobile bone will occur because the muscle attaches on-axis (i.e., it does not wrap around to attach onto the bone to either side of the axis). Figure 1.14C is an oblique view of another hypothetical muscle that attaches onto the mobile bone; however, this muscle attaches **off-axis** (i.e., it wraps around the bone to attach off to the side of the long axis of the mobile bone). When this muscle contracts and shortens, it can move the mobile bone toward the fixed bone; it can also rotate the mobile bone as demonstrated by the red arrow. Figure 1.14D shows a similar muscle attaching onto the mobile bone off-axis to the other side and shows the rotation that this muscle would produce when contracting and shortening. (Note: The two muscles in Figure 1.14C and D attach off-axis on the opposite sides of the long axis from each other; therefore, they produce rotation actions that are opposite to each other.)
- Using the *off-axis attachment method* to determine the rotation action of a muscle necessitates that one visualizes the long axis of a bone. If a muscle attaches onto the bone on-axis (i.e., such that its attachment is directly over the axis), it has no possible rotation action. However, if it attaches onto the bone off-axis (i.e., off the axis to either side), it can create a rotation action.

SECTION 1.9 TRANSFERRING THE FORCE OF A MUSCLE'S CONTRACTION TO ANOTHER JOINT

In Section 1.3, we stated two rules about muscle contractions:

- Rule 1: If a muscle crosses a joint, it can have an action at that joint[5] (if the joint allows movement along the line of pull of the muscle).
- Rule 2: If a muscle does not cross a joint, it cannot have an action at that joint.
- Although rule 1 is true, rule 2 is usually, but not always, true. Sometimes the force of a muscle's contraction can be transferred to a joint that the muscle does not cross.[5]
- An example of this is lateral rotation of the arm at the GH joint with the distal end of the upper extremity fixed (i.e., closed-chain). Usually when the lateral rotators of the arm contract, the humerus rotates laterally relative to the scapula at the GH joint, and the bones of the forearm and hand "go along for the ride," maintaining their relative positions to each other. However, when the distal end of the upper extremity is fixed, the hand cannot go along for the ride; and because the

hand is fixed, the radius is also fixed and cannot move (with regard to rotation motion, because the wrist joint does not allow rotation). In this scenario, when the lateral rotators of the humerus contract and shorten, the humerus laterally rotates. Because the elbow joint does not allow rotation, this rotation force is transferred to the ulna, which then *rotates laterally* relative to the fixed radius. This motion causes the ulna to cross over the radius. When the ulna and radius cross, the motion is defined as pronation of the forearm. Although it is possible for pronators of the forearm to create this action of forearm pronation, in this instance the force for forearm pronation came from lateral rotators of the humerus at the GH joint (whose force was transferred to the radioulnar joints). Hence, even though these lateral rotator muscles of the GH joint do not cross the radioulnar joints, they were able to create radioulnar joint motion because the force of their contraction was transferred to the radioulnar joints (Figure 1.15). (Note: This concept could work in the reverse manner. If pronation musculature [e.g., pronator quadratus] were to contract, the force would transfer across the elbow joint to the humerus, causing lateral rotation of the humerus at the GH joint.)

- Note: Whenever the distal end of an extremity is fixed, the activity is termed a *closed-chain* activity. An open-chain activity is one wherein the distal end of the extremity is free to move.[5] With pronation of the forearm, the radius is usually considered to move and cross over a fixed ulna. When the radius is fixed and the ulna is mobile, moving and crossing over the radius, it is still defined as pronation; however, it is an example of a reverse action in which the ulna moves instead of the radius (at the radioulnar joints).
- Another example of the force of a muscle being transferred to a joint that it does not cross is contraction of shoulder joint adductor muscles with the distal end of the upper extremity fixed. In this scenario movement of the humerus is transferred across the elbow joint to create extension of the forearm at the elbow joint (Figure 1.16).
- The force of a muscle's contraction is often transferred to another joint in the human body. This force transference usually occurs when the distal end of an extremity is fixed and does not allow for free motion of the distal body part (closed chain). As a result, when the distal attachment of the contracting muscle moves, it forces motion to occur at another joint—in other words, its force is transferred to another joint that it does not cross.[4]
- Note: Transferring the force of a muscle contraction to another joint that the muscle does not cross is not the same as another body part simply *going along for the ride*. When other body parts go along for the ride, they

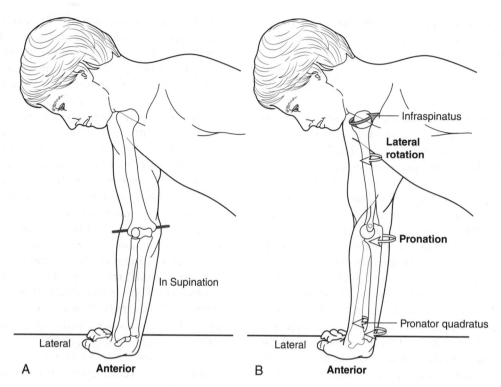

Figure 1.15 A, Person whose glenohumeral (GH) joint is medially rotated; forearm is supinated. **B,** Person contracts the lateral rotator musculature of the GH joint (e.g., infraspinatus).

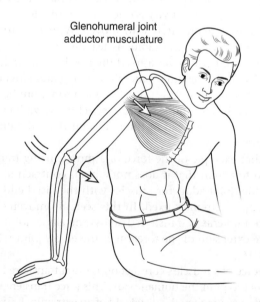

Figure 1.16 Person who is seated with the elbow joint partially flexed and the hand fixed to a tabletop. This person is contracting the shoulder joint adductor muscles. This results in elbow joint extension.

always maintain their relative position to each other at the other joints that were not crossed by the contracting muscle; the only relative joint position change is at the joint that is crossed by the muscle that contracted. When the force of a muscle's contraction is transferred

to another joint, a change in the relative position of body parts takes place at the other joint that is not crossed by the muscle that contracted. (To better visualize this, see Figures 1.15 and 1.16.)

- Many other scenarios exist in which the force of a muscle's contraction is transferred to a joint that it does not cross. One is the ability of the hamstrings to extend the knee joint in a person who is standing with the feet fixed to the ground; another is the lateral rotation force of the gluteus maximus causing the feet to supinate/invert at the subtalar tarsal joint if a person is standing with the feet fixed to the ground; and yet another is the ability of the ankle plantarflexors to create extension at the metatarsophalangeal joints when a person is standing. Try these scenarios for yourself.

SECTION 1.10 MUSCLE ACTIONS THAT CHANGE

Can a Muscle's Action Change?

- Yes. A muscle's action is dependent on its line of pull *relative* to the joint that it crosses; therefore, if the relationship of the muscle's line of pull to the joint changes, the muscle's action changes. This relationship can change if the position of the joint changes.[5]
- Some kinesiologists use the term **anatomic action** of a muscle to describe a muscle's action when the body is in anatomic position. This verbiage implicitly recognizes

that a muscle's action on the body when the body is not in anatomic position may well be different from the action of the muscle when the body is in anatomic position.

- Example 1: Clavicular head of the pectoralis major
  - The clavicular head of the pectoralis major is considered to be an adductor of the arm at the GH joint. This is because its line of pull is from medial to lateral, below the center of the GH joint.
  - However, if the arm is abducted to approximately 100 degrees or more, the orientation of the

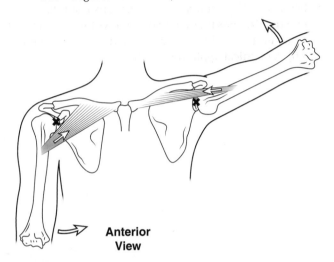

Anterior View

Figure 1.17 Orientation of the fibers of the clavicular head of the pectoralis major to the glenohumeral (GH) joint when the GH joint is in two different positions. Person's right arm is in anatomic position. The person's left arm is abducted approximately 100 degrees at the GH joint. (Note: The center of the shoulder joint on both sides is indicated by an X.)

clavicular head of the pectoralis major relative to the GH joint changes from being below the center of the joint to being above the center of the joint (Figure 1.17). Like any muscle that crosses above the center of the GH joint (e.g., deltoid, supraspinatus), the clavicular head of the pectoralis major can now abduct the arm at the GH joint.[10]

- It stands to reason that if the line of pull relative to the joint changes, the action of the muscle changes. In anatomic position, the clavicular head of the pectoralis major is an adductor of the arm at the GH joint. However, with the arm abducted to 100 degrees or more, the clavicular head of the pectoralis major changes to become an abductor.
- More specifically, a muscle's action is dependent on its line of pull relative to the *axis of motion* of the joint that it crosses. In Figure 1.17, the "x," representing the "center of the joint" more specifically represents the anteroposterior axis for frontal-plane motion.
- Note: This change in action becomes very useful. As the supraspinatus and deltoid muscles become functionally weaker with the arm in a great deal of abduction, the pectoralis major steps in to become an additional abductor, adding strength to this joint action.
- Example 2: Adductor longus
  - The adductor longus is considered to be a flexor (in addition to being an adductor) of the thigh at the hip joint because it passes anteriorly to the hip joint with a vertical direction to its fibers. All flexors of the thigh have their lines of pull anterior to the hip joint (Figure 1.18B). However, when the thigh

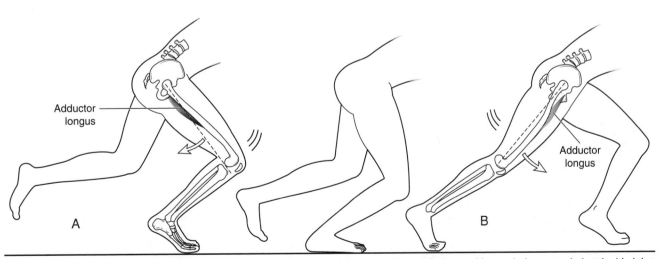

Adductor longus

Adductor longus

A

B

Figure 1.18 Illustration of a person who is running. **A,** Person's right thigh is in a position of flexion and is now being extended at the hip joint, helping to propel him forward. **B,** Person's right thigh is in a position of extension and is now beginning to flex at the hip joint. (Note: In both figures the dashed line represents the axis for motion of the thigh at the hip joint.)

is first flexed to approximately 60 degrees or more, the line of pull of the adductor longus lies posterior to the hip joint and the adductor longus becomes an extensor of the thigh at the hip joint (see Figure 1.18A). Except for the posterior head of the adductor magnus, which is always an extensor at the hip joint, this change in action is true for the other adductors of the thigh at the hip joint.[3] (Note: The *members of the adductors of the thigh group* are the pectineus, adductor longus, gracilis, adductor brevis, and adductor magnus.)

- Note: This change in action becomes very useful. While running, when we are in a position of extension, the adductors aid in flexing the thigh at the hip joint. However, when we are in a position of flexion, they aid in extending the thigh at the hip joint. This dual use may also explain why these muscles are so often injured.
- A muscle's action often changes when its line of pull relative to the joint changes[3] (because of a change in the position of the joint).
- For this reason, a certain amount of flexibility is needed when learning the actions of muscles. If one memorizes that a certain muscle does a certain action, it may or may not be true depending on the position of the joint. This is another reason why memorizing muscle actions is not recommended.
- Being able to reason a muscle's actions from its line of pull requires less brain memory, allows for a deeper and easier understanding of muscles' actions, and facilitates a better clinical application of this information!

Review Questions

Answers to the following review questions appear on the Evolve website accompanying this book at: http://evolve.elsevier.com/Muscolino/anatomycoloring/

1. When a muscle contracts, does it always succeed in shortening?

2. What is the name given to a shortening contraction of a muscle?

3. What are the three possible scenarios that can occur when a muscle contracts and shortens?

4. What is the name given to the attachment of a muscle that moves and to the attachment of a muscle that does not move?

5. Describe and give an example of a *reverse action*.

6. What are the five steps of the five-step approach to learning muscles?

7. What are the questions that must be asked and answered in step 3 of the five-step approach to learning muscles?

8. What determines the action(s) of a muscle?

9. Other than the reverse action(s), how many actions will a muscle have if it is has one line of pull and that line of pull is oriented within a cardinal plane?

10. How does one determine the action(s) of a muscle that has its line of pull within an oblique plane?

11. Can a multijoint muscle create movement at every one of the joints that it crosses?

12. What is the importance of using the *functional group approach* to learning muscles?

13. Give an example of a muscle that has more than one line of pull.

14. Muscles that belong to a flexor functional mover group are usually located in what plane?

15. Muscles that belong to an abductor functional mover group are usually located in what plane?

16. Muscles that belong to a rotation functional mover group are usually located in what plane?

17. How is the long axis of a bone determined?

18. Describe how the off-axis attachment method is used to determine the rotation action of a muscle.

_____

_____

_____

_____

19. Give an example of and explain how a muscle can create a joint action at a joint that it does not cross.

_____

_____

_____

_____

20. Give an example of and explain how a muscle can change its action at a joint based on a change in the position of that joint.

_____

_____

_____

_____

_____

REFERENCES

1. Soames RW, Palastanga N: *Anatomy and Human Movement: Structure and Function*, 7th ed., London, 2019, Elsevier.
2. Nordin M, Frankel VH: *Basic Biomechanics of the Musculoskeletal System*, 5th ed., Philadelphia, PA, 2022, Wolters Kluwer.
3. Houglum PA, Bertoti DB: *Brunnstrom's Clinical Kinesiology*, 6th ed., Philadelphia, PA, 2012, F.A. Davis.
4. Patton KT, Thibodeau GA: *Anatomy & Physiology*, St. Louis, MO, 2019, Elsevier.
5. Neumann DA: *Kinesiology of the Musculoskeletal System: Foundations for Rehabilitation*, 3rd ed., St. Louis, MO, 2017, Elsevier.
6. Levangie PK, Norkin CC, Lewek MD: *Joint Structure and Function: A Comprehensive Analysis*, 6th ed., Philadelphia, PA, 2019, F.A. Davis Company.
7. Hamill J, Knutzen KM, Derrick TR: *Biomechanical Basis of Human Movement*, 5th ed., Philadelphia, PA, 2022, Wolters Kluwer.
8. Watkins J: *Structure and Function of the Musculoskeletal System*, 2nd ed., Champaign, IL, 2010, Human Kinetics.
9. Enoka RM: *Neuromechanics of Human Movement*, 5th ed., Champaign, IL, 2015, Human Kinetics.
10. Muscolino JE: *The Muscular System Manual: The Skeletal Muscles of the Human Body*, 4th ed., St. Louis, MO, 2017, Elsevier.

The Skeletal System 2

An asterisk (*) following a number indicates that the structure is a bony landmark rather than a bone. Answers to labeling exercises are on p. 480.

⊕ **More review activities on Evolve at: http://evolve.elsevier.com/Muscolino/anatomycoloring/**

ANTERIOR VIEW OF THE BONES AND BONY LANDMARKS OF THE HEAD

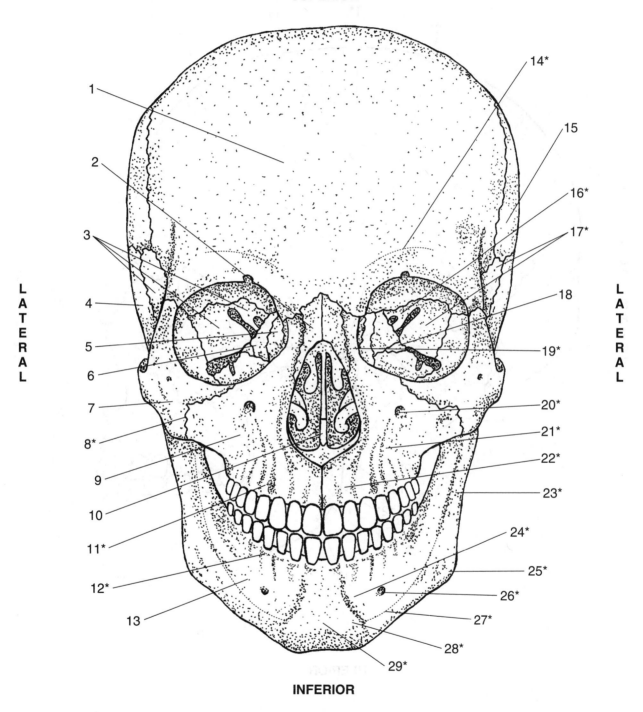

SUPERIOR

LATERAL

LATERAL

INFERIOR

LATERAL VIEW OF THE BONES AND BONY LANDMARKS OF THE HEAD

SUPERIOR

POSTERIOR

ANTERIOR

INFERIOR

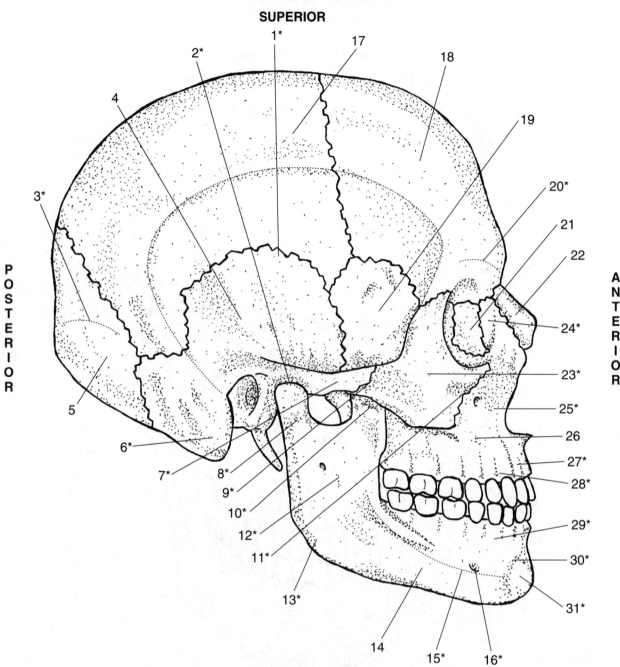

INFERIOR VIEW OF THE BONES AND BONY LANDMARKS OF THE HEAD

ANTERIOR

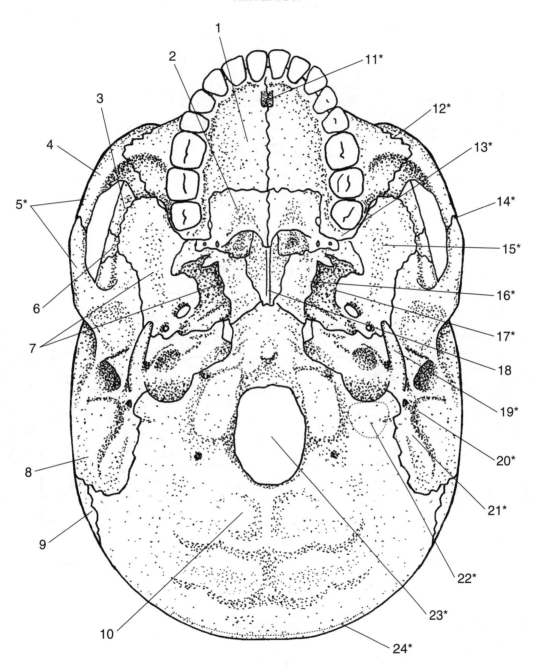

POSTERIOR

ANTERIOR VIEW OF THE BONES AND BONY LANDMARKS OF THE NECK

SUPERIOR

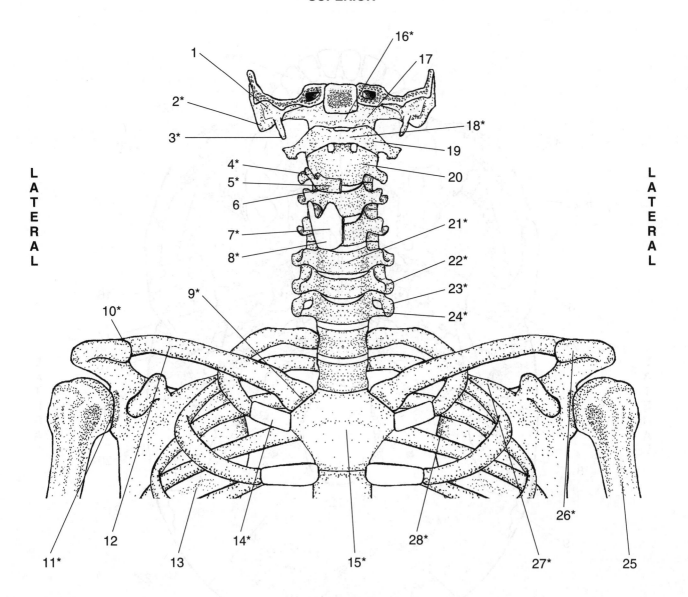

LATERAL

LATERAL

INFERIOR

POSTERIOR VIEW OF THE BONES AND BONY LANDMARKS OF THE NECK

SUPERIOR

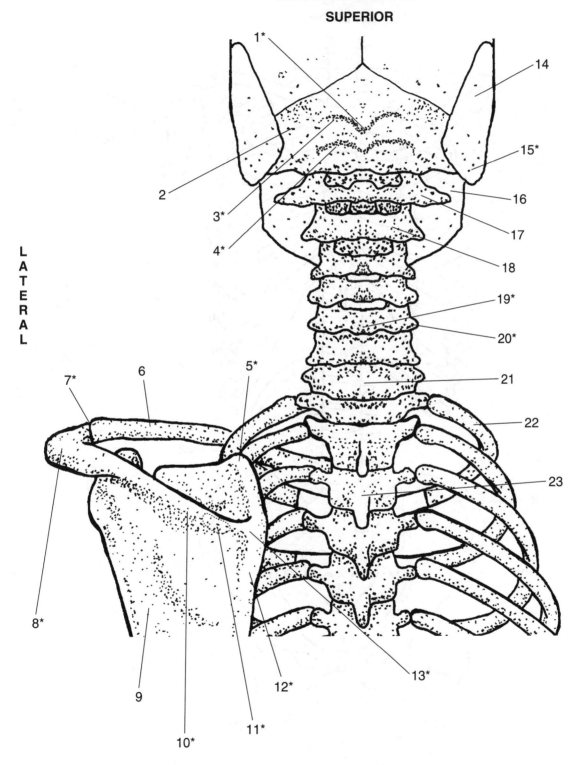

LATERAL

LATERAL

INFERIOR

ANTERIOR VIEW OF THE BONES AND BONY LANDMARKS OF THE TRUNK

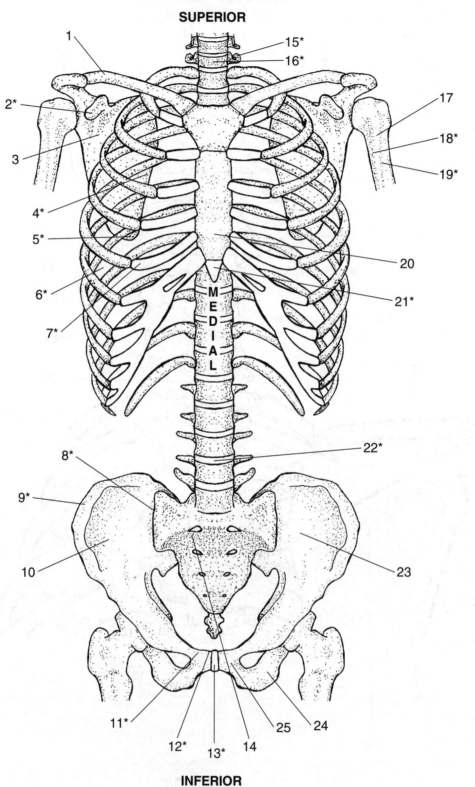

SUPERIOR

1

15*

16*

2*

17

3

18*

19*

4*

5*

20

6*

21*

7*

LATERAL

LATERAL

MEDIAL

22*

8*

9*

10

23

11*

25   24

12*   13*   14

INFERIOR

POSTERIOR VIEW OF THE BONES AND BONY LANDMARKS OF THE TRUNK

SUPERIOR

LATERAL

LATERAL

MEDIAL

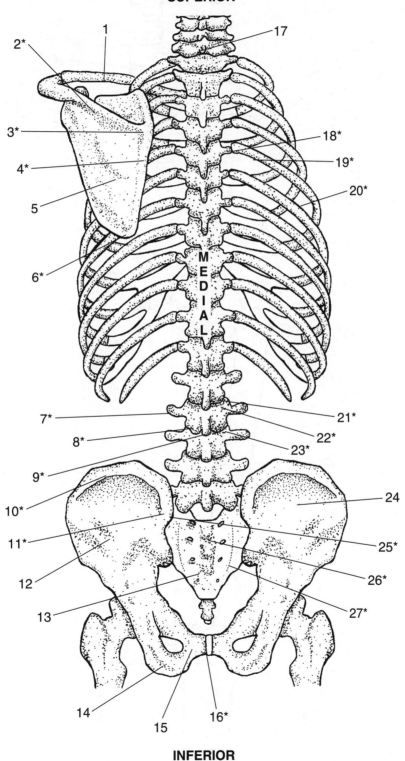

INFERIOR

ANTERIOR VIEW OF THE BONES AND BONY LANDMARKS OF THE RIGHT PELVIS AND THIGH

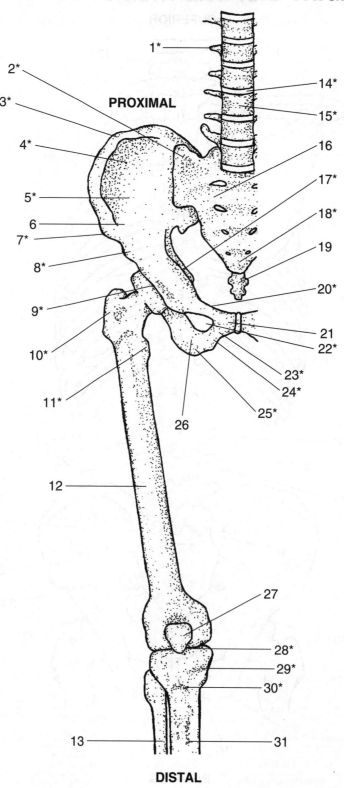

PROXIMAL

LATERAL

MEDIAL

DISTAL

POSTERIOR VIEW OF THE BONES AND BONY LANDMARKS OF THE RIGHT PELVIS AND THIGH

PROXIMAL

1*
2
3*
4*
5
6*
7
8*
9*
10*
11
12*
13*
14*
15*
16
17*
18*
19*
20

21*
22*
23*
24
25*
26*
27*
28*
29*
30*
31*
32*
33*
34*
35*
36*
37*
38*
39*
40*
41

MEDIAL

LATERAL

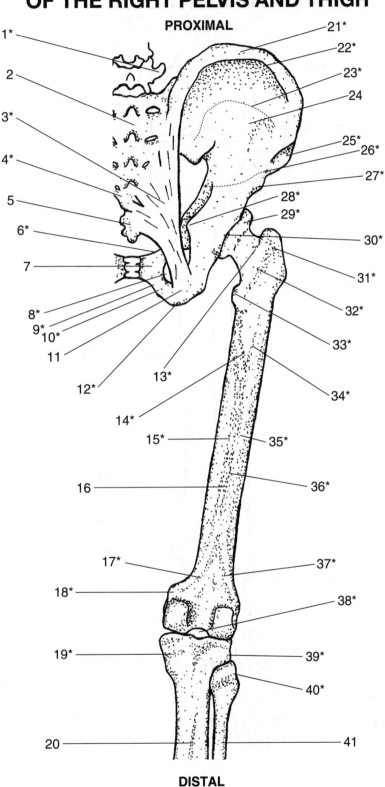

DISTAL

ANTERIOR VIEW OF THE BONES AND BONY LANDMARKS OF THE RIGHT LEG

PROXIMAL

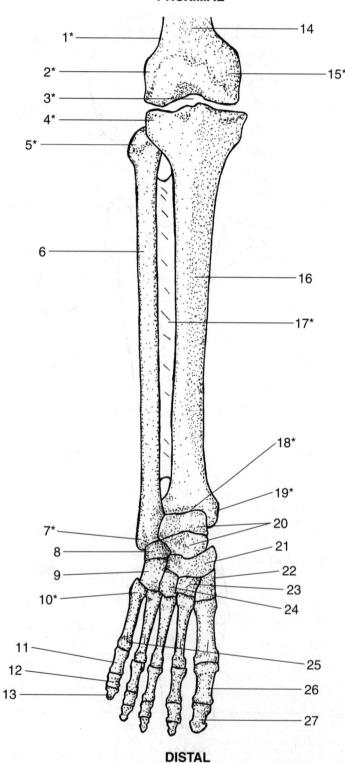

L
A
T
E
R
A
L

M
E
D
I
A
L

1*

2*

3*

4*

5*

6

7*

8

9

10*

11

12

13

14

15*

16

17*

18*

19*

20

21

22

23

24

25

26

27

DISTAL

POSTERIOR VIEW OF THE BONES AND BONY LANDMARKS OF THE RIGHT LEG

PROXIMAL

MEDIAL

LATERAL

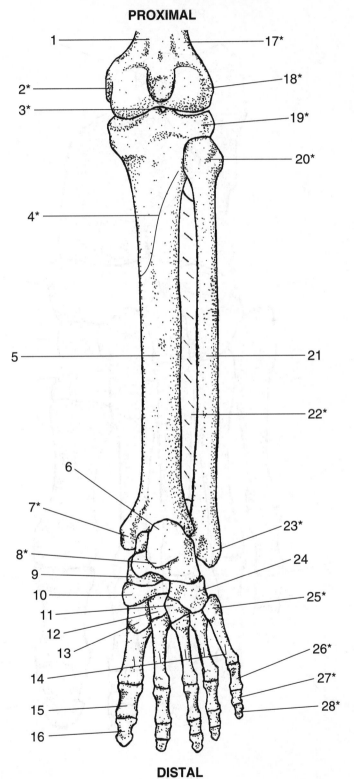

DISTAL

DORSAL VIEW OF THE BONES AND BONY LANDMARKS OF THE RIGHT FOOT

PROXIMAL

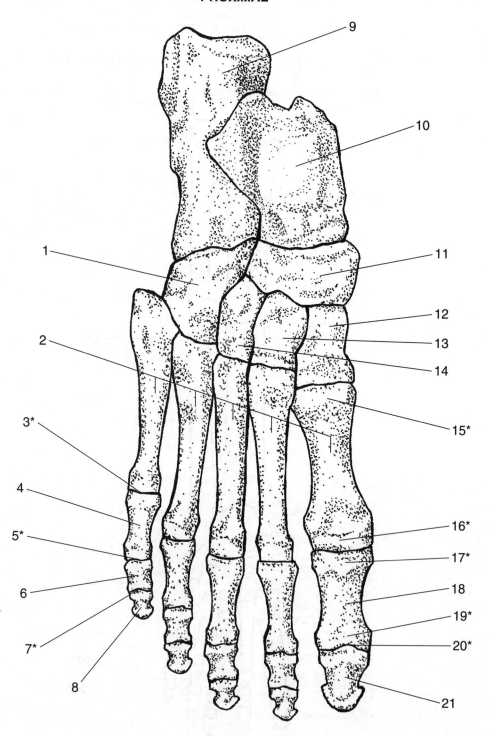

LATERAL

MEDIAL

DISTAL

PLANTAR VIEW OF THE BONES AND BONY LANDMARKS OF THE RIGHT FOOT

PROXIMAL

MEDIAL

LATERAL

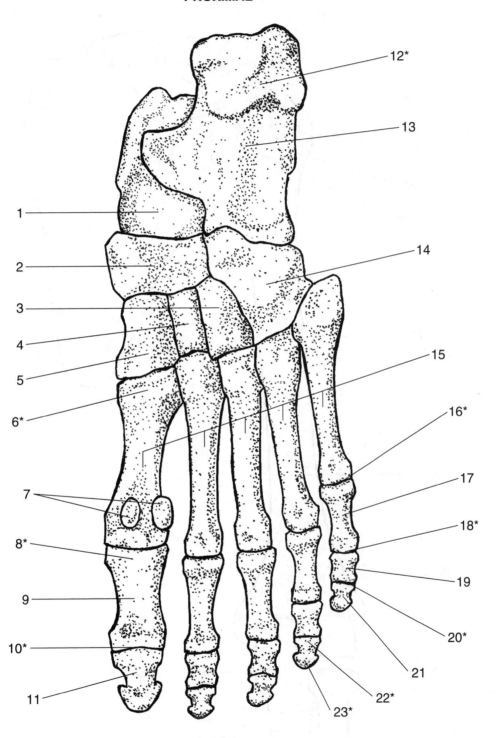

DISTAL

ANTERIOR VIEW OF THE BONES AND BONY LANDMARKS OF THE RIGHT SCAPULA/ARM

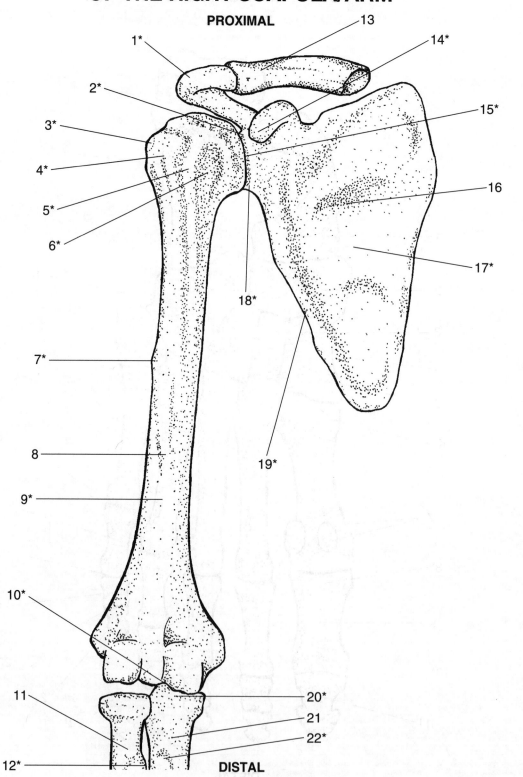

PROXIMAL

1*
13
14*
2*
15*
3*
4*
16
5*
6*
17*

LATERAL

MEDIAL

7*

18*

8

9*

19*

10*

11

20*
21
22*

12*

DISTAL

POSTERIOR VIEW OF THE BONES AND BONY LANDMARKS OF THE RIGHT SCAPULA/ARM

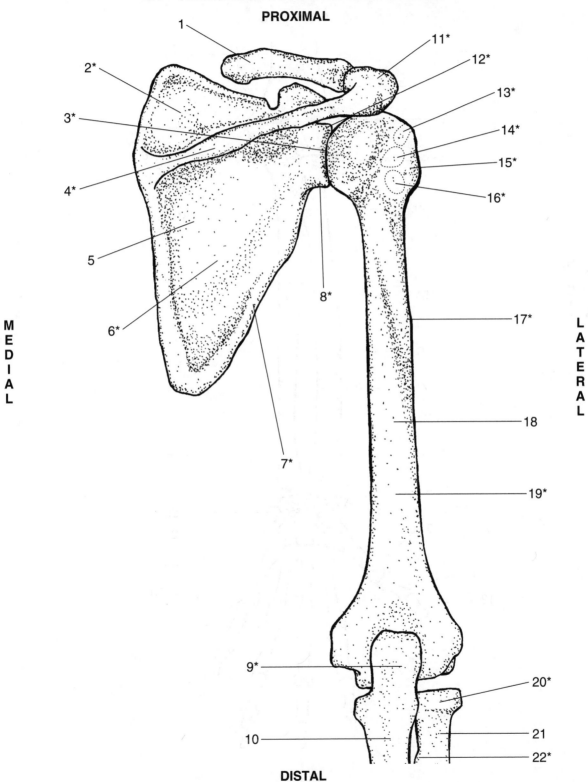

PROXIMAL

1

11*

12*

2*

13*

3*

14*

15*

4*

16*

5

6*

8*

MEDIAL

7*

17*

LATERAL

18

19*

9*

20*

10

21

22*

DISTAL

ANTERIOR VIEW OF THE BONES AND BONY LANDMARKS OF THE RIGHT FOREARM

PROXIMAL

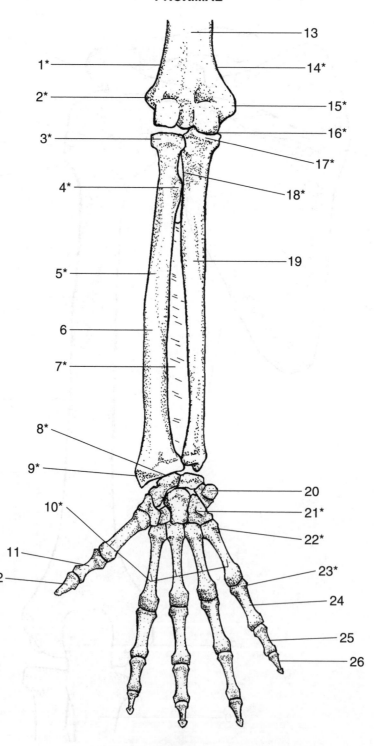

1*
2*
3*
4*
5*
6
7*
8*
9*
10*
11
12

13
14*
15*
16*
17*
18*
19
20
21*
22*
23*
24
25
26

LATERAL RADIAL

ULNAR MEDIAL

DISTAL

POSTERIOR VIEW OF THE BONES AND BONY LANDMARKS OF THE RIGHT FOREARM

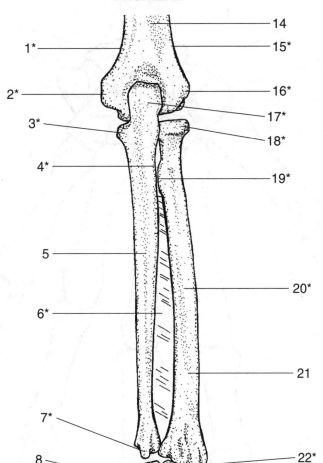

PROXIMAL

1*

2*

3*

4*

5

6*

7*

8

9*

10*

11

12

13

14

15*

16*

17*

18*

19*

20*

21

22*

23*

24

25

MEDIAL

ULNAR

RADIAL

LATERAL

DISTAL

PALMAR VIEW OF THE BONES AND BONY LANDMARKS OF THE RIGHT HAND

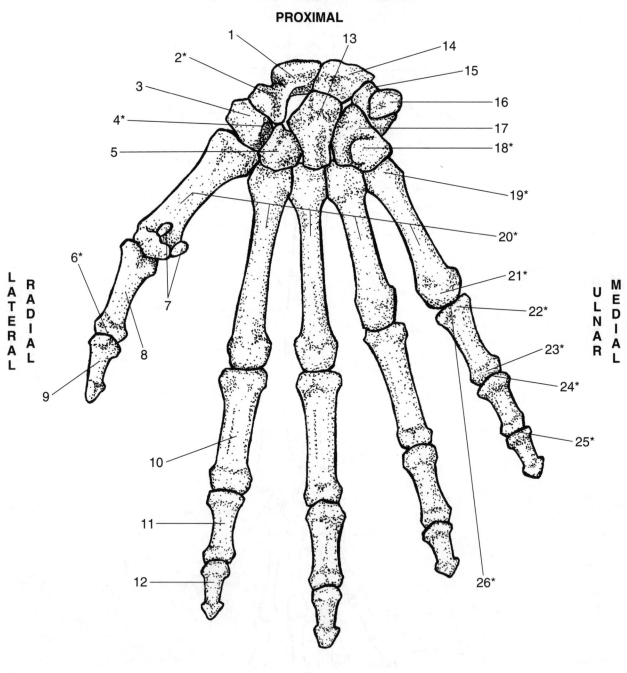

PROXIMAL

DISTAL

LATERAL

RADIAL

ULNAR

MEDIAL

DORSAL VIEW OF THE BONES AND BONY LANDMARKS OF THE RIGHT HAND

PROXIMAL

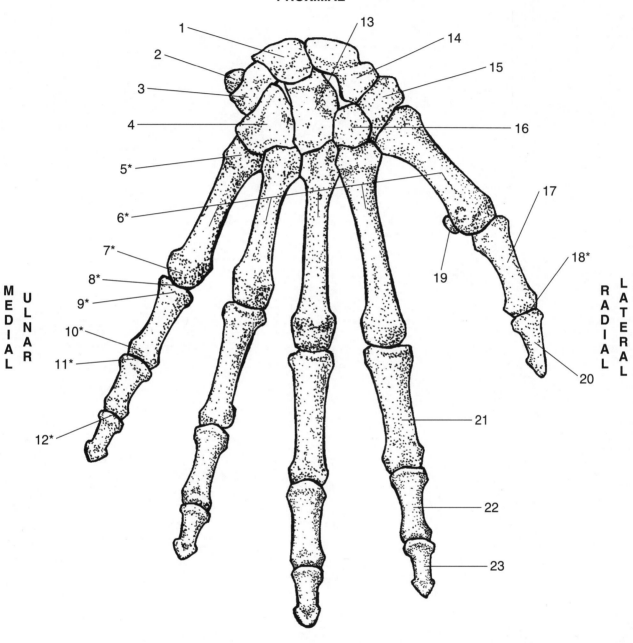

MEDIAL

ULNAR

RADIAL

LATERAL

DISTAL

Muscles of the Head 3

Note: Throughout this chapter, muscle attachments are indicated by italics.

⊕ **More review activities on Evolve at: http://evolve.elsevier.com/Muscolino/anatomycoloring/**

ANTERIOR VIEW OF THE HEAD

SUPERIOR

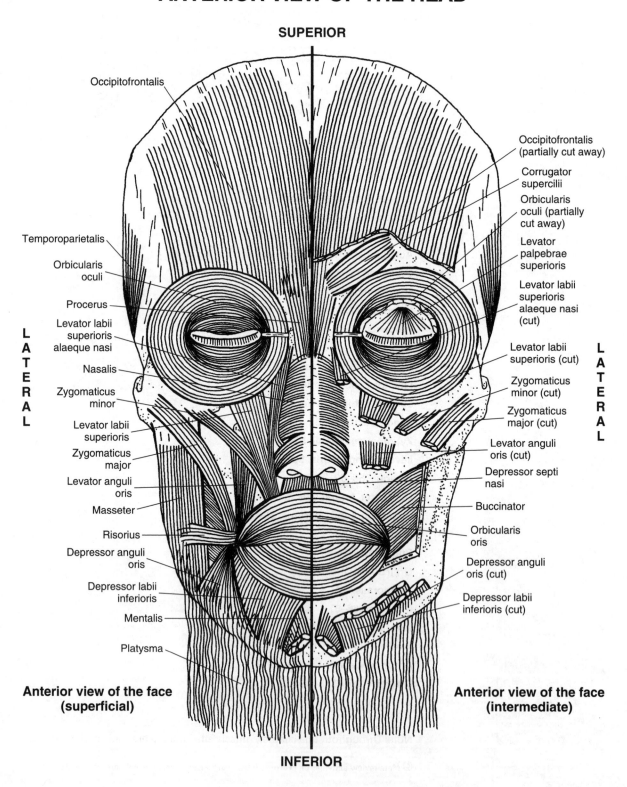

Occipitofrontalis

Occipitofrontalis (partially cut away)

Corrugator supercilii

Orbicularis oculi (partially cut away)

Levator palpebrae superioris

Levator labii superioris alaeque nasi (cut)

Levator labii superioris (cut)

Zygomaticus minor (cut)

Zygomaticus major (cut)

Levator anguli oris (cut)

Depressor septi nasi

Buccinator

Orbicularis oris

Depressor anguli oris (cut)

Depressor labii inferioris (cut)

Temporoparietalis

Orbicularis oculi

Procerus

Levator labii superioris alaeque nasi

Nasalis

Zygomaticus minor

Levator labii superioris

Zygomaticus major

Levator anguli oris

Masseter

Risorius

Depressor anguli oris

Depressor labii inferioris

Mentalis

Platysma

L A T E R A L

L A T E R A L

Anterior view of the face (superficial)

Anterior view of the face (intermediate)

INFERIOR

LATERAL VIEW OF THE HEAD

SUPERIOR

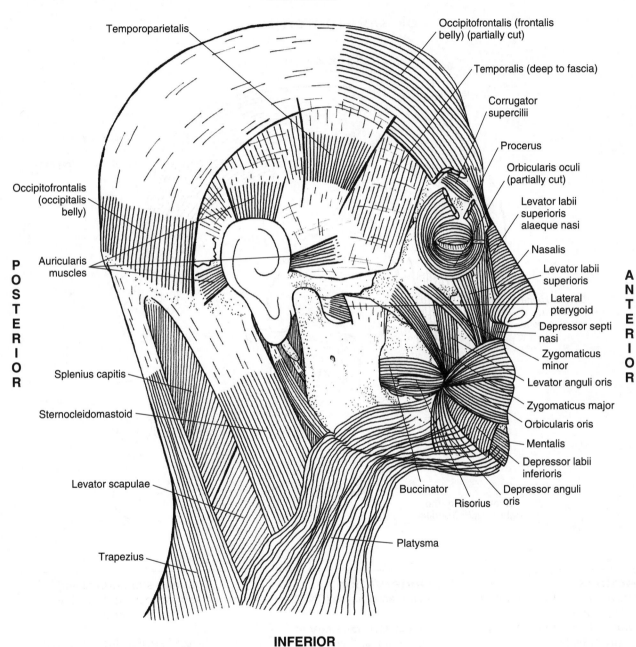

Temporoparietalis

Occipitofrontalis (frontalis belly) (partially cut)

Temporalis (deep to fascia)

Corrugator supercilii

Procerus

Orbicularis oculi (partially cut)

Occipitofrontalis (occipitalis belly)

Levator labii superioris alaeque nasi

Auricularis muscles

Nasalis

Levator labii superioris

Lateral pterygoid

P O S T E R I O R

A N T E R I O R

Depressor septi nasi

Zygomaticus minor

Levator anguli oris

Splenius capitis

Zygomaticus major

Sternocleidomastoid

Orbicularis oris

Mentalis

Depressor labii inferioris

Levator scapulae

Buccinator

Depressor anguli oris

Risorius

Platysma

Trapezius

INFERIOR

OCCIPITOFRONTALIS
(PART OF THE EPICRANIUS)

ok-**sip**-i-to-fron-**ta**-lis

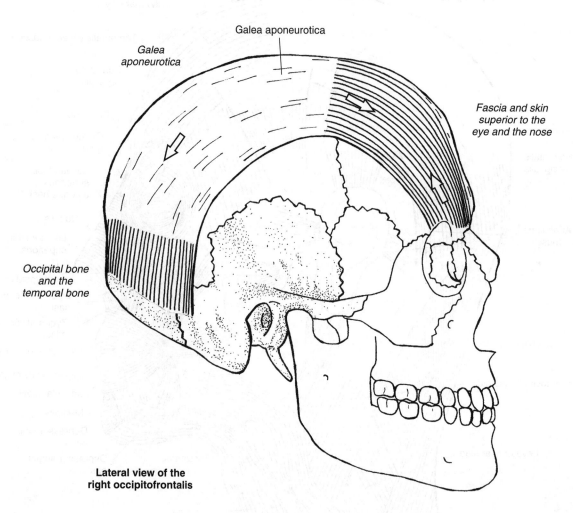

Galea aponeurotica

Galea aponeurotica

Fascia and skin superior to the eye and the nose

Occipital bone and the temporal bone

Lateral view of the right occipitofrontalis

Actions	**Innervation**	Frontalis: supraorbital and

Actions
Draws the scalp posteriorly (occipitalis)
Draws the scalp anteriorly (frontalis)
Elevates the eyebrows (frontalis)

Innervation
The facial nerve (CN VII)

Arterial Supply
Occipitalis: the occipital and posterior auricular arteries

Frontalis: supraorbital and supratrochlear branches of the ophthalmic artery

Myofascial Meridians
Superficial back line

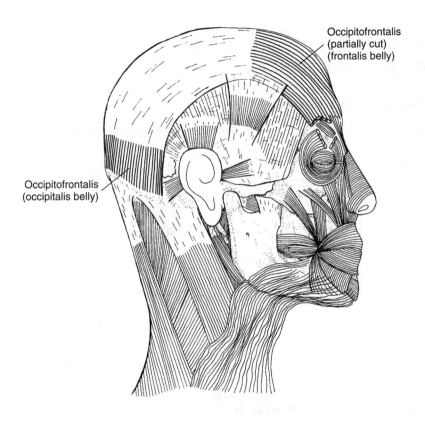

Occipitofrontalis
(partially cut)
(frontalis belly)

Occipitofrontalis
(occipitalis belly)

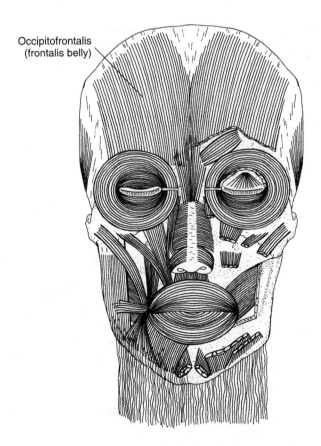

Occipitofrontalis
(frontalis belly)

DID
YOU ?
KNOW

The occipitofrontalis is often involved in tension headaches.

DID
YOU ?
KNOW

The occipitofrontalis can contribute to the expression of surprise or fright.

TEMPOROPARIETALIS
(PART OF THE EPICRANIUS)

tem-po-ro-pa-ri-i-tal-is

Actions
Elevates the ear
Tightens the scalp

Innervation
The facial nerve (CN VII)

Arterial Supply
The superficial temporal and posterior auricular
    arteries

Myofascial Meridians
Deep front line

The temporoparietalis and
occipitofrontalis attach into the Galea
aponeurotica.

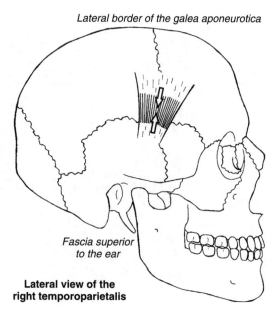

Lateral border of the galea aponeurotica

*Fascia superior
to the ear*

**Lateral view of the
right temporoparietalis**

AURICULARIS ANTERIOR, SUPERIOR, AND POSTERIOR

aw-rik-u-la-ris an-tee-ri-or, sue-pee-ri-or, pos-tee-ri-or

Actions
Draws the ear anteriorly (auricularis
    anterior)
Elevates the ear (auricularis
    superior)
Draws the ear posteriorly
    (auricularis posterior)
Tightens and moves the scalp
    (auricularis anterior and superior)

Innervation
The facial nerve (CN VII)

Arterial Supply
The superficial temporal and
    posterior auricular arteries

Myofascial Meridians
Deep front line

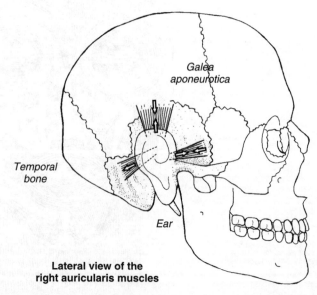

*Galea
aponeurotica*

*Temporal
bone*

Ear

**Lateral view of the
right auricularis muscles**

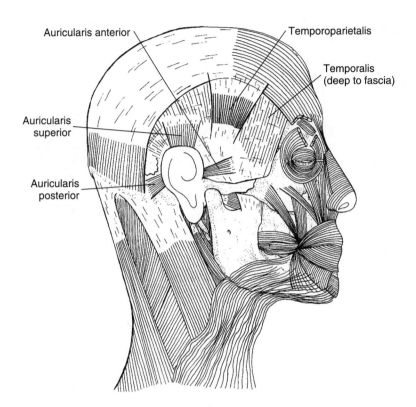

Auricularis anterior

Temporoparietalis

Temporalis
(deep to fascia)

Auricularis
superior

Auricularis
posterior

DID YOU KNOW?

The temporoparietalis is located superficial to the temporalis.

DID YOU KNOW?

The auricularis muscles are extremely well developed in dogs.

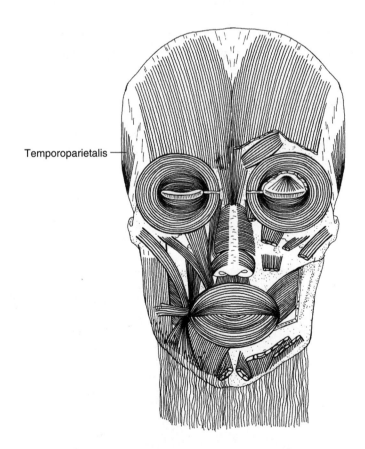

Temporoparietalis

DID YOU KNOW?

The actions of moving the ear that are created by the auricularis muscles are largely vestigial and are nonfunctional in many people.

ORBICULARIS OCULI

or-**bik**-you-la-ris **ok**-you-lie

Actions
Closes and squints the eye
  (orbital part)
Depresses the upper eyelid
  (palpebral part)
Elevates the lower eyelid
  (palpebral part)
Assists tear transport and
  drainage (lacrimal part)

Innervation
The facial nerve (CN VII)

Arterial Supply
The branches of the facial
  artery and superficial
  temporal artery

Myofascial Meridians
Deep front line

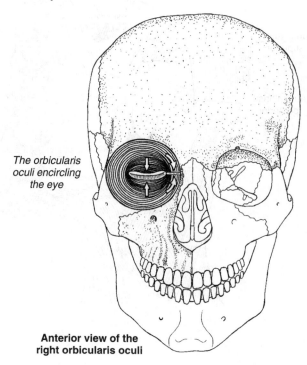

The orbicularis
oculi encircling
the eye

**Anterior view of the
right orbicularis oculi**

LEVATOR PALPEBRAE SUPERIORIS

le-vay-tor pal-**pee**-bree su-**pee**-ri-**or**-is

Action
Elevates the upper eyelid

Innervation
The oculomotor nerve (CN III)

Arterial Supply
The ophthalmic artery

Myofascial Meridians
Deep front line

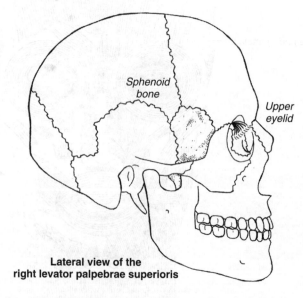

Sphenoid
bone

Upper
eyelid

**Lateral view of the
right levator palpebrae superioris**

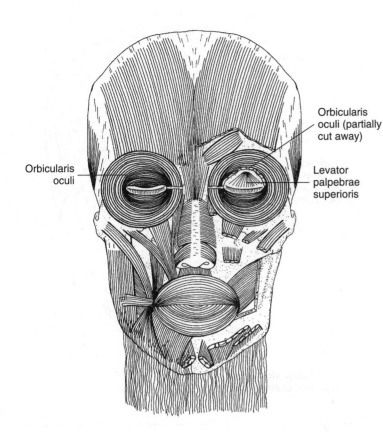

Orbicularis oculi (partially cut away)

Orbicularis oculi

Levator palpebrae superioris

The portion of the orbicularis oculi located in the eyelids is under both conscious control to blink the eye voluntarily and unconscious control to blink the eye involuntarily (as part of a reflex to protect the eye from possible damage).

Contraction of the orbicularis oculi can help to protect the eye from excessive sunlight.

Levator palpebrae superioris

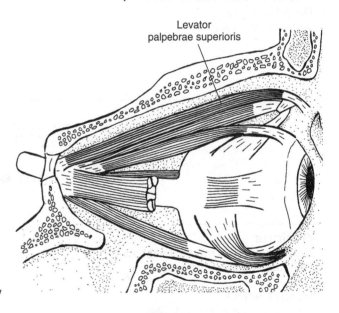

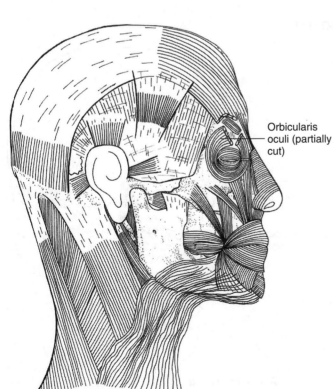

Orbicularis oculi (partially cut)

The levator palpebrae superioris is located within the socket of the eye and the upper eyelid.

By elevating the upper eyelid, the levator palpebrae can create the expression of surprise or shock.

CORRUGATOR SUPERCILII

kor-u-gay-tor su-per-**sil**-i-eye

Action
Draws eyebrow inferiorly and
   medially

Innervation
The facial nerve (CN VII)

Arterial Supply
The supratrochlear and
   supraorbital arteries

Myofascial Meridians
Deep front line
Superficial back line

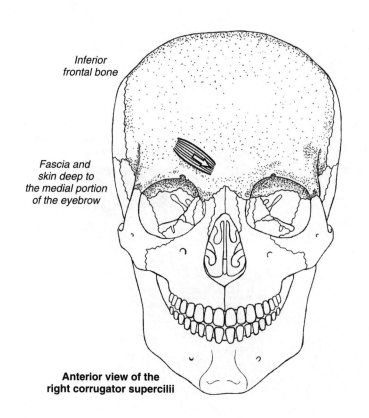

Inferior
frontal bone

Fascia and
skin deep to
the medial portion
of the eyebrow

**Anterior view of the
right corrugator supercilii**

PROCERUS

pro-**se**-rus

Actions
Draws down the medial eyebrow
Wrinkles the skin of the nose

Innervation
The facial nerve (CN VII)

Arterial Supply
The facial artery

Myofascial Meridians
Deep front line
Superficial back line

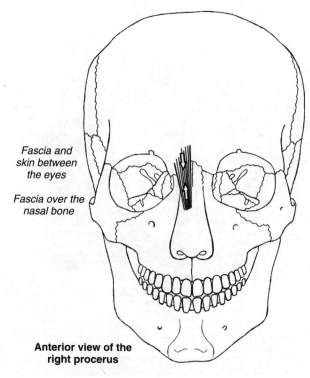

Fascia and
skin between
the eyes

Fascia over the
nasal bone

**Anterior view of the
right procerus**

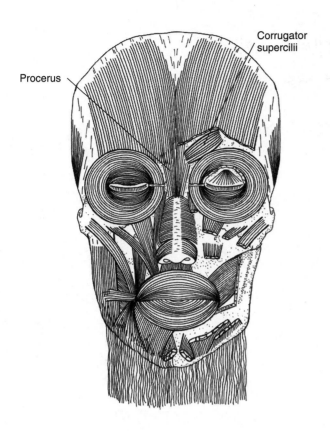

Corrugator
supercilii

Procerus

Contraction of the corrugator supercilii contributes to frowning and also assists in shielding the eyes from bright sunlight.

Contraction of the corrugator supercilii creates vertical wrinkles superior and medial to the eye (think "corrugated" cardboard).

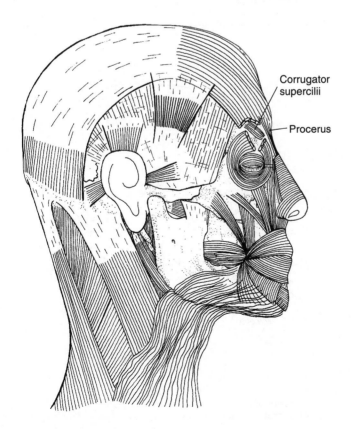

Corrugator
supercilii

Procerus

Procerus in Latin means "chief noble" or "prince"; hence the action of the procerus creates an expression that conveys a look of superiority.

Contraction of the procerus also helps to protect the eye from bright sunlight.

NASALIS

nay-**sa**-lis

Action
Flares the nostril (alar part)
Constricts the nostril
(transverse part)

Innervation
The facial nerve (CN VII)

Arterial Supply
The facial artery

Myofascial Meridians
Deep front line
Superficial back line

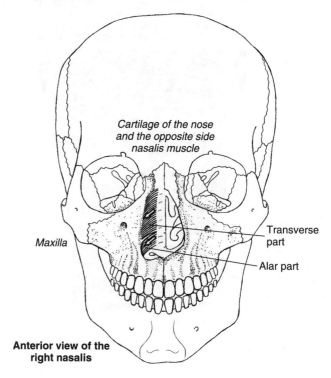

*Cartilage of the nose
and the opposite side
nasalis muscle*

Maxilla

Transverse part

Alar part

**Anterior view of the
right nasalis**

DEPRESSOR SEPTI NASI

dee-**pres**-or **sep**-ti **nay**-zi

Action
Constricts the nostril

Innervation
The facial nerve (CN VII)

Arterial Supply
The facial artery

Myofascial Meridians
Deep front line

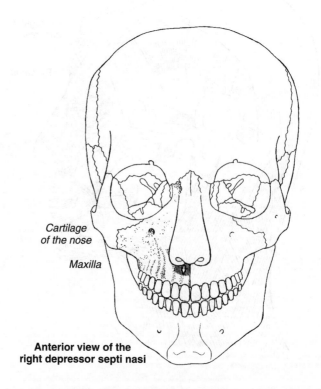

*Cartilage
of the nose*

Maxilla

**Anterior view of the
right depressor septi nasi**

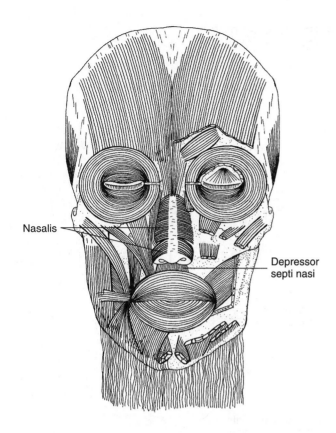

Nasalis

Depressor
septi nasi

The nasalis has two parts: a transverse
part and an alar part.

The action of flaring the nostril by
the nasalis opens the aperture for
breathing and can be important for
conveying emotional states.

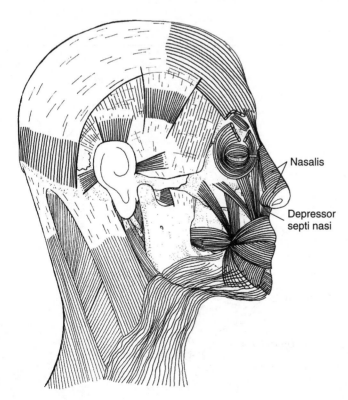

Nasalis

Depressor
septi nasi

The action of constricting the nostril
by the depressor septi nasi closes the
aperture for breathing and can also be
involved in facial expressions.

The depressor septi nasi is sometimes
considered to be part of the nasalis
muscle.

LEVATOR LABII SUPERIORIS ALAEQUE NASI

le-**vay**-tor **lay**-be-eye

soo-**pee**-ri-o-ris

a-**lee**-kwe **nay**-si

Actions
Elevates the upper lip
Flares the nostril
Everts the upper lip

Innervation
The facial nerve (CN VII)

Arterial Supply
The infraorbital artery

Myofascial Meridians
Deep front line

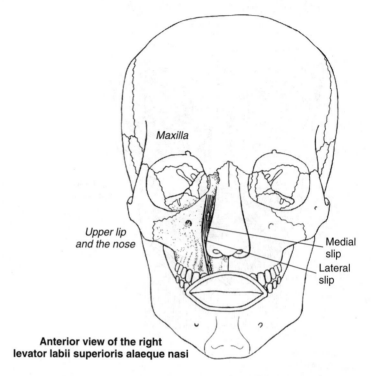

**Anterior view of the right
levator labii superioris alaeque nasi**

LEVATOR LABII SUPERIORIS

le-**vay**-tor **lay**-be-eye

soo-**pee**-ri-**o**-ris

Actions
Elevates the upper lip
Everts the upper lip

Innervation
The facial nerve (CN VII)

Arterial Supply
The facial artery

Myofascial Meridians
Deep front line

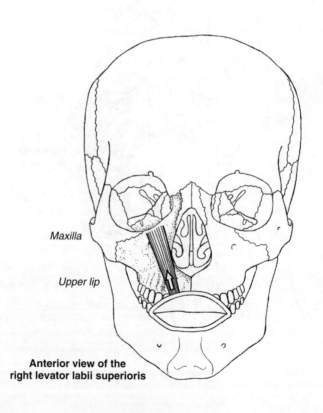

**Anterior view of the
right levator labii superioris**

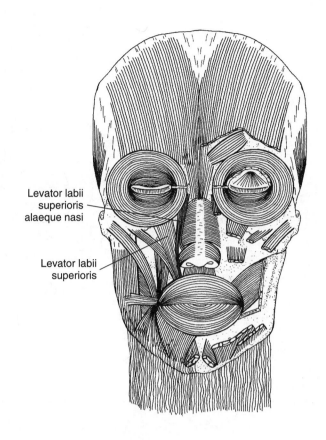

Levator labii
superioris
alaeque nasi

Levator labii
superioris

The levator labii superioris alaeque nasi is a muscle of facial expression that, as its name describes, can move both the mouth and the nose.

The levator labii superioris alaeque nasi is sometimes considered to be part of the levator labii superioris muscle.

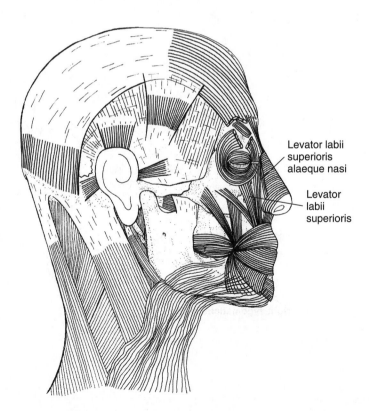

Levator labii
superioris
alaeque nasi

Levator
labii
superioris

Contraction of the levator labii superioris muscles lifts the upper lip, which exposes the upper teeth. This action can contribute to a number of facial expressions, including happiness, smugness, or disdain.

ZYGOMATICUS MINOR

zi-go-**mat**-ik-us **my**-nor

Actions
Elevates the upper lip
Everts the upper lip

Innervation
The facial nerve (CN VII)

Arterial Supply
The facial artery

Myofascial Meridians
Deep front line

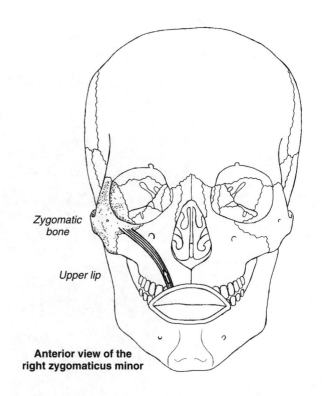

Zygomatic bone

Upper lip

Anterior view of the right zygomaticus minor

ZYGOMATICUS MAJOR

zi-go-**mat**-ik-us **may**-jor

Actions
Elevates the angle of the mouth
Draws laterally the angle of the mouth

Innervation
The facial nerve (CN VII)

Arterial Supply
The facial artery

Myofascial Meridians
Deep front line

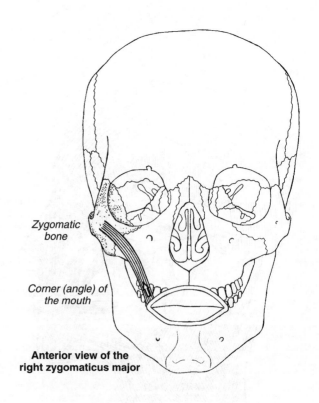

Zygomatic bone

Corner (angle) of the mouth

Anterior view of the right zygomaticus major

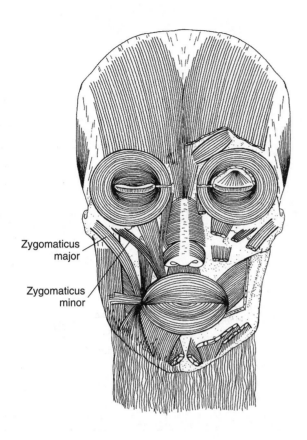

Zygomaticus
major

Zygomaticus
minor

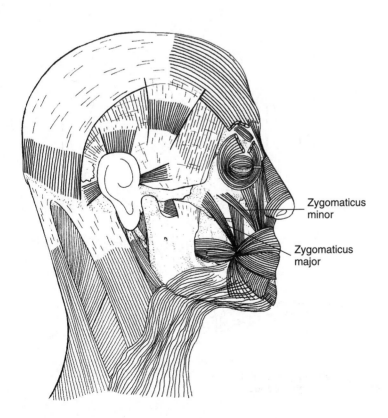

Zygomaticus
minor

Zygomaticus
major

DID
YOU
KNOW

As the name zygomaticus implies, both zygomaticus muscles attach onto the zygomatic bone.

DID
YOU
KNOW

Contraction of the zygomaticus minor alone will expose your upper teeth. Contraction of the zygomaticus major alone will widen your smile.

LEVATOR ANGULI ORIS

le-**vay**-tor **ang**-you-lie **o**-ris

Action
Elevates the angle of the mouth

Action
Elevates the angle of the mouth

Innervation
The facial nerve (CN VII)

Arterial Supply
The facial artery

Myofascial Meridians
Deep front line

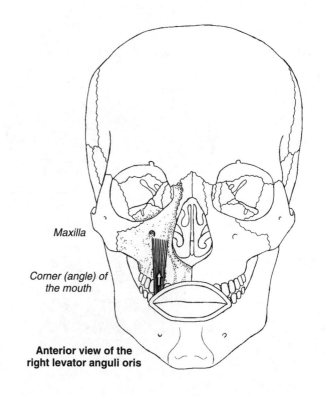

Maxilla

Corner (angle) of
the mouth

**Anterior view of the
right levator anguli oris**

RISORIUS

ri-**so**-ri-us

Action
Draws laterally the angle of
the mouth

Innervation
The facial nerve (CN VII)

Arterial Supply
The facial artery

Myofascial Meridians
Deep front line

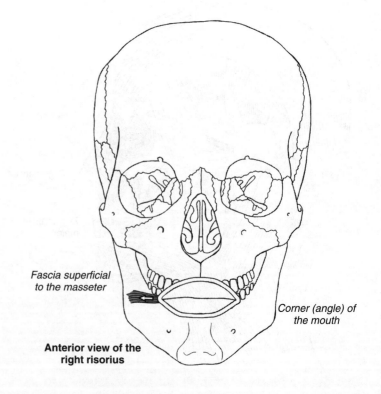

Fascia superficial
to the masseter

Corner (angle) of
the mouth

**Anterior view of the
right risorius**

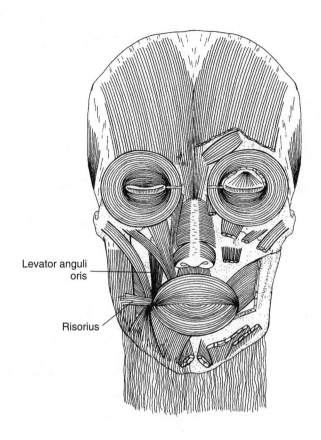

Levator anguli oris

Risorius

DID
YOU
KNOW

The levator anguli oris is also known as the caninus because contraction of this muscle results in the typical "Dracula" expression wherein the canine teeth are exposed.

DID
YOU
KNOW

The levator anguli oris can contribute to the expression of a smile or a sneer.

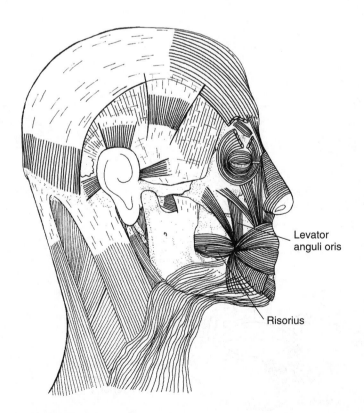

Levator anguli oris

Risorius

DID
YOU
KNOW

The name risorius means "laughing" in Latin; the risorius draws the angle of the mouth laterally, which occurs during laughter.

DID
YOU
KNOW

The risorius also contributes to grinning and smiling.

DEPRESSOR ANGULI ORIS

dee-**pres**-or **ang**-you-lie **o**-ris

Actions
Depresses the angle of the mouth
Draws laterally the angle of the mouth

Innervation
The facial nerve (CN VII)

Arterial Supply
The facial artery

Myofascial Meridians
Deep front line

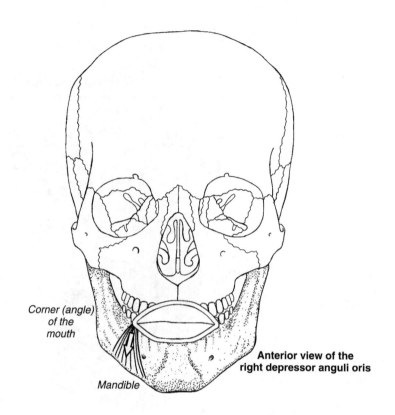

Corner (angle) of the mouth

Mandible

Anterior view of the right depressor anguli oris

DEPRESSOR LABII INFERIORIS

dee-**pres**-or **lay**-be-eye in-**fee**-ri-**o**-ris

Actions
Depresses the lower lip
Draws laterally the lower lip
Everts the lower lip

Innervation
The facial nerve (CN VII)

Arterial Supply
The facial artery

Myofascial Meridians
Deep front line

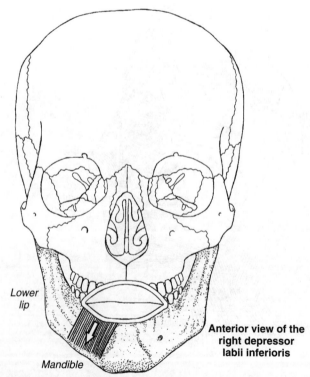

Lower lip

Mandible

Anterior view of the right depressor labii inferioris

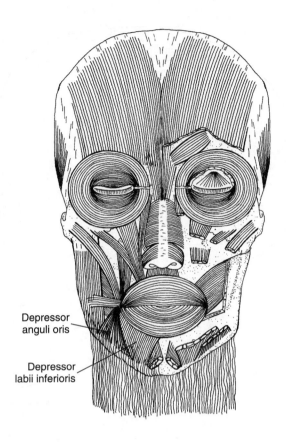

Depressor
anguli oris

Depressor
labii inferioris

**DID
YOU
KNOW**

*Contraction of the depressor anguli oris
and depressor labii inferioris muscles
contributes to facial expressions of
sadness, doubt, and uncertainty.*

**DID
YOU
KNOW**

*Both of these muscles attach onto the
inferior aspect of the mandible.*

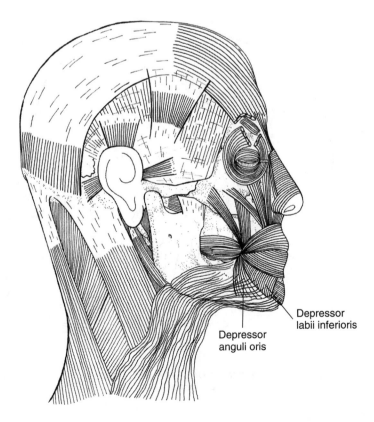

Depressor
labii inferioris

Depressor
anguli oris

MENTALIS

men-**ta**-lis

Actions
Elevates the lower lip
Everts and protracts the lower lip
Wrinkles the skin of the chin

Innervation
The facial nerve (CN VII)

Arterial Supply
The facial artery

Myofascial Meridians
Deep front line

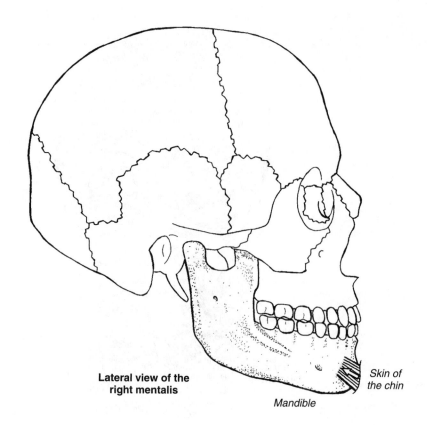

**Lateral view of the
right mentalis**

*Skin of
the chin*

Mandible

BUCCINATOR

buk-sin-**a**-tor

Action
Compresses the cheeks
(against the teeth)

Innervation
The facial nerve (CN VII)

Arterial Supply
The maxillary and facial
arteries

Myofascial Meridians
Deep front line

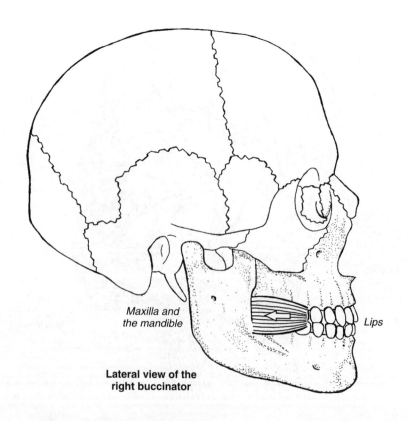

*Maxilla and
the mandible*

Lips

**Lateral view of the
right buccinator**

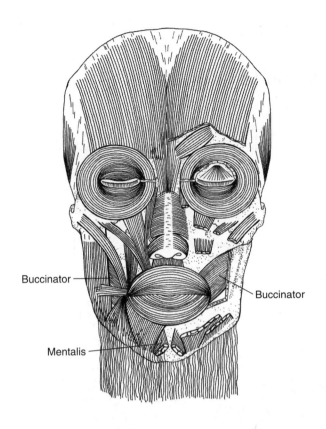

Buccinator

Buccinator

Mentalis

Strong contraction of the mentalis muscles can make the lower lip stick out, creating the facial expression of pouting.

Contraction of the mentalis to evert and protract the lower lip is useful when drinking.

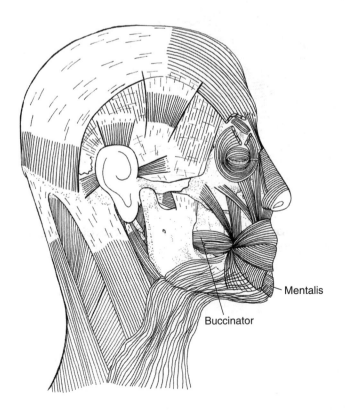

Mentalis

Buccinator

The buccinator attaches into the mandible and the maxilla.

Contraction of the buccinator muscles is necessary for whistling, blowing up a balloon, and blowing into a brass or woodwind instrument.

ORBICULARIS ORIS

or-**bik**-you-**la**-ris **o**-ris

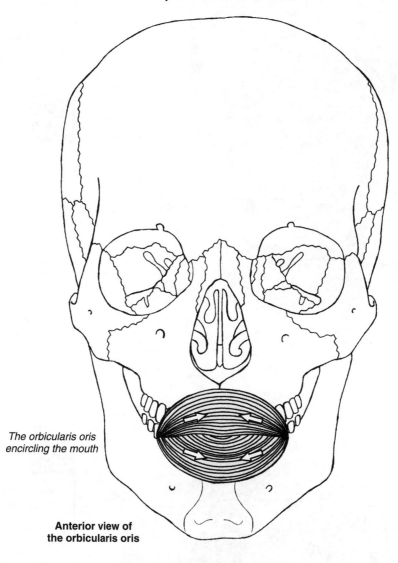

The orbicularis oris encircling the mouth

Anterior view of the orbicularis oris

Actions	**Arterial Supply**	**Myofascial Meridians**
Closes the mouth	The facial artery	Deep front line
Protracts the lips		

Innervation
The facial nerve (CN VII)

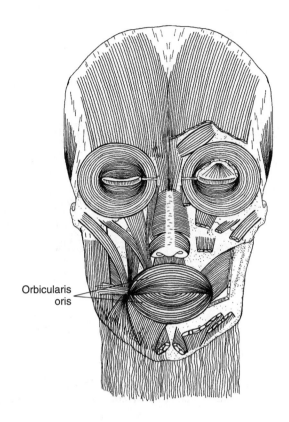

Orbicularis
oris

DID YOU KNOW ?

Contraction of the orbicularis oris causes the lips to close and protrude as in puckering the lips or whistling.

DID YOU KNOW ?

Because the orbicularis oris puckers the lips, it is sometimes called "the kissing muscle."

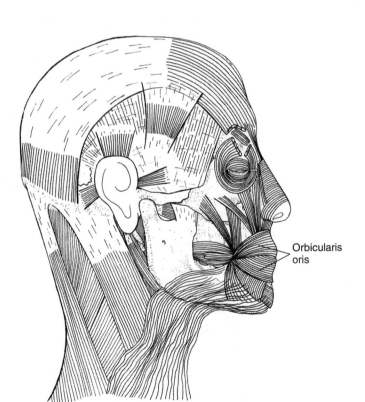

Orbicularis
oris

TEMPORALIS

tem-po-**ra**-lis

Actions
Elevates the mandible at the
   temporomandibular joints
Retracts the mandible at the
   temporomandibular joints

Innervation
The trigeminal nerve (CN V)

Arterial Supply
The maxillary and superficial
temporal arteries

Myofascial Meridians
Deep front line

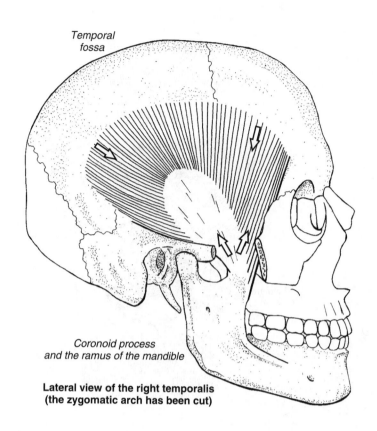

Temporal
fossa

Coronoid process
and the ramus of the mandible

**Lateral view of the right temporalis
(the zygomatic arch has been cut)**

MASSETER

ma-sa-ter

Actions
Elevates the mandible at the
   temporomandibular joints
Protracts the mandible at the
   temporomandibular joints
Retracts the mandible at the
   temporomandibular joints

Innervation
The trigeminal nerve (CN V)

Arterial Supply
The maxillary artery

Myofascial Meridians
Deep front line

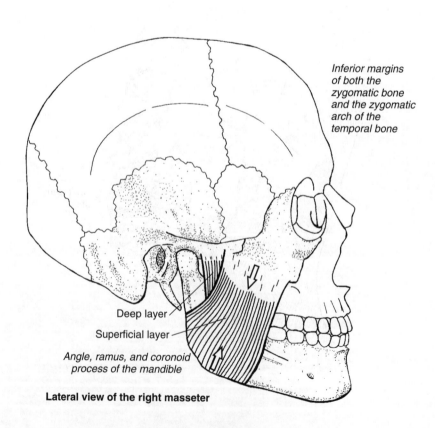

Inferior margins
of both the
zygomatic bone
and the zygomatic
arch of the
temporal bone

Deep layer

Superficial layer

Angle, ramus, and coronoid
process of the mandible

Lateral view of the right masseter

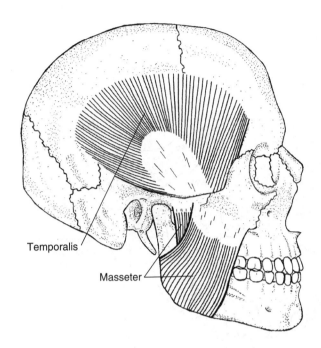

Temporalis

Masseter

DID
YOU
KNOW

The temporalis fossa attachment of the temporalis overlies a number of cranial bones.

DID
YOU
KNOW

The temporalis is often involved in tension headaches and temporomandibular joint (TMJ) dysfunction.

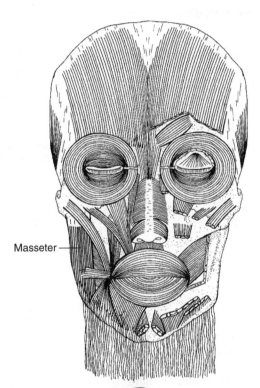

Masseter

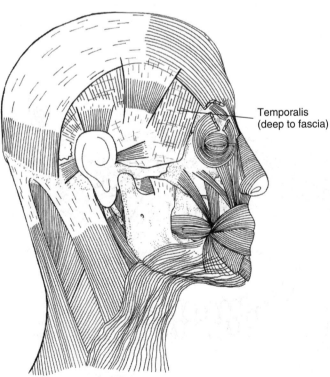

Temporalis
(deep to fascia)

(Masseter not shown
in this view)

DID
YOU
KNOW

The masseter has two layers: the larger superficial layer and the smaller deep layer.

DID
YOU
KNOW

Proportional to its size, the masseter is considered to be the strongest muscle in the human body.

LATERAL PTERYGOID

lat-er-al **ter**-i-goyd

Actions
Protracts the mandible at the
   temporomandibular joints
Contralaterally deviates
   the mandible at the
   temporomandibular joints

Innervation
The trigeminal nerve (CN V)

Arterial Supply
The maxillary artery

Myofascial Meridians
Deep front line

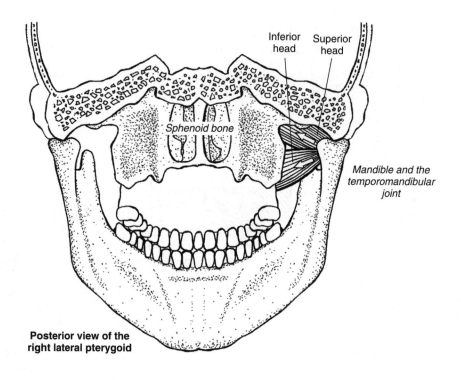

Inferior head

Superior head

Sphenoid bone

Mandible and the temporomandibular joint

Posterior view of the right lateral pterygoid

MEDIAL PTERYGOID

mee-dee-al **ter**-i-goyd

Actions
Elevates the mandible at the
   temporomandibular joints
Protracts the mandible at the
   temporomandibular joints
Contralaterally deviates
   the mandible at the
   temporomandibular joints

Innervation
The trigeminal nerve (CN V)

Arterial Supply
The maxillary artery

Myofascial Meridians
Deep front line

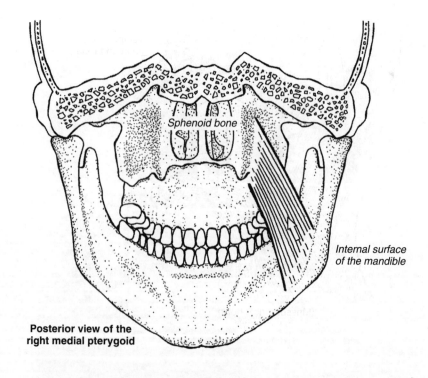

Sphenoid bone

Internal surface of the mandible

Posterior view of the right medial pterygoid

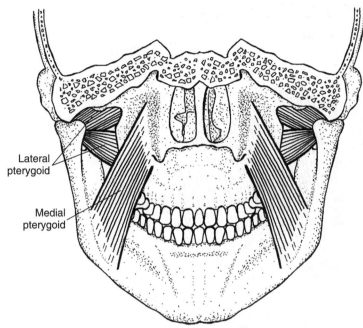

Lateral pterygoid

Medial pterygoid

The lateral pterygoid has two heads: a superior head and an inferior head.

The lateral pterygoid has an attachment directly into the capsule and articular disc of the TMJ, making this muscle likely to be involved in TMJ dysfunction.

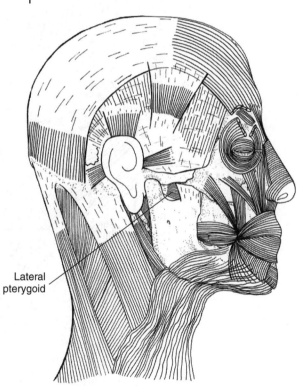

Lateral pterygoid

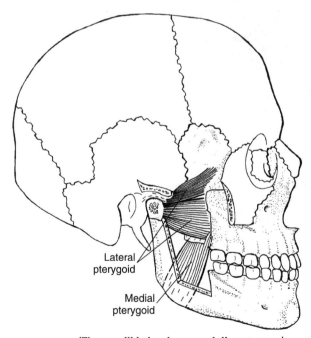

Lateral pterygoid

Medial pterygoid

(The mandible has been partially cut away.)

The direction of fibers of the medial pterygoid is essentially identical to the masseter, except that the medial pterygoid is deep to the mandible and the masseter is superficial to the mandible.

The medial pterygoid is sometimes known as the internal pterygoid.

ANTERIOR VIEW OF THE HEAD

SUPERIOR

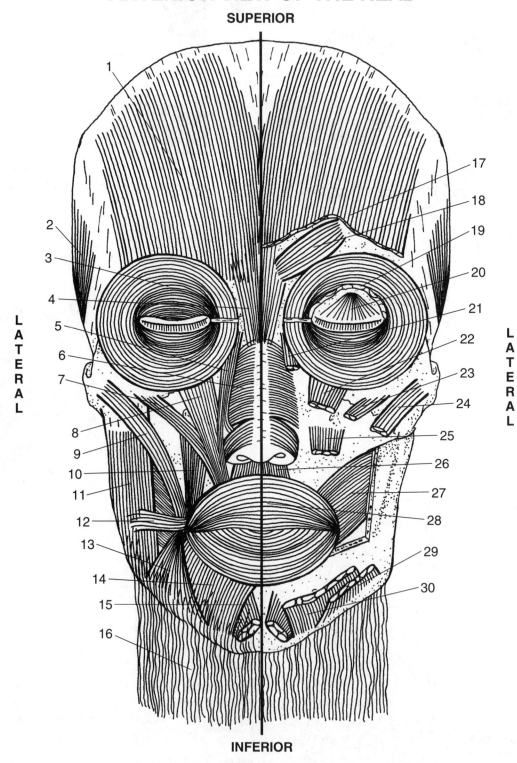

LATERAL

LATERAL

INFERIOR

LATERAL VIEW OF THE HEAD

SUPERIOR

POSTERIOR

ANTERIOR

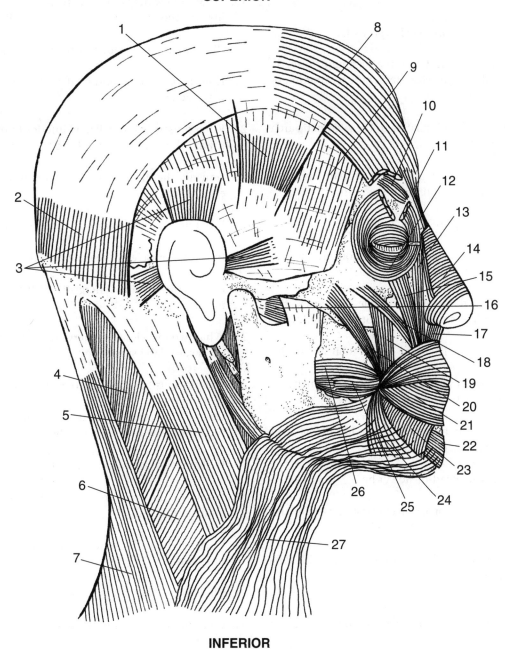

INFERIOR

Review Questions

Muscles of the Head
Answers to these questions are found on page 483.

1. What muscle of mastication has attachments directly into the capsule and articular disc of the temporomandibular joint?

2. Where is the temporalis relative to the zygomatic arch of the temporal bone?

3. What muscle of facial expression is primarily responsible for making the expression of pouting?

4. What muscles comprise the epicranius?

5. How many muscles of facial expression elevate the angle of the mouth?

6. Where they overlap, which muscle is deeper, the depressor anguli oris or the depressor labii inferioris?

7. What muscle lies medial to the levator labii superioris?

8. How are the depressor labii inferioris and mentalis antagonistic to each other?

9. What muscle of the mouth and nose lies medial and inferior to the orbicularis oculi?

10. What two muscles evert the lower lip?

11. How many muscles of facial expression elevate the upper lip?

12. Which scalp muscle is likely most involved with tension headaches?

13. What happens to the length of the right lateral pterygoid if the mandible laterally deviates to the right?

14. What muscle is located immediately inferior to the orbicularis oris?

15. What three muscles elevate the mandible at the temporomandibular joint?

16. How is the levator anguli oris synergistic with the zygomaticus major?

17. What muscle is synergistic with the nasalis?

18. Where they overlap, which muscle is superficial, the temporalis or the masseter?

19. What muscle helps to close the mouth by bringing the lips together without moving the mandible?

20. What are the two bellies of the occipitofrontalis?

21. How are the lateral and medial pterygoids synergistic with each other?

22. What muscle is immediately inferior to the occipitalis toward the midline of the head?

23. How are the digastric and temporalis antagonistic to each other?

24. What muscle is antagonistic to the nasalis?

25. Into what muscle of the nose does the frontalis blend?

26. How is the risorius synergistic with the zygomaticus major?

27. What two muscles are synergistic with both actions of the levator labii superioris?

28. The procerus lies superior to what muscle?

29. What is the name of the sheet of fascia that connects the frontalis with the occipitalis?

30. What muscle is antagonistic to the auricularis anterior?

31. What two muscles are immediately superior to the orbicularis oculi?

32. What muscle is antagonistic to the corrugator supercilii?

33. What muscle lies lateral to the levator labii superioris?

34. What muscle's superior attachment is located deep to the zygomaticus minor?

35. What muscle of facial expression creates the typical "Dracula" expression?

36. What muscle is immediately deep to the lateral attachment of the risorius?

37. What muscle attaches to the angle of the mouth and is located inferiorly to the risorius?

38. How are the depressor labii inferioris and mentalis synergistic with each other?

39. What two muscles are located immediately lateral to the orbicularis oris?

40. The depressor anguli oris and depressor labii inferioris both attach into what bone?

41. What muscle is synergistic with the corrugator supercilii?

42. What muscle is a muscle of facial expression of the mouth and nose?

43. What three muscles elevate the upper lip?

44. Which muscle is deeper, the temporoparietalis or the temporalis?

45. What muscle closes and squints the eye?

46. Where they overlap, which muscle is deeper, the depressor labii inferioris or the mentalis?

47. Which muscle is more medial, the zygomaticus major or minor?

48. What muscle of facial expression is primarily used when whistling?

49. What happens to the length of the orbicularis oris when the lips are puckered?

50. What are the two parts of the nasalis?

51. What two muscles lie superficial to the buccinator?

52. What muscle lies superior to the levator labii superioris?

53. What two muscles elevate the ear?

54. What muscle is located immediately medial to the zygomaticus minor?

55. What are the four major muscles of mastication?

56. What is similar and different about the orientation of the masseter and medial pterygoid?

57. What muscle lies immediately lateral to the nasalis?

58. The majority of the corrugator supercilii lies deep to what muscle?

59. What muscle of the nose attaches into only skin and fascia?

60. Name the auricularis muscles.

61. What muscle is superficial to the mentalis?

62. What muscle is located immediately superior to the orbicularis oris at the midline?

63. What muscle of the face is a sphincter muscle?

64. What muscle of facial expression is primarily used when blowing up a balloon?

65. What muscle is immediately inferior to the depressor septi nasi?

66. Which auricularis muscle attaches into the Galea aponeurotica?

67. What muscle of facial expression lies primarily within the eye socket?

68. What muscle of mastication attaches to the internal surface of the angle of the mandible?

69. What does the name risorius mean in Latin?

70. What muscle is antagonistic to the levator palpebrae superioris?

71. What action does the occipitofrontalis have upon the eyebrow?

72. Where they overlap, what is the relationship of the auricularis muscles to the temporalis?

73. What five muscles of facial expression attach into the mandible?

74. What happens to the length of the depressor anguli oris if the angle of the mouth is elevated?

75. The name of what facial muscle is derived from the Latin word for prince?

76. What happens to the length of the temporalis when the mandible depresses at the temporomandibular joints?

77. What muscle attaches between the two parts of the nasalis?

78. How many muscles of facial expression draw laterally the angle of the mouth?

Muscles of the Neck 4

Note: Throughout this chapter, muscle attachments are indicated by italics.

☻ More review activities on Evolve at: http://evolve.elsevier.com/Muscolino/anatomycoloring/

ANTERIOR VIEW OF THE NECK (SUPERFICIAL)

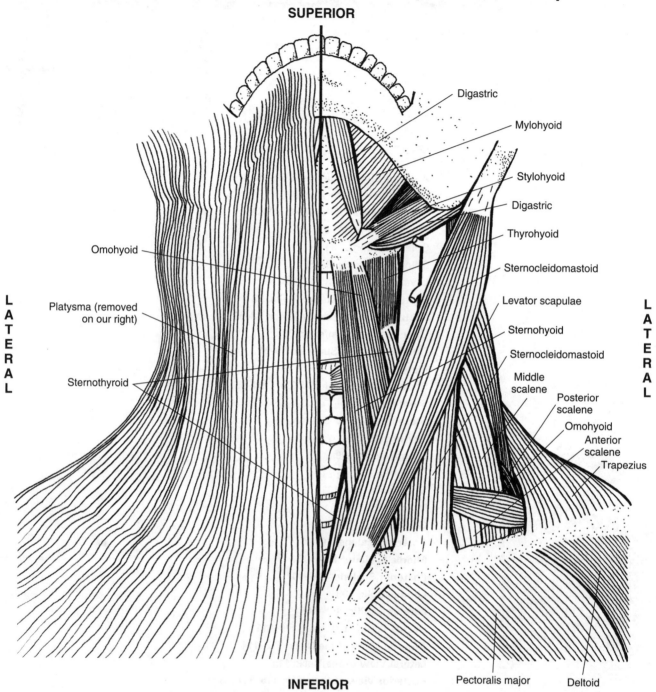

SUPERIOR

Digastric

Mylohyoid

Stylohyoid

Digastric

Thyrohyoid

Sternocleidomastoid

Levator scapulae

Sternohyoid

Sternocleidomastoid

Middle scalene

Posterior scalene

Omohyoid

Anterior scalene

Trapezius

Omohyoid

Platysma (removed on our right)

Sternothyroid

LATERAL

LATERAL

Pectoralis major

Deltoid

INFERIOR

ANTERIOR VIEW OF THE NECK (INTERMEDIATE)

SUPERIOR

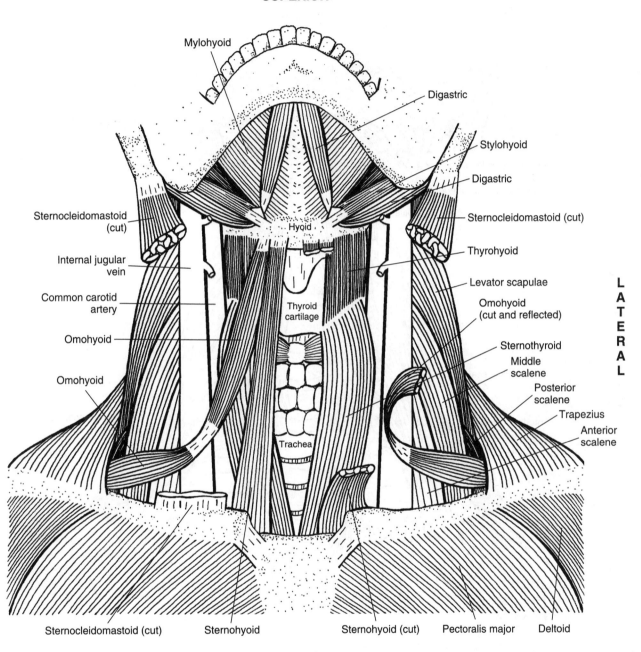

Mylohyoid

Digastric

Stylohyoid

Digastric

Sternocleidomastoid (cut)

Sternocleidomastoid (cut)

Internal jugular vein

Hyoid

Thyrohyoid

Common carotid artery

Thyroid cartilage

Levator scapulae

Omohyoid

Omohyoid (cut and reflected)

Omohyoid

Sternothyroid

Middle scalene

Posterior scalene

Trapezius

Trachea

Anterior scalene

LATERAL

LATERAL

Sternocleidomastoid (cut)   Sternohyoid   Sternohyoid (cut)   Pectoralis major   Deltoid

INFERIOR

ANTERIOR VIEW OF THE NECK (DEEP)

SUPERIOR

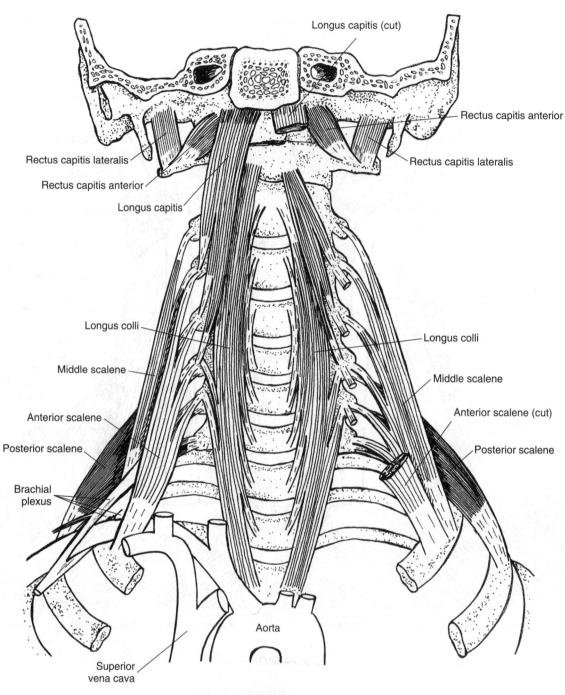

Longus capitis (cut)

Rectus capitis anterior

Rectus capitis lateralis

Rectus capitis lateralis

Rectus capitis anterior

Longus capitis

LATERAL

LATERAL

Longus colli

Longus colli

Middle scalene

Middle scalene

Anterior scalene

Anterior scalene (cut)

Posterior scalene

Posterior scalene

Brachial plexus

Aorta

Superior vena cava

INFERIOR

LATERAL VIEW OF THE NECK

SUPERIOR

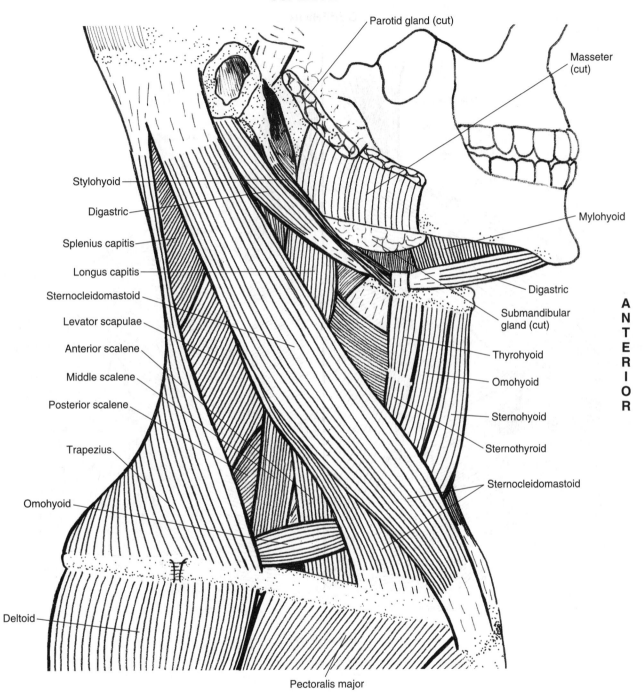

Parotid gland (cut)

Masseter (cut)

Stylohyoid

Digastric

Splenius capitis

Longus capitis

Sternocleidomastoid

Levator scapulae

Anterior scalene

Middle scalene

Posterior scalene

Trapezius

Omohyoid

Deltoid

Mylohyoid

Digastric

Submandibular gland (cut)

Thyrohyoid

Omohyoid

Sternohyoid

Sternothyroid

Sternocleidomastoid

P O S T E R I O R

A N T E R I O R

Pectoralis major

INFERIOR

POSTERIOR VIEW OF THE NECK
(SUPERFICIAL AND INTERMEDIATE)

SUPERIOR

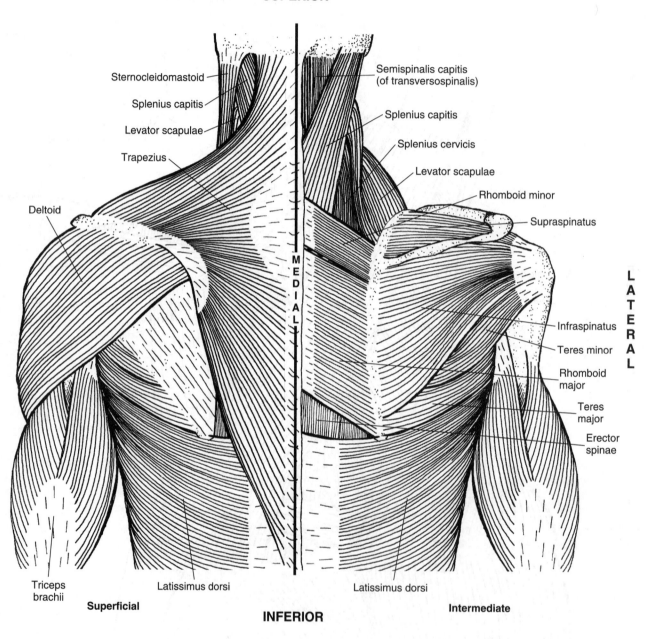

Sternocleidomastoid

Splenius capitis

Levator scapulae

Trapezius

Deltoid

LATERAL

Triceps brachii

Superficial

Latissimus dorsi

MEDIAL

Semispinalis capitis
(of transversospinalis)

Splenius capitis

Splenius cervicis

Levator scapulae

Rhomboid minor

Supraspinatus

Infraspinatus

Teres minor

Rhomboid major

Teres major

Erector spinae

LATERAL

Latissimus dorsi

Intermediate

INFERIOR

POSTERIOR VIEW OF THE NECK
(INTERMEDIATE AND DEEP)

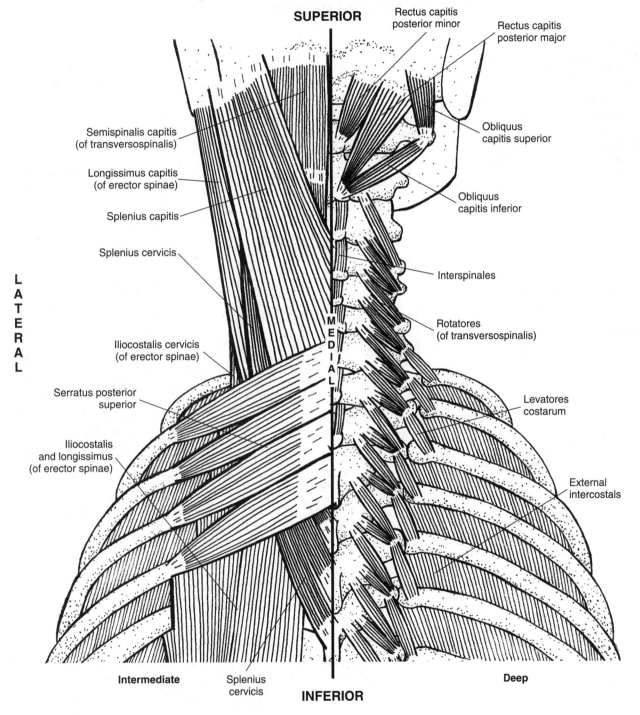

SUPERIOR

Rectus capitis
posterior minor

Rectus capitis
posterior major

Semispinalis capitis
(of transversospinalis)

Obliquus
capitis superior

Longissimus capitis
(of erector spinae)

Splenius capitis

Obliquus
capitis inferior

Splenius cervicis

Interspinales

Iliocostalis cervicis
(of erector spinae)

Rotatores
(of transversospinalis)

Serratus posterior
superior

Levatores
costarum

Iliocostalis
and longissimus
(of erector spinae)

External
intercostals

LATERAL

LATERAL

MEDIAL

Intermediate

Splenius
cervicis

Deep

INFERIOR

TRAPEZIUS ("TRAP")

tra-**pee**-zee-us

Actions
Lateral flexion of the neck and
the head at the spinal joints
(upper)
Extension of the neck and the
head at the spinal joints
(upper)
Contralateral rotation of the
neck and the head at the
spinal joints (upper)
Elevation of the scapula at the
scapulocostal joint (upper)
Retraction (adduction) of the
scapula at the scapulocostal
joint (entire muscle)
Depression of the scapula at the
scapulocostal joint (lower)
Upward rotation of the scapula
at the scapulocostal joint
(upper and lower)
Extension of the trunk at the
spinal joints (middle and
lower)

Innervation
Spinal accessory nerve (CN XI)

Arterial Supply
The transverse cervical artery
and the dorsal scapular artery

Myofascial Meridians
Superficial back line

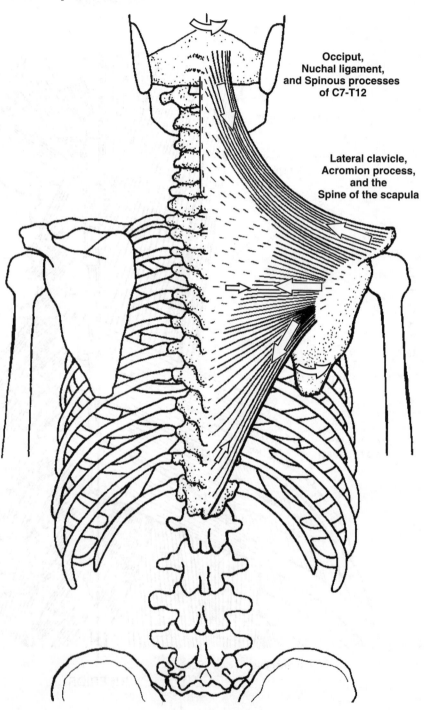

Occiput,
Nuchal ligament,
and Spinous processes
of C7-T12

Lateral clavicle,
Acromion process,
and the
Spine of the scapula

**Posterior view of the
right trapezius**

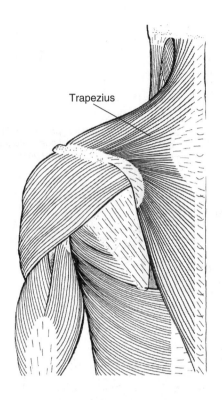

Trapezius

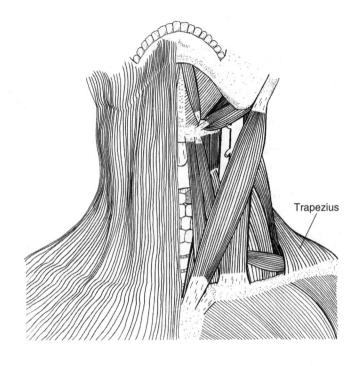

Trapezius

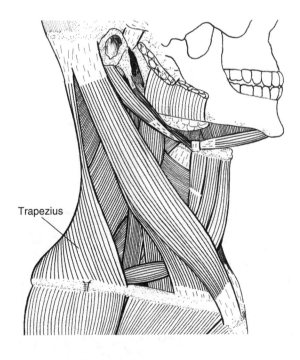

Trapezius

The trapezius is considered to have three functional parts: upper, middle, and lower. This muscle is extremely important, as it is involved in both postural stabilization and active movement of the head, neck, trunk, and shoulder girdle.

The distal attachments of the trapezius are the same as the proximal attachments of the deltoid.

SPLENIUS CAPITIS

splee-nee-us **kap**-i-tis

Actions
Extension of the head and the neck at the spinal joints
Lateral flexion of the head and the neck at the spinal joints
Ipsilateral rotation of the head and the neck at the spinal joints

Innervation
Cervical spinal nerves

Arterial Supply
The occipital artery

Myofascial Meridians
Lateral line
Spiral line

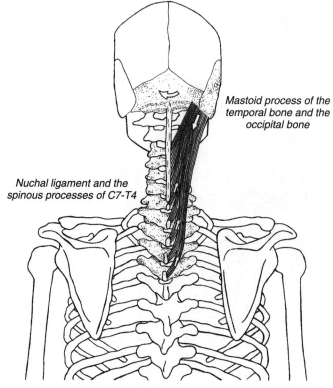

Mastoid process of the temporal bone and the occipital bone

Nuchal ligament and the spinous processes of C7-T4

Posterior view of the right splenius capitis

SPLENIUS CERVICIS

splee-nee-us **ser**-vi-sis

Actions
Extension of the neck at the spinal joints
Lateral flexion of the neck at the spinal joints
Ipsilateral rotation of the neck at the spinal joints

Innervation
Cervical spinal nerves

Arterial Supply
The occipital artery and the dorsal branches of the upper posterior intercostal arteries

Myofascial Meridians
Spiral line

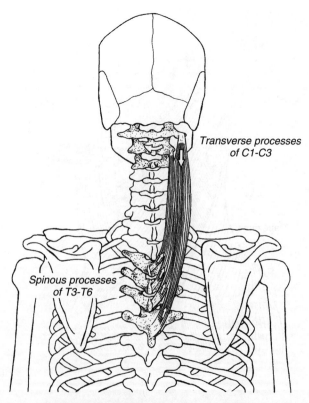

Transverse processes of C1-C3

Spinous processes of T3-T6

Posterior view of the right splenius cervicis

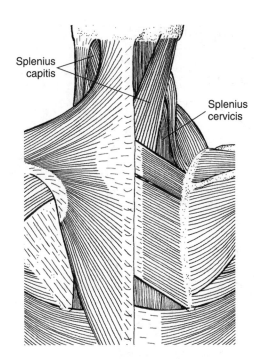

Splenius capitis

Splenius cervicis

Because of their "V" shape, the left and right splenius capitis muscles are sometimes called the "golf tee" muscles.

The word "splenius" means bandage.

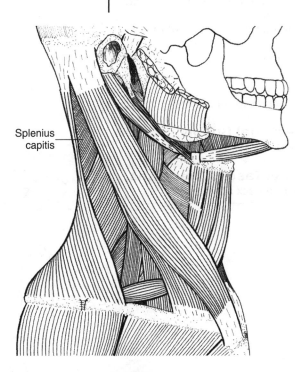

Splenius capitis

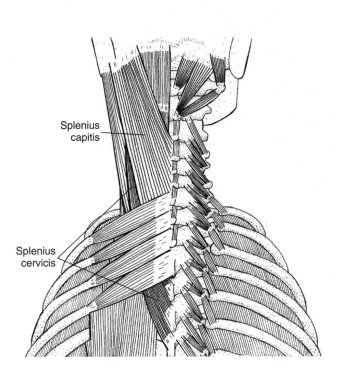

Splenius capitis

Splenius cervicis

The left and right splenius cervicis muscles also form a "V" shape.

Most of the splenius cervicis lies deep to the splenius capitis.

LEVATOR SCAPULAE

le-**vay**-tor **skap**-you-lee

Actions
Elevation of the scapula at the scapulocostal joint

Extension of the neck at the spinal joints

Lateral flexion of the neck at the spinal joints

Ipsilateral rotation of the neck at the spinal joints

Downward rotation of the scapula at the scapulocostal joint

Retraction (adduction) of the scapula at the scapulocostal joint

Innervation
Dorsal scapular nerve

Arterial Supply
The dorsal scapular artery

Myofascial Meridians
Deep back arm line

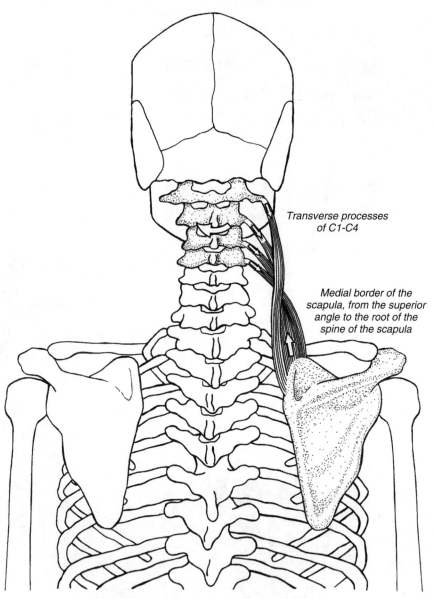

Transverse processes of C1-C4

Medial border of the scapula, from the superior angle to the root of the spine of the scapula

Posterior view of the right levator scapulae

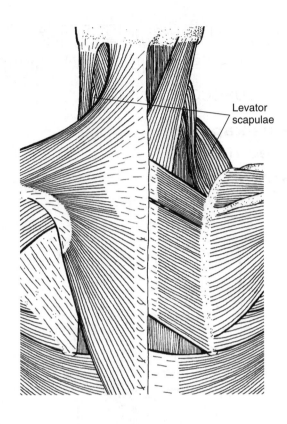

Levator
scapulae

DID YOU KNOW?

The levator scapulae has a twist in its fibers so that the most superior fibers on the scapula attach the most inferiorly on the spine, and vice versa.

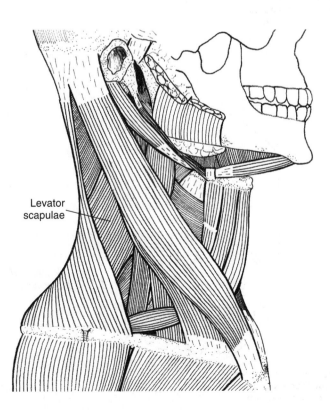

Levator
scapulae

DID YOU KNOW?

Regarding the neck, the levator scapulae and upper trapezius are synergistic with respect to sagittal-plane extension and frontal-plane lateral flexion, but are antagonistic with respect to transverse plane rotation.

Actions
Extension of the head at the atlanto-occipital joint

Lateral flexion of the head at the atlanto-occipital joint

Ipsilateral rotation of the head at the atlanto-occipital joint

Extension and ipsilateral rotation of the atlas at the atlantoaxial joint

Innervation
The suboccipital nerve

Arterial Supply
The occipital artery and the deep cervical artery

Myofascial Meridians
Superficial back line

RECTUS CAPITIS POSTERIOR MAJOR
(OF THE SUBOCCIPITAL GROUP)

rek-tus **kap**-i-tis
pos-**tee**-ri-or
may-jor

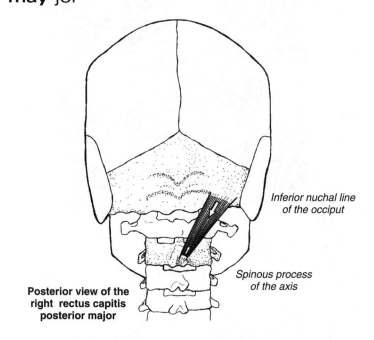

Inferior nuchal line of the occiput

Spinous process of the axis

Posterior view of the right rectus capitis posterior major

RECTUS CAPITIS POSTERIOR MINOR
(OF THE SUBOCCIPITAL GROUP)

rek-tus **kap**-i-tis pos-**tee**-ri-or **my**-nor

Action
Protraction of the head at the atlanto-occipital joint

Extension of the head at the atlanto-occipital joint

Innervation
The suboccipital nerve

Arterial Supply
The occipital artery and muscular branches of the vertebral artery

Myofascial Meridians
Superficial back line

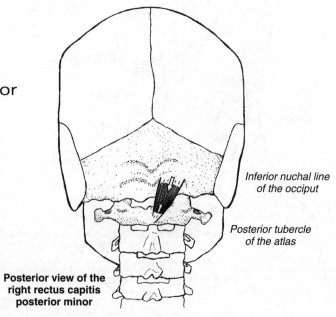

Inferior nuchal line of the occiput

Posterior tubercle of the atlas

Posterior view of the right rectus capitis posterior minor

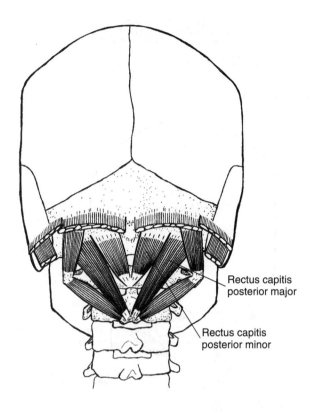

Rectus capitis
posterior major

Rectus capitis
posterior minor

*The rectus capitis posterior major is
the largest of the suboccipital group.
The suboccipital group is primarily
important as the postural stabilizer of
the head.*

*The rectus capitis posterior major and
rectus capitis posterior minor both
attach onto the inferior nuchal line of
the occiput.*

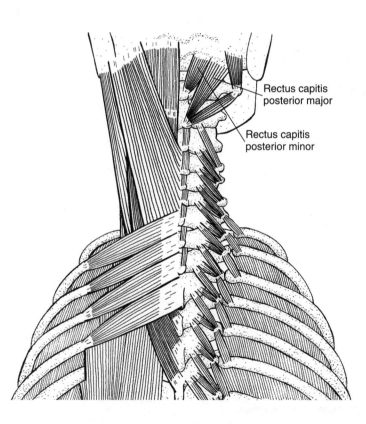

Rectus capitis
posterior major

Rectus capitis
posterior minor

*The rectus capitis posterior minor has
an additional attachment that asserts
its pull into the dura mater, making
this muscle extremely likely to cause
headaches when it is tight.*

*The rectus capitis posterior minor
is locked short (tight) in people with
forward head posture.*

OBLIQUUS CAPITIS INFERIOR

(OF THE SUBOCCIPITAL GROUP)

ob-**lee**-kwus **kap**-i-tis in-**fee**-ri-or

Action
Ipsilateral rotation of the atlas at the
   atlantoaxial joint

Innervation
The suboccipital nerve

Arterial Supply
The deep cervical artery and the
   descending branch of the occipital
   artery

Myofascial Meridians
Superficial back line

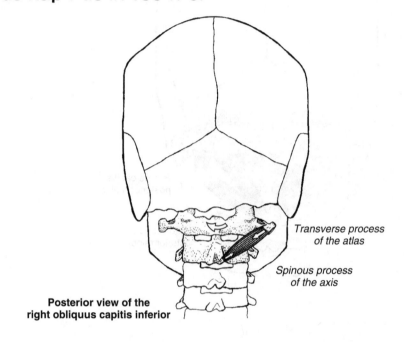

Transverse process
of the atlas

Spinous process
of the axis

**Posterior view of the
right obliquus capitis inferior**

OBLIQUUS CAPITIS SUPERIOR

(OF THE SUBOCCIPITAL GROUP)

ob-**lee**-kwus **kap**-i-tis sue-**pee**-ri-or

Actions
Protraction of the head at the atlanto-
   occipital joint
Extension of the head at the atlanto-
   occipital joint
Lateral flexion of the head at the atlanto-
   occipital joint

Innervation
The suboccipital nerve

Arterial Supply
The occipital artery and the deep cervical
   artery

Myofascial Meridians
Superficial back line
Lateral line

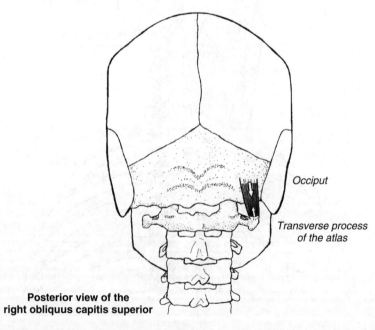

Occiput

Transverse process
of the atlas

**Posterior view of the
right obliquus capitis superior**

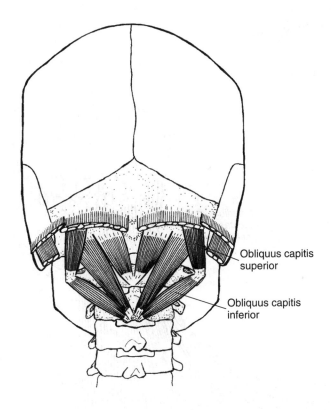

Obliquus capitis
superior

Obliquus capitis
inferior

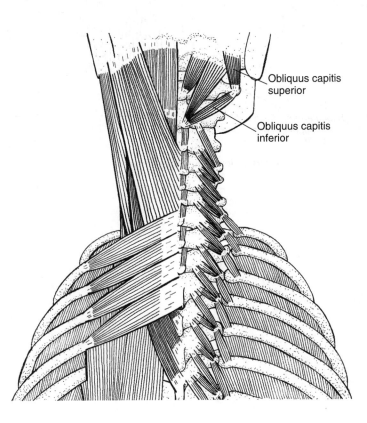

Obliquus capitis
superior

Obliquus capitis
inferior

The obliquus capitis inferior is the only one of the four suboccipital muscles that does not cross the atlanto-occipital joint to attach onto the head; therefore its name is a misnomer.

The obliquus capitis inferior is misnamed because it has the word "capitis" in its name, but it does not attach onto the head.

Of the four suboccipital muscles, the obliquus capitis superior attaches the most superiorly on the occiput.

The obliquus capitis superior, obliquus capitis inferior, and rectus capitis posterior major enclose a space known as the suboccipital triangle.

PLATYSMA

pla-**tiz**-ma

Actions
Draws up the skin of the superior
chest and neck, creating ridges
of skin in the neck
Depresses and draws the lower lip
laterally
Depression of the mandible at the
temporomandibular joint

Innervation
Facial nerve (CN VII)

Arterial Supply
The facial artery

Myofascial Meridians
Involved: Superficial back line
Involved: Superficial front arm line

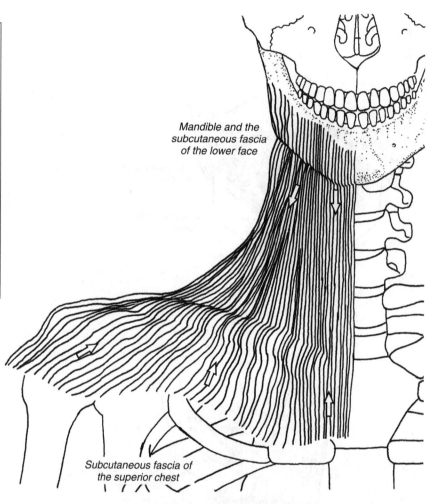

Mandible and the
subcutaneous fascia
of the lower face

Subcutaneous fascia of
the superior chest

Anterior view of the right platysma

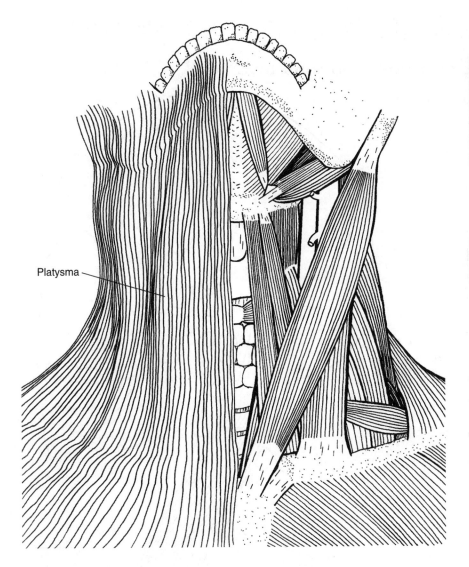

Platysma

The platysma creates wrinkles on the neck that are reminiscent of the creature from the film, The Creature from the Black Lagoon.

The platysma is considered to be a muscle of facial expression.

STERNOCLEIDOMASTOID ("SCM")

ster-no-**kli**-do-**mas**-toyd

Actions
Flexion of the neck at the
  spinal joints
Lateral flexion of the neck and
  the head at the spinal joints
Contralateral rotation of the
  neck and the head at the
  spinal joints
Extension of the head at the
  atlanto-occipital joint
Elevation of the sternum and
  the clavicle

Innervation
Spinal accessory nerve (CN XI)

Arterial Supply
The occipital and posterior
  auricular arteries

Myofascial Meridians
Superficial front line
Lateral line

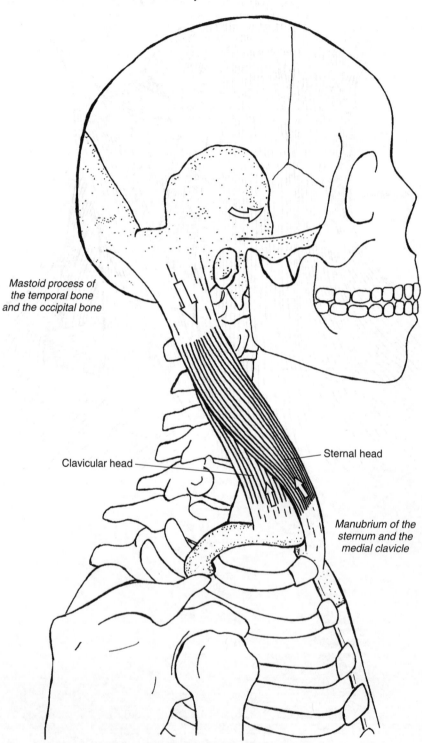

*Mastoid process of
the temporal bone
and the occipital bone*

Clavicular head ———

——— Sternal head

*Manubrium of the
sternum and the
medial clavicle*

Lateral view of the right sternocleidomastoid

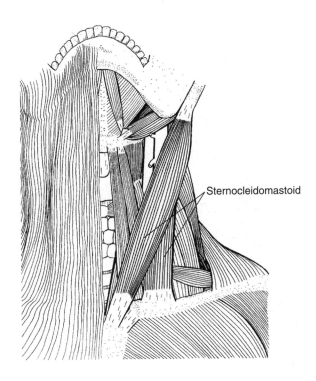

Sternocleidomastoid

The sternocleidomastoid is unusual in that it flexes the neck at the spinal joints, but it extends the head at the atlanto-occipital joint.

Sternocleidomastoid

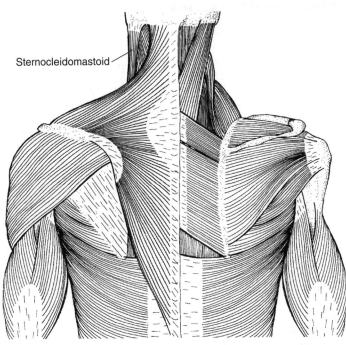

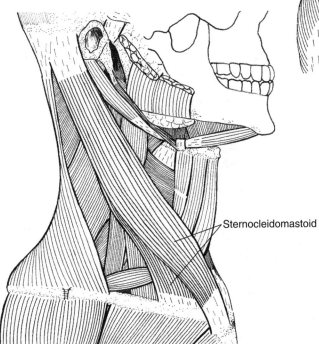

Sternocleidomastoid

Because of its occipital bone attachment, the sternocleidomastoid is sometimes known as the sterno-cleido-masto-occipitalis.

STERNOHYOID
(OF THE HYOID GROUP)
ster-no-hi-oyd

Action
Depression of the hyoid

Innervation
The cervical plexus

Arterial Supply
The superior thyroid artery

Myofascial Meridians
Deep front line

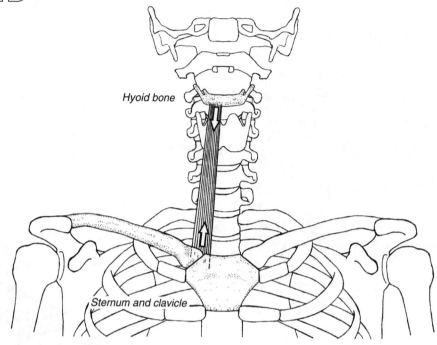

Hyoid bone

Sternum and clavicle

Anterior view of the right sternohyoid

STERNOTHYROID
(OF THE HYOID GROUP)

ster-no-thi-royd

Action
Depression of the thyroid cartilage

Innervation
The cervical plexus

Arterial Supply
The superior thyroid artery

Myofascial Meridians
Deep front line

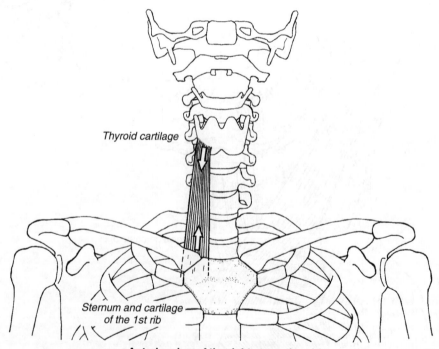

Thyroid cartilage

Sternum and cartilage of the 1st rib

Anterior view of the right sternothyroid

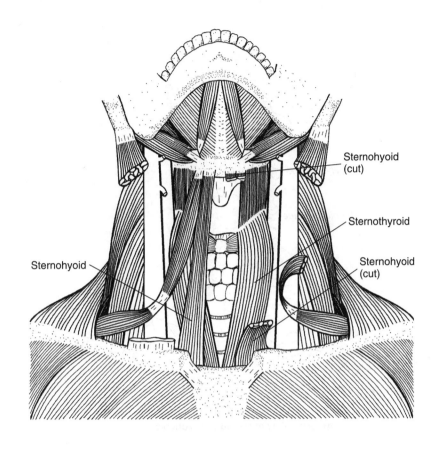

Sternohyoid (cut)

Sternothyroid

Sternohyoid (cut)

Sternohyoid

The sternohyoid attaches to the posterior surface of both the manubrium of the sternum and the medial clavicle.

The sternohyoid overlies the sternothyroid and thyrohyoid.

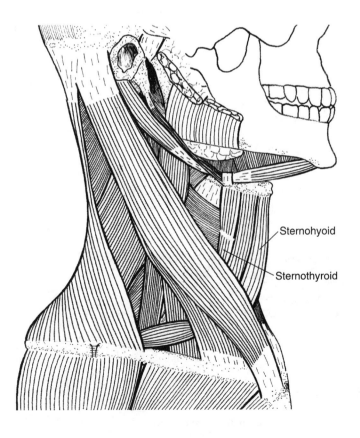

Sternohyoid

Sternothyroid

The sternothyroid attaches to the posterior surface of both the manubrium of the sternum and the costal cartilage of the 1st rib.

The sternothyroid and thyrohyoid together can function as one continuous muscle from the sternum to the hyoid bone.

THYROHYOID
(OF THE HYOID GROUP)

thi-ro-hi-oyd

Actions
Depression of the hyoid
Elevation of the thyroid
   cartilage

Innervation
The hypoglossal nerve (CN
XII)

Arterial Supply
The superior thyroid artery

Myofascial Meridians
Deep front line

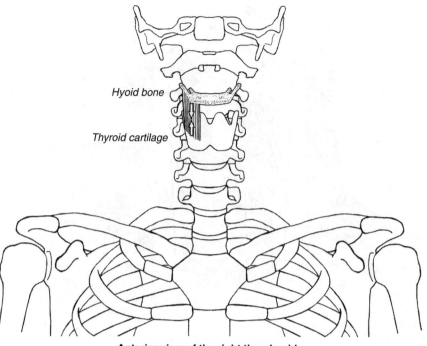

Anterior view of the right thyrohyoid

OMOHYOID
(OF THE HYOID GROUP)

o-mo-hi-oyd

Action
Depression of the hyoid

Innervation
The cervical plexus

Arterial Supply
The superior thyroid artery
   and the transverse
   cervical artery

**Myofascial
Meridians**
Deep front line

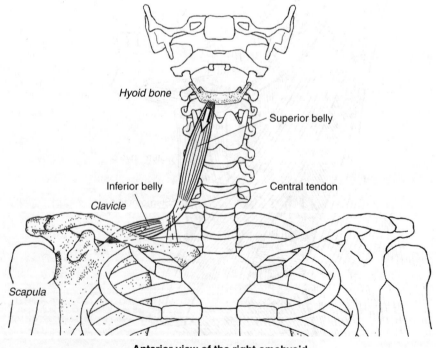

Anterior view of the right omohyoid

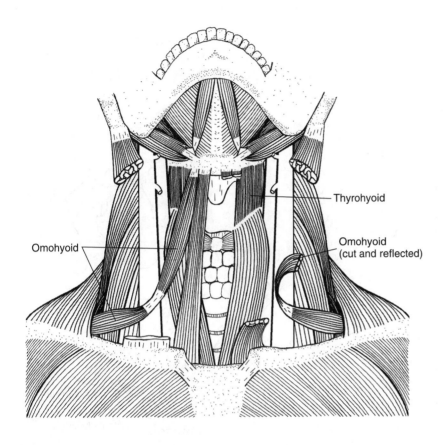

Thyrohyoid

Omohyoid

Omohyoid
(cut and reflected)

The thyrohyoid can be considered to be an upward continuation of the sternothyroid muscle.

A major function of all infrahyoid musculature is to stabilize the hyoid bone downward as the suprahyoid musculature depresses the mandible.

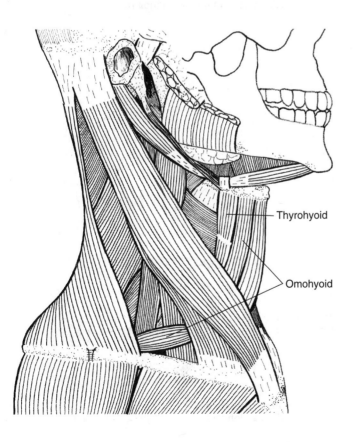

Thyrohyoid

Omohyoid

The omohyoid has two bellies separated by a central tendon that attaches to the clavicle by a fibrous sling of tissue.

The omohyoid attaches onto the scapula. "Omo" is Greek for shoulder.

DIGASTRIC
(OF THE HYOID GROUP)

di-**gas**-trik

Actions
Elevation of the hyoid
Depression of the mandible at the
   temporomandibular joints
Retraction of the mandible at the
   temporomandibular joints

Innervation
The trigeminal (CN V) and the facial
   nerve (CN VII)

Arterial Supply
The occipital, posterior auricular,
   and facial arteries

Myofascial Meridians
Deep front line

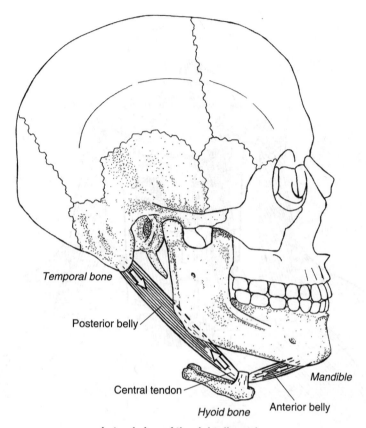

Temporal bone

Posterior belly

Central tendon
Hyoid bone

Mandible

Anterior belly

Lateral view of the right digastric

STYLOHYOID
(OF THE HYOID GROUP)

sti-lo-**hi**-oyd

Action
Elevation of the hyoid

Innervation
The facial nerve (CN VII)

Arterial Supply
The occipital, posterior
   auricular, and facial arteries

Myofascial Meridians
Deep front line

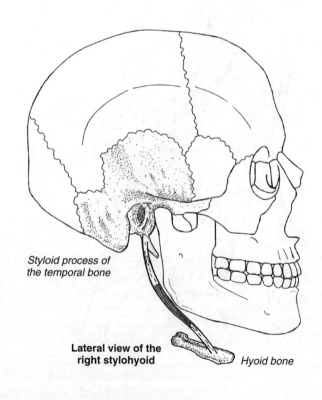

*Styloid process of
the temporal bone*

**Lateral view of the
right stylohyoid**

Hyoid bone

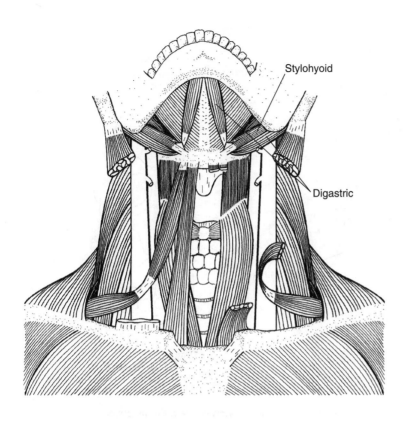

Stylohyoid

Digastric

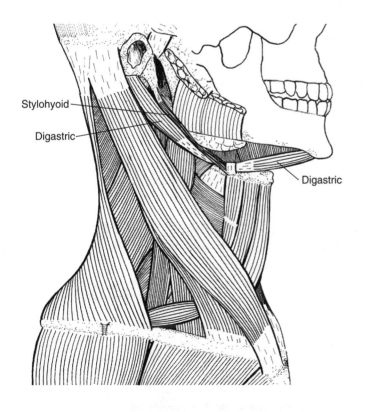

Stylohyoid

Digastric

Digastric

DID YOU KNOW?

The digastric has two bellies that are separated by a central tendon that attaches to the hyoid bone by a fibrous sling of tissue. In fact, the name digastric means "two bellies" in Greek.

DID YOU KNOW?

The digastric is considered to be the prime mover of depression of the mandible at the temporomandibular joints.

DID YOU KNOW?

The attachment of the stylohyoid onto the hyoid bone is perforated by the central tendon of the digastric.

DID YOU KNOW?

The stylohyoid is the only infrahyoid muscle that does not attach onto the mandible.

MYLOHYOID
(OF THE HYOID GROUP)

my-lo-**hi**-oyd

Actions
Elevation of the hyoid
Depression of the mandible at the
  temporomandibular joints

Innervation
The trigeminal nerve (CN V)

Arterial Supply
The inferior alveolar artery

Myofascial Meridians
Deep front line

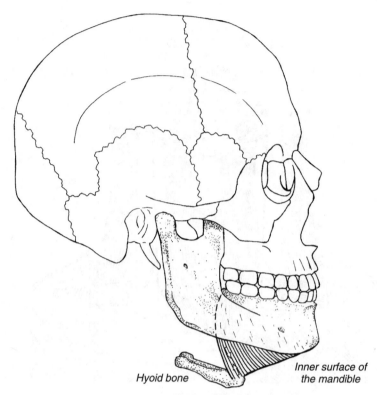

Hyoid bone   *Inner surface of
                       the mandible*

Lateral view of the right mylohyoid

GENIOHYOID
(OF THE HYOID GROUP)

jee-nee-o-**hi**-oyd

Actions
Elevation of the hyoid
Depression of the mandible at the
  temporomandibular joints

Innervation
The hypoglossal nerve (CN XII)

Arterial Supply
The lingual artery

Myofascial Meridians
Deep front line

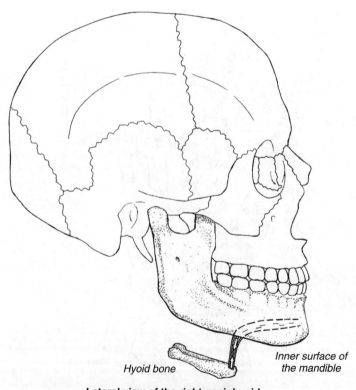

Hyoid bone   *Inner surface of
                       the mandible*

Lateral view of the right geniohyoid

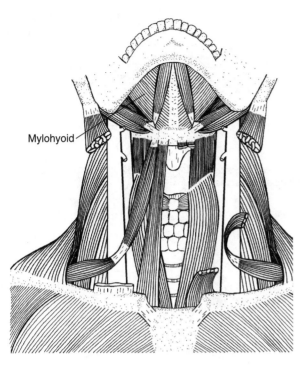

Mylohyoid

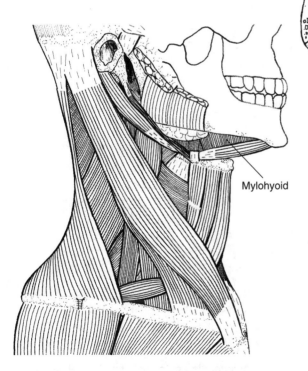

Mylohyoid

One function of the mylohyoid is to elevate the floor of the mouth during the first stage of swallowing.

"Mylo" is Greek for molar. The mylohyoid attaches onto the mandible near the molar teeth.

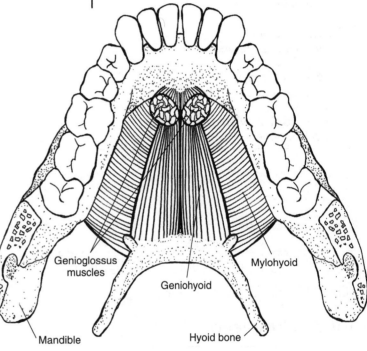

Genioglossus muscles

Mylohyoid

Geniohyoid

Mandible

Hyoid bone

Superior view of the floor of the mouth

The geniohyoid muscles are two pencil-thin muscles located between the mylohyoids and the genioglossus muscles of the tongue.

"Genio" is Greek for chin. The geniohyoid attaches onto the mandible in the region of the chin.

ANTERIOR SCALENE
(OF THE SCALENE GROUP)

an-**tee**-ri-or **skay**-leen

Actions
Flexion of the neck at the spinal joints
Lateral flexion of the neck at the spinal
    joints
Elevation of the 1st rib at the
    sternocostal and costovertebral joints
Contralateral rotation of the neck at the
    spinal joints

Innervation
Cervical spinal nerves

Arterial Supply
The ascending cervical artery

Myofascial Meridians
Deep front line

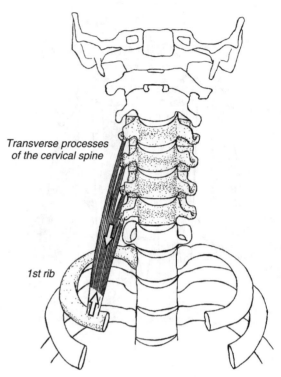

*Transverse processes
of the cervical spine*

1st rib

Anterior view of the right anterior scalene

MIDDLE SCALENE
(OF THE SCALENE GROUP)

mi-dil **skay**-leen

Actions
Lateral flexion of the neck at
    the spinal joints
Flexion of the neck at the
    spinal joints
Elevation of the 1st rib at
    the sternocostal and
    costovertebral joints

Innervation
Cervical spinal nerves

Arterial Supply
The transverse cervical artery

Myofascial Meridians
Deep front line

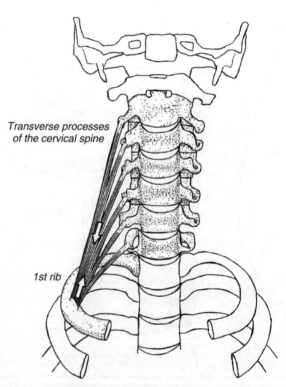

*Transverse processes
of the cervical spine*

1st rib

Anterior view of the right middle scalene

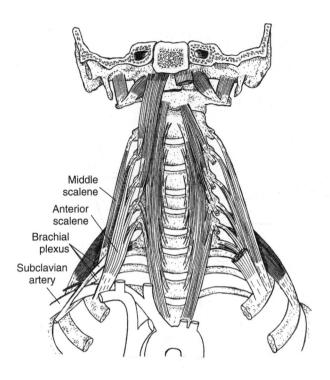

Middle scalene

Anterior scalene

Brachial plexus

Subclavian artery

The brachial plexus of nerves and subclavian artery run between the anterior and middle scalenes and can be compressed if these muscles are tight. When this occurs, it is called anterior scalene syndrome, a type of thoracic outlet syndrome.

The anterior scalene attaches onto the anterior tubercles of the transverse processes of the cervical spine.

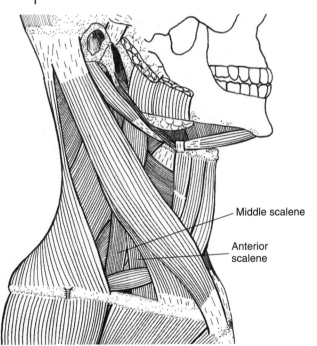

Middle scalene

Anterior scalene

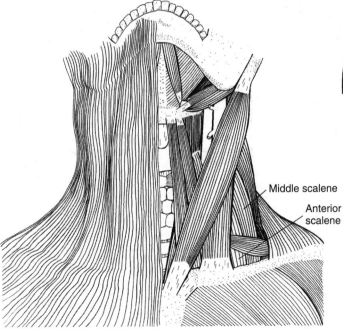

Middle scalene

Anterior scalene

The middle scalene is the largest of the three scalene muscles.

The middle scalene attaches onto the posterior tubercles of the transverse processes of the cervical spine.

POSTERIOR SCALENE
(OF THE SCALENE GROUP)

pos-**tee**-ri-or **skay**-leen

Actions
Lateral flexion of the neck at
 the spinal joints
Elevation of the 2nd rib
 at the sternocostal and
 costovertebral joints

Innervation
Cervical spinal nerves

Arterial Supply
The transverse cervical artery

Myofascial Meridians
Deep front line

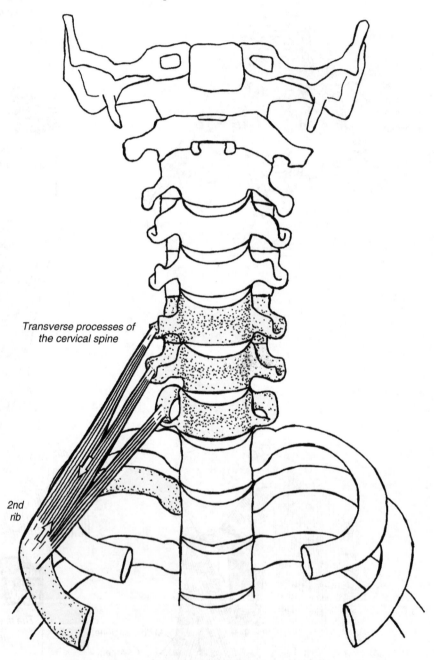

Transverse processes of
the cervical spine

2nd
rib

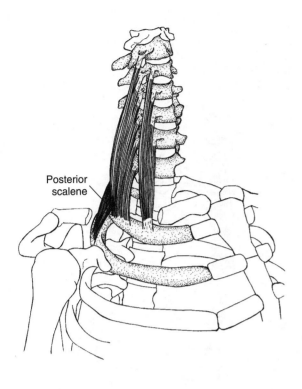

Posterior
scalene

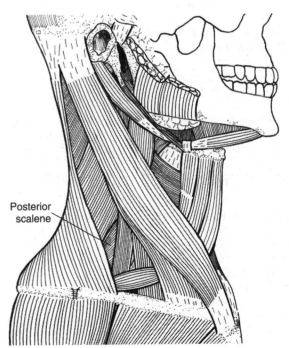

Posterior
scalene

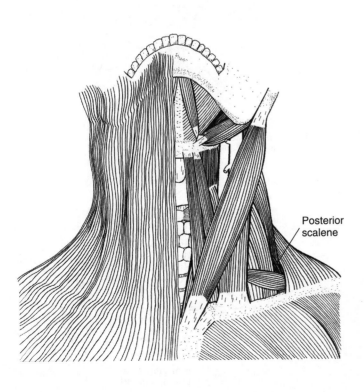

Posterior
scalene

LONGUS COLLI
(OF THE PREVERTEBRAL GROUP)

long-us kol-eye

Actions
Flexion of the neck at the spinal joints
Lateral flexion of the neck at the spinal joints
Contralateral rotation of the neck at the spinal joints

Innervation
Cervical spinal nerves

Arterial Supply
The inferior thyroid artery and the vertebral artery

Myofascial Meridians
Deep front line

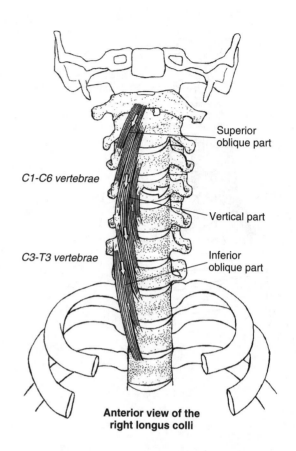

C1-C6 vertebrae

C3-T3 vertebrae

Superior oblique part

Vertical part

Inferior oblique part

Anterior view of the right longus colli

LONGUS CAPITIS
(OF THE PREVERTEBRAL GROUP)

long-us kap-i-tis

Actions
Flexion of the head and the neck at the spinal joints
Lateral flexion of the head and the neck at the spinal joints

Innervation
Cervical spinal nerves

Arterial Supply
The inferior thyroid artery and the vertebral artery

Myofascial Meridians
Deep front line

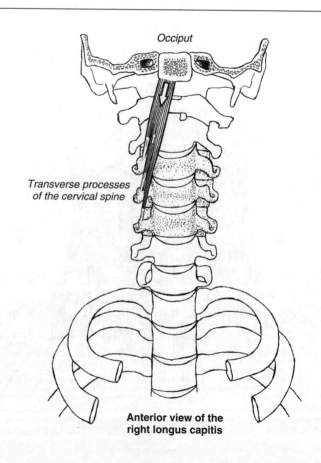

Occiput

Transverse processes of the cervical spine

Anterior view of the right longus capitis

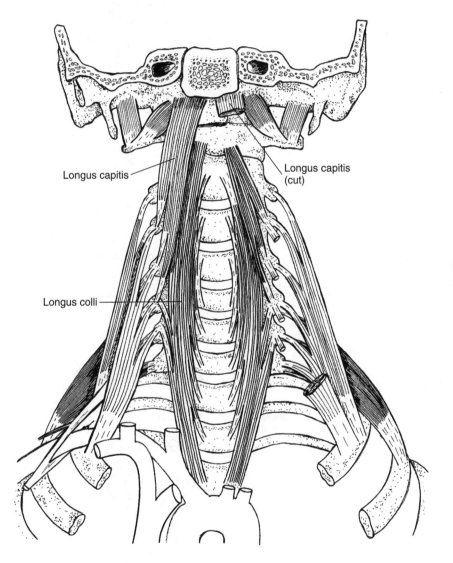

Longus capitis

Longus capitis (cut)

Longus colli

DID YOU KNOW?

When the longus colli and longus capitis muscles are tight, it can hurt to swallow and feel like a sore throat.

DID YOU KNOW?

The longus colli and longus capitis lie very close to the common carotid artery, so palpation and soft tissue manipulation of these muscles must be done very carefully.

RECTUS CAPITIS ANTERIOR

(OF THE PREVERTEBRAL GROUP)

rek-tus **kap**-i-tis an-**tee**-ri-or

Action
Flexion of the head at the
atlanto-occipital joint

Innervation
Cervical spinal nerves

Arterial Supply
The vertebral artery

Myofascial Meridians
Deep front line

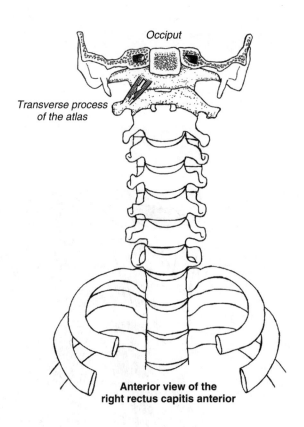

Occiput

*Transverse process
of the atlas*

**Anterior view of the
right rectus capitis anterior**

RECTUS CAPITIS LATERALIS

(OF THE PREVERTEBRAL GROUP)

rek-tus **kap**-i-tis la-ter-**a**-lis

Action
Lateral flexion of the head at
the atlanto-occipital joint

Innervation
Cervical spinal nerves

Arterial Supply
The vertebral artery and the
occipital artery

Myofascial Meridians
Involved: Deep front line
Involved: Lateral line
Involved: Deep back arm line

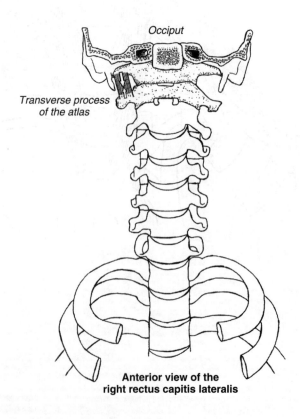

Occiput

*Transverse process
of the atlas*

**Anterior view of the
right rectus capitis lateralis**

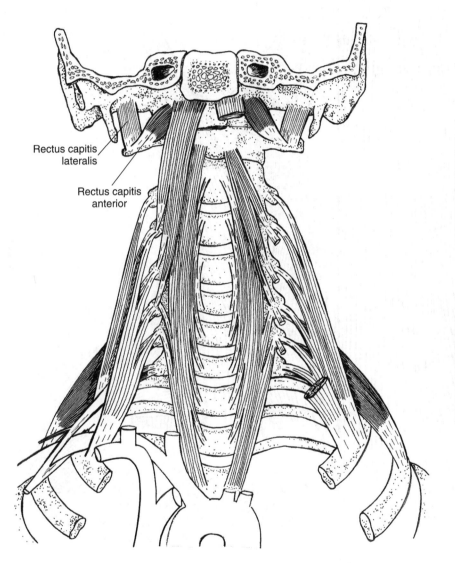

Rectus capitis
lateralis

Rectus capitis
anterior

**DID
YOU
KNOW**

*The rectus capitis anterior and
rectus capitis lateralis are generally
considered to be more important as
postural stabilization muscles of the
head than as movers.*

**DID
YOU
KNOW**

*Both the rectus capitis anterior and the
rectus capitis lateralis attach from the
transverse process of the atlas to the
occiput.*

ANTERIOR VIEW OF THE NECK (SUPERFICIAL)

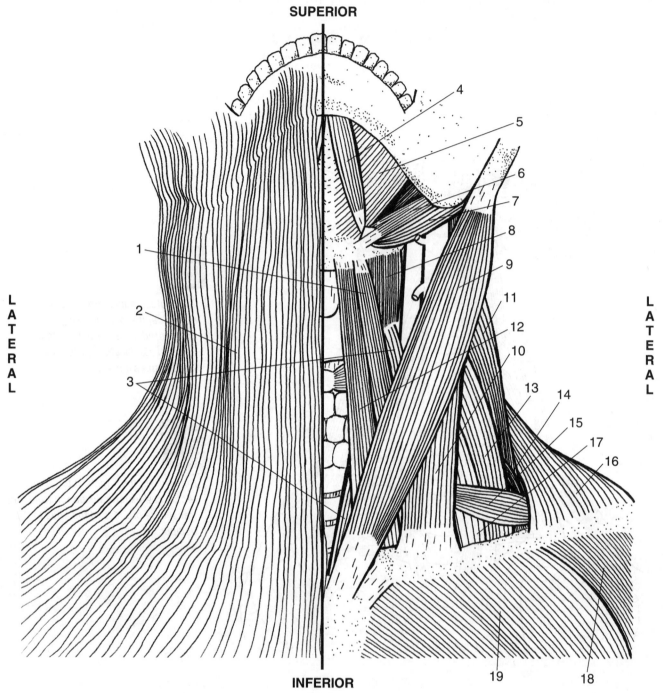

SUPERIOR

LATERAL

LATERAL

INFERIOR

Answers to labeling exercises are on p. 483.

ANTERIOR VIEW OF THE NECK (INTERMEDIATE)

SUPERIOR

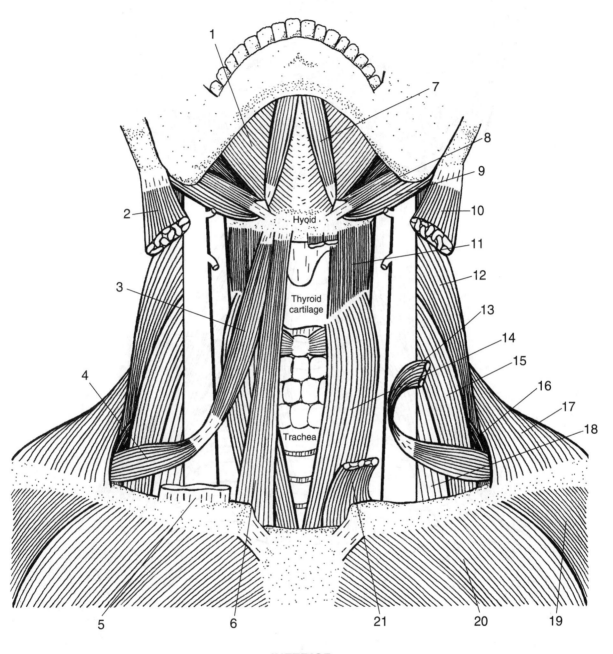

LATERAL

LATERAL

Hyoid

Thyroid
cartilage

Trachea

INFERIOR

ANTERIOR VIEW OF THE NECK (DEEP)

SUPERIOR

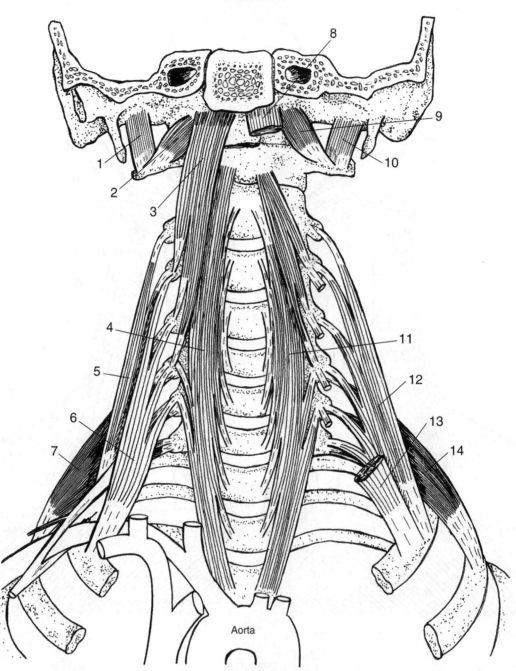

LATERAL

LATERAL

Aorta

INFERIOR

LATERAL VIEW OF THE NECK

SUPERIOR

POSTERIOR

ANTERIOR

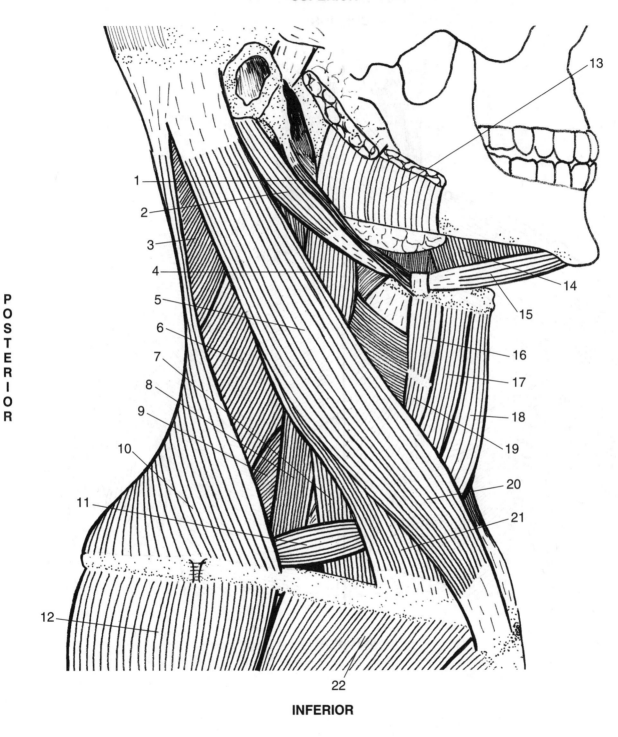

INFERIOR

POSTERIOR VIEW OF THE NECK (SUPERFICIAL AND INTERMEDIATE)

SUPERIOR

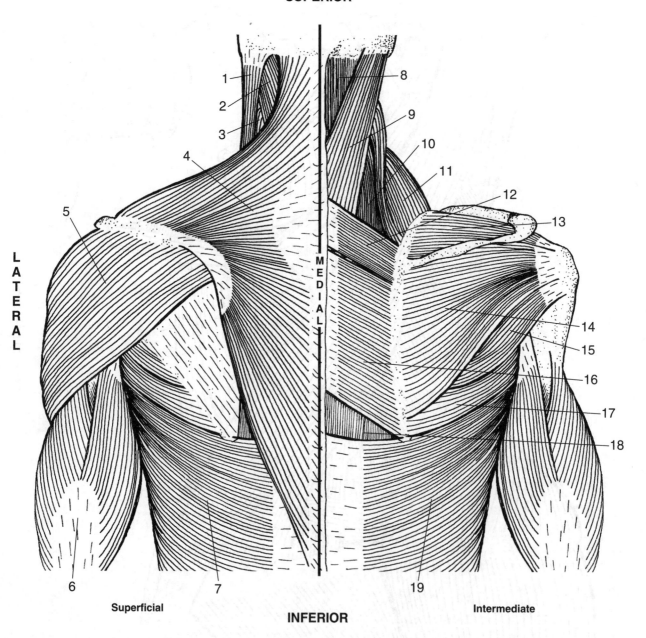

LATERAL

MEDIAL

LATERAL

Superficial

Intermediate

INFERIOR

POSTERIOR VIEW OF THE NECK (INTERMEDIATE AND DEEP)

SUPERIOR

LATERAL

LATERAL

MEDIAL

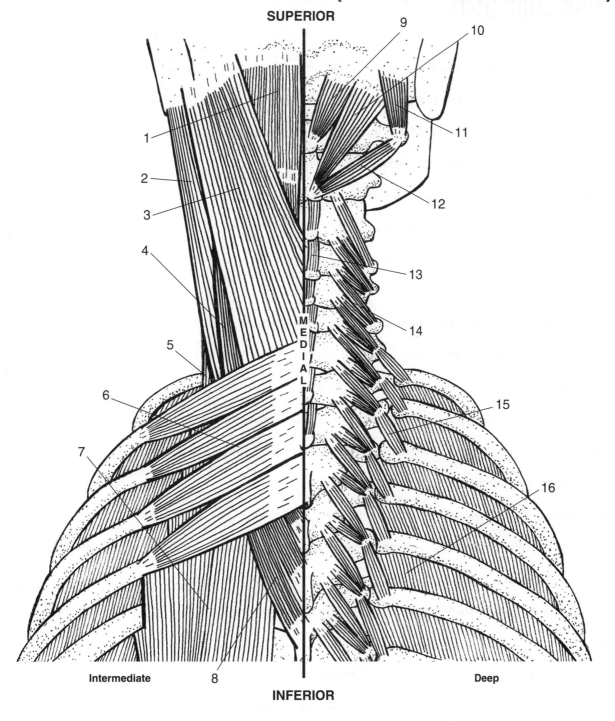

Intermediate 8 Deep

INFERIOR

Review Questions

Muscles of the Neck
Answers to these questions are found on page 484.

1. What type of neck and head rotation does the right upper trapezius do?

2. What muscle is immediately superficial to the rectus capitis posterior major and minor?

3. At its scapular attachment, the levator scapulae is deep to what muscle?

4. What passive joint action of the mandible would shorten and slacken the mylohyoid?

5. What does the name *digastric* literally mean?

6. What muscle perforates the attachment of the stylohyoid onto the hyoid bone?

7. What action would lengthen and stretch the sternohyoid?

8. What muscle can be considered to be an upward extension of the sternothyroid?

9. How are the right and left obliquus capitis inferior muscles antagonistic to each other?

10. What are the names of the two bellies of the omohyoid?

11. If the left posterior scalene is eccentrically contracting, what spinal joint motion is occurring?

12. What muscles are immediately deep to the middle trapezius in the interscapular region?

13. What muscle is superficial to the sternocleidomastoid?

14. Why is the stylohyoid antagonistic to the sternohyoid?

15. What effect would right rotation of the neck at the spinal joints have upon the right sternocleidomastoid?

16. What two suboccipital muscles attach to the inferior nuchal line of the occiput?

17. What is the only hyoid muscle that does not attach to the hyoid bone?

18. From underneath the mandible, what muscle is immediately superficial to the mylohyoid?

19. What motion would lengthen and stretch the omohyoid?

20. What passive ranges of motion would shorten and slacken the right splenius capitis?

21. Besides the rectus capitis posterior major, what other suboccipital muscle attaches to the spinous process of C2?

22. What muscles attach to the medial border of the scapula?

23. From underneath the mandible, which suprahyoid muscle is deeper, the mylohyoid or the geniohyoid?

24. Name a muscle that is antagonistic to the scapular downward rotation action of the levator scapulae.

25. What four muscles comprise the suprahyoid group?

26. What happens to the length of the right posterior scalene if the neck is left laterally flexed?

27. How are the left upper trapezius and the left posterior scalene synergistic with each other?

28. What three muscles comprise the scalene group?

29. Which muscle attaches to cervical transverse processes and is directly posterior to the posterior scalene?

30. Which scalene is the largest?

31. What happens to the length of the longus colli muscles if the neck is thrown back into extension?

32. What passive joint motion would shorten and slacken both longus colli muscles?

33. How are the right longus colli and the left sternocleidomastoid muscles synergistic with each other?

34. Which muscle attaches more superiorly, the longus colli or the longus capitis?

35. What muscle group is directly lateral to the longus colli?

36. At what spinal levels do the longus colli and capitis overlap?

37. What passive joint motion would lengthen and stretch the right rectus capitis lateralis?

38. What four muscles comprise the prevertebral group?

39. If the rectus capitis anterior concentrically contracts, what joint motion would occur?

40. What inferior attachment is shared by the rectus capitis anterior and lateralis?

41. What muscle is directly medial to the rectus capitis anterior?

42. What superior attachment is shared by the rectus capitis anterior and lateralis?

43. What attachment is shared by the sternothyroid and the thyrohyoid?

44. How is the left sternocleidomastoid synergistic with the left upper trapezius?

45. How are the digastric and masseter antagonistic to each other?

46. What joint actions would lengthen and stretch the right splenius cervicis?

47. What four muscles comprise the suboccipital group?

48. What effect would passive depression of the mandible at the temporomandibular joints have upon the platysma?

49. Which one of the following passive joint motions of the head would shorten and slacken the right rectus capitis posterior major? left lateral flexion / right lateral flexion

50. What joint action is common to all three scalenes?

51. What joint motion of the head is occurring if both rectus capitis posterior major muscles are eccentrically contracting at the same time?

52. What four muscles comprise the infrahyoid group?

53. Which scalene muscle attaches the highest on the cervical spine?

54. What two muscles attach to the lateral clavicle, acromion process, and spine of the scapula?

55. If both anterior scalene muscles contract at the same time, what spinal joint action would occur?

56. Which two suboccipital muscles attach to the transverse process of the atlas?

57. Name a synergistic to the digastric with respect to motion of the hyoid bone?

58. What muscle is superficial to nearly the entire splenius capitis?

59. What effect would right rotation of the neck at the spinal joints have upon the right sterno-cleidomastoid?

60. What action is common to all four infrahyoid muscles?

61. What muscle is immediately deep to the superior attachment of the sternocleidomastoid?

62. How are the right sternocleidomastoid and upper trapezius muscles synergistic with each other?

63. What happens to the length of the mylohyoid if the temporalis muscle contracts and shortens?

64. What two muscles are immediately deep to the inferior aspect of the sternocleidomastoid's clavicular head?

65. What joint actions would lengthen and stretch the digastric?

66. What passive motion would shorten and slacken the omohyoid?

67. What muscles have the same superior attachment as the splenius capitis?

68. Besides the digastric, what other hyoid muscle has a central tendon?

69. Name a synergist to the scapular elevation action of the levator scapulae?

70. Which scalene muscle is the smallest?

71. What happens to the length of the right anterior scalene if the left posterior scalene contracts and shortens?

72. Which one of the following joint actions of the neck would lengthen and stretch the left levator scapulae? extension / right lateral flexion / left rotation

73. What type of neck and head rotation does the left splenius capitis do?

74. How many hyoid muscles attach onto the mandible?

75. Which two suboccipital muscles attach to the spinous process of the axis?

76. What is the only suboccipital muscle that does not attach to the head?

77. Which is more superficial, the omohyoid or the scalenes?

78. What joint actions would lengthen and stretch the left lower trapezius?

79. What joint action is shared by all three parts of the trapezius?

80. What is the nickname for the splenius capitis muscles?

81. How are the omohyoid and sternohyoid synergistic with each other?

82. What joint action would lengthen and stretch the left obliquus capitis inferior?

83. From a posterior perspective, what muscle is superficial to the levator scapulae at its spinal attachment?

84. Where is the brachial plexus of nerves found relative to the scalene muscles?

Muscles of the Trunk 5

GET READY TO EXPLORE:

Note: Throughout this chapter, muscle attachments are indicated by italics.

☺ More review activities on Evolve at: http://evolve.elsevier.com/Muscolino/anatomycoloring/

POSTERIOR VIEW OF THE TRUNK (SUPERFICIAL AND INTERMEDIATE)

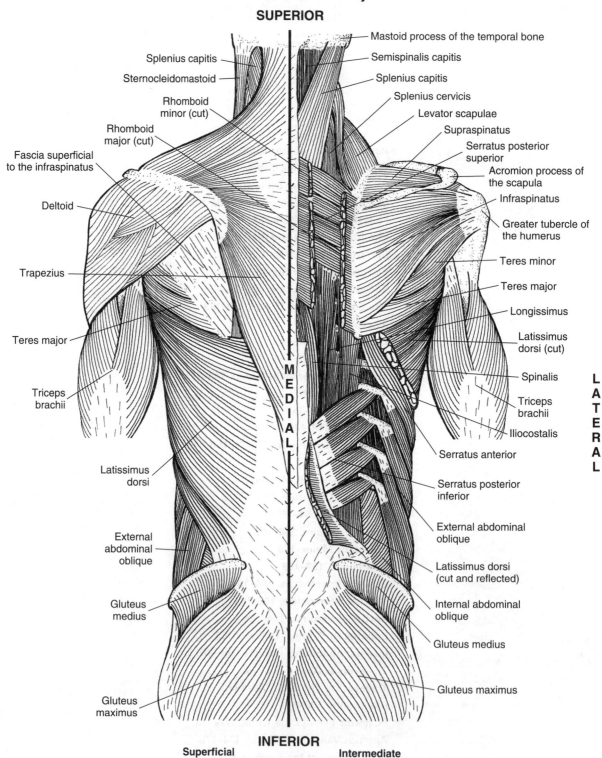

SUPERIOR

Splenius capitis

Sternocleidomastoid

Rhomboid minor (cut)

Rhomboid major (cut)

Fascia superficial to the infraspinatus

Deltoid

Trapezius

Teres major

Triceps brachii

Latissimus dorsi

External abdominal oblique

Gluteus medius

Gluteus maximus

Mastoid process of the temporal bone

Semispinalis capitis

Splenius capitis

Splenius cervicis

Levator scapulae

Supraspinatus

Serratus posterior superior

Acromion process of the scapula

Infraspinatus

Greater tubercle of the humerus

Teres minor

Teres major

Longissimus

Latissimus dorsi (cut)

Spinalis

Triceps brachii

Iliocostalis

Serratus anterior

Serratus posterior inferior

External abdominal oblique

Latissimus dorsi (cut and reflected)

Internal abdominal oblique

Gluteus medius

Gluteus maximus

LATERAL

LATERAL

MEDIAL

INFERIOR

Superficial

Intermediate

POSTERIOR VIEW OF THE TRUNK (DEEP LAYERS)

SUPERIOR

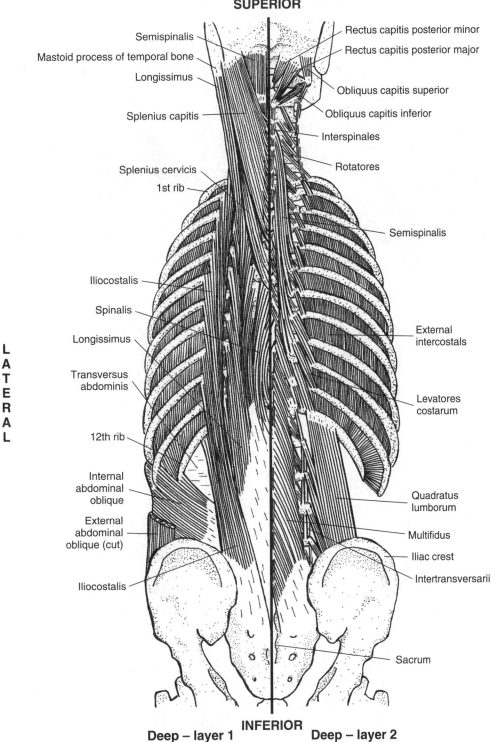

Semispinalis

Mastoid process of temporal bone

Longissimus

Splenius capitis

Splenius cervicis

1st rib

Iliocostalis

Spinalis

Longissimus

Transversus abdominis

12th rib

Internal abdominal oblique

External abdominal oblique (cut)

Iliocostalis

Rectus capitis posterior minor

Rectus capitis posterior major

Obliquus capitis superior

Obliquus capitis inferior

Interspinales

Rotatores

Semispinalis

External intercostals

Levatores costarum

Quadratus lumborum

Multifidus

Iliac crest

Intertransversarii

Sacrum

LATERAL

LATERAL

INFERIOR

Deep – layer 1   **Deep – layer 2**

ANTERIOR VIEW OF THE TRUNK (SUPERFICIAL AND INTERMEDIATE)

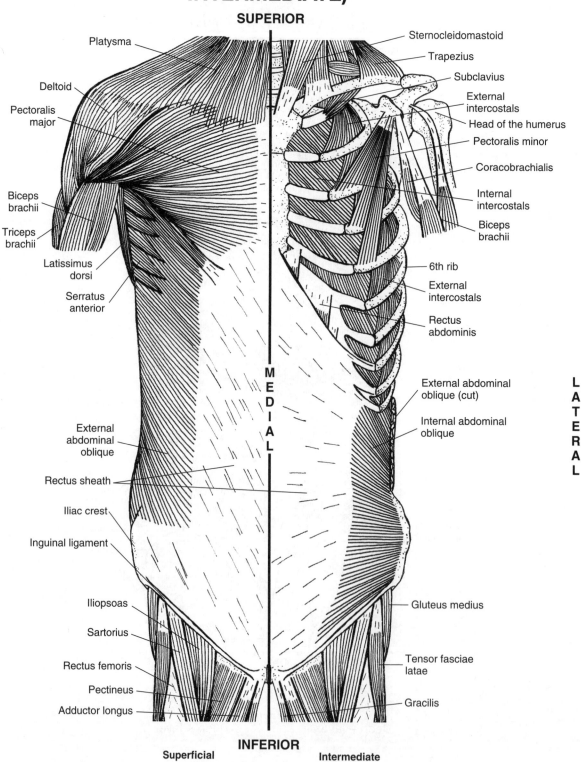

SUPERIOR

Platysma

Deltoid

Pectoralis major

Biceps brachii

Triceps brachii

Latissimus dorsi

Serratus anterior

External abdominal oblique

Rectus sheath

Iliac crest

Inguinal ligament

Iliopsoas

Sartorius

Rectus femoris

Pectineus

Adductor longus

Sternocleidomastoid

Trapezius

Subclavius

External intercostals

Head of the humerus

Pectoralis minor

Coracobrachialis

Internal intercostals

Biceps brachii

6th rib

External intercostals

Rectus abdominis

External abdominal oblique (cut)

Internal abdominal oblique

Gluteus medius

Tensor fasciae latae

Gracilis

LATERAL

MEDIAL

LATERAL

INFERIOR

Superficial

Intermediate

ANTERIOR VIEW OF THE TRUNK (INTERMEDIATE AND DEEP)

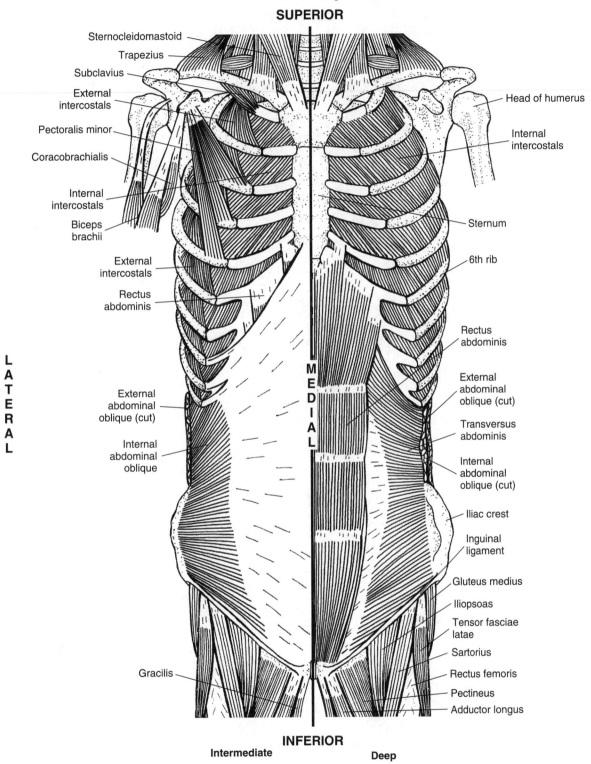

SUPERIOR

Sternocleidomastoid

Trapezius

Subclavius

External intercostals

Pectoralis minor

Coracobrachialis

Internal intercostals

Biceps brachii

External intercostals

Rectus abdominis

External abdominal oblique (cut)

Internal abdominal oblique

Gracilis

Head of humerus

Internal intercostals

Sternum

6th rib

Rectus abdominis

External abdominal oblique (cut)

Transversus abdominis

Internal abdominal oblique (cut)

Iliac crest

Inguinal ligament

Gluteus medius

Iliopsoas

Tensor fasciae latae

Sartorius

Rectus femoris

Pectineus

Adductor longus

LATERAL **MEDIAL** **LATERAL**

INFERIOR

Intermediate   Deep

LATERAL VIEW OF THE TRUNK

SUPERIOR

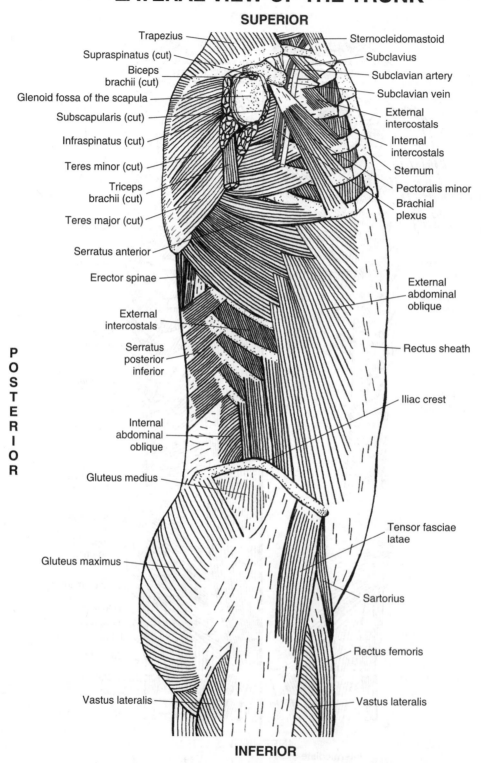

Trapezius

Supraspinatus (cut)

Biceps brachii (cut)

Glenoid fossa of the scapula

Subscapularis (cut)

Infraspinatus (cut)

Teres minor (cut)

Triceps brachii (cut)

Teres major (cut)

Serratus anterior

Erector spinae

External intercostals

Serratus posterior inferior

Internal abdominal oblique

Gluteus medius

Gluteus maximus

Vastus lateralis

Sternocleidomastoid

Subclavius

Subclavian artery

Subclavian vein

External intercostals

Internal intercostals

Sternum

Pectoralis minor

Brachial plexus

External abdominal oblique

Rectus sheath

Iliac crest

Tensor fasciae latae

Sartorius

Rectus femoris

Vastus lateralis

POSTERIOR

ANTERIOR

INFERIOR

CROSS SECTION VIEWS OF THE TRUNK

ANTERIOR

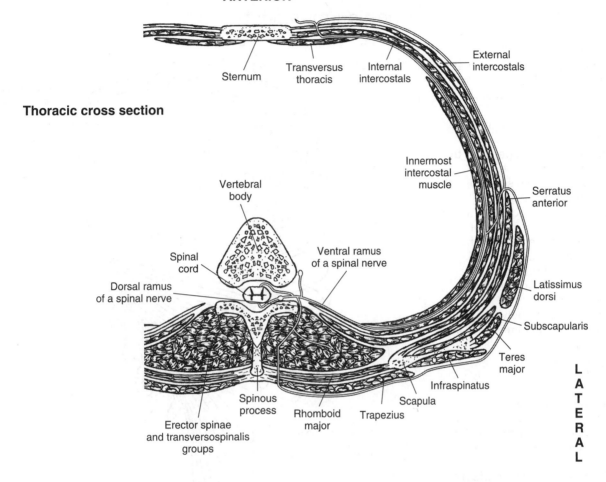

Thoracic cross section

Sternum

Transversus thoracis

Internal intercostals

External intercostals

Innermost intercostal muscle

Serratus anterior

Vertebral body

Ventral ramus of a spinal nerve

Latissimus dorsi

Spinal cord

Subscapularis

Dorsal ramus of a spinal nerve

Teres major

Spinous process

Infraspinatus

Rhomboid major

Scapula

Trapezius

Erector spinae and transversospinalis groups

LATERAL

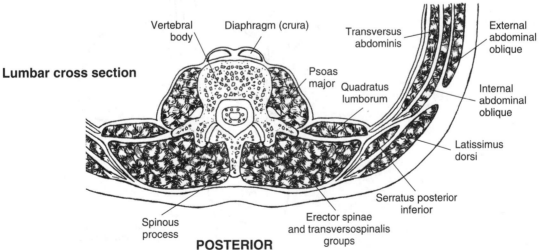

Vertebral body

Diaphragm (crura)

Transversus abdominis

External abdominal oblique

Lumbar cross section

Psoas major

Quadratus lumborum

Internal abdominal oblique

Latissimus dorsi

Serratus posterior inferior

Spinous process

Erector spinae and transversospinalis groups

POSTERIOR

LATISSIMUS DORSI ("LAT")

la-**tis**-i-mus **door**-si

Actions
Medial rotation of the arm at the shoulder joint
Adduction of the arm at the shoulder joint
Extension of the arm at the shoulder joint
Anterior tilt of the pelvis at the lumbosacral joint
Depression of the scapula at the scapulocostal joint
Lateral deviation of the trunk at the scapulo-costal joint
Elevation of the trunk at the scapulocostal joint
Contralateral rotation of the trunk at the scapulocostal joint
Elevation of the pelvis at the lumbosacral joint

Innervation
The thoracodorsal nerve

Arterial Supply
The thoracodorsal artery and the dorsal branches of the posterior intercostal arteries

Myofascial Meridians
Superficial front arm line
Back functional line

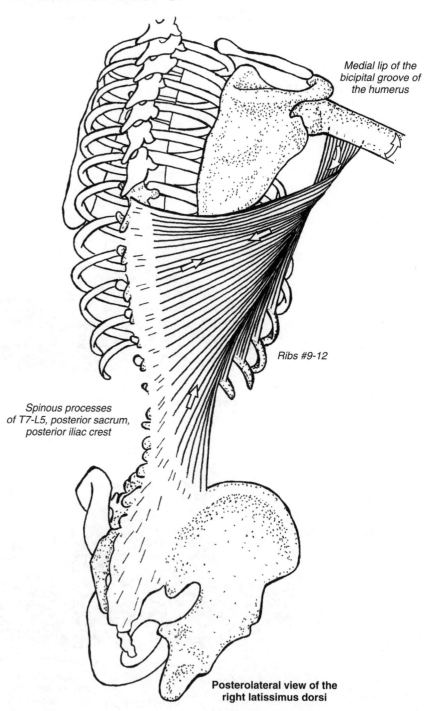

Medial lip of the bicipital groove of the humerus

Ribs #9-12

Spinous processes of T7-L5, posterior sacrum, posterior iliac crest

Posterolateral view of the right latissimus dorsi

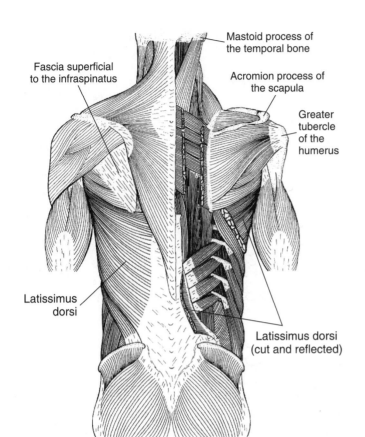

Mastoid process of
the temporal bone

Fascia superficial
to the infraspinatus

Acromion process of
the scapula

Greater
tubercle
of the
humerus

Latissimus
dorsi

Latissimus dorsi
(cut and reflected)

DID YOU KNOW

The latissimus dorsi (and the teres major) make up
the majority of the posterior axillary fold of tissue,
which borders the armpit posteriorly.

DID YOU KNOW

There is a twist in the latissimus dorsi such that the
most superior axial body fibers attach the most distally
on the humerus, and the most inferior axial body fibers
attach the most proximally on the humerus.

Latissimus
dorsi

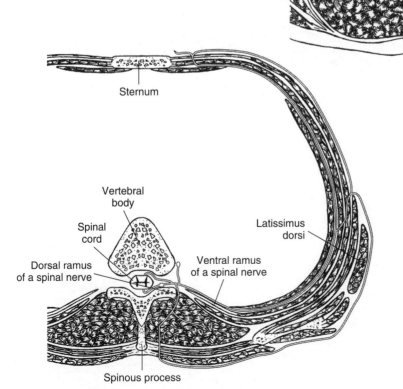

Sternum

Vertebral
body

Spinal
cord

Latissimus
dorsi

Dorsal ramus
of a spinal nerve

Ventral ramus
of a spinal nerve

Spinous process

RHOMBOIDS MAJOR AND MINOR

rom-boyd **may**-jor, **my**-nor

Actions
Retraction (adduction) of the
    scapula at the scapulocostal
    joint
Elevation of the scapula at the
    scapulocostal joint
Downward rotation of the
    scapula at the scapulocostal
    joint
Contralateral rotation of the
    trunk at the spinal joints

Innervation
The dorsal scapular nerve

Arterial Supply
The dorsal scapular artery

Myofascial Meridians
Spiral line
Deep back arm line

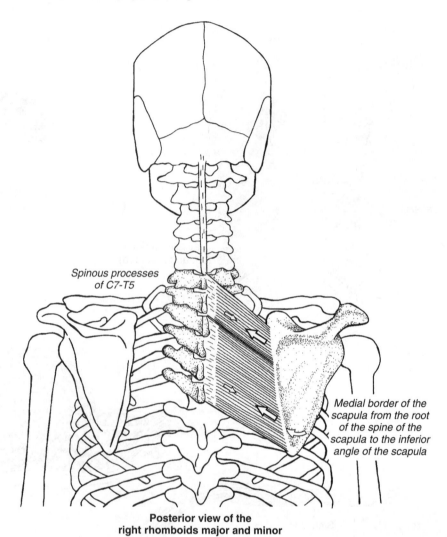

Spinous processes
of C7-T5

Medial border of the
scapula from the root
of the spine of the
scapula to the inferior
angle of the scapula

**Posterior view of the
right rhomboids major and minor**

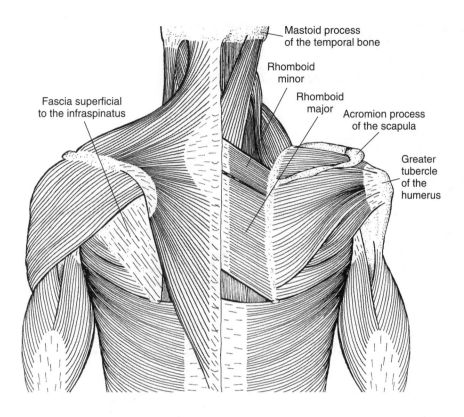

Mastoid process
of the temporal bone

Rhomboid
minor

Rhomboid
major

Acromion process
of the scapula

Greater
tubercle
of the
humerus

Fascia superficial
to the infraspinatus

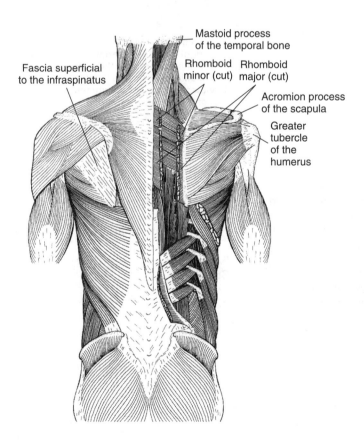

Mastoid process
of the temporal bone

Rhomboid   Rhomboid
minor (cut) major (cut)

Acromion process
of the scapula

Greater
tubercle
of the
humerus

Fascia superficial
to the infraspinatus

DID YOU KNOW

The rhomboids are sometimes known as the "Christmas tree" muscles. When you look at them bilaterally with the spine between them, they look like a Christmas tree.

DID YOU KNOW

The word "rhomboid" comes from the word "rhombus," which means diamond-shape.

SERRATUS ANTERIOR

ser-**a**-tus an-**tee**-ri-or

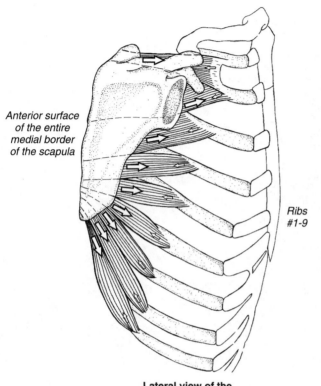

Anterior surface
of the entire
medial border
of the scapula

Ribs
#1-9

**Lateral view of the
right serratus anterior**

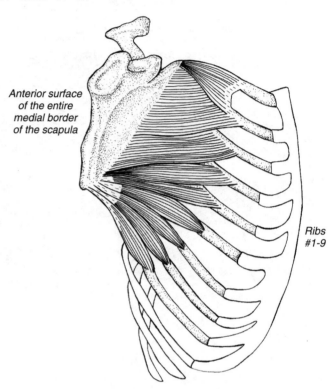

Anterior surface
of the entire
medial border
of the scapula

Ribs
#1-9

**Lateral view of the
right serratus anterior
(with the lateral border of the scapula
pulled away from the trunk
to view the scapular attachment
of the serratus anterior)**

Actions
Protraction (abduction) of the
    scapula at the scapulocostal
    joint
Upward rotation of the scapula at
    the scapulocostal joint

Elevation of the scapula at the
    scapulocostal joint
Depression of the scapula at the
    scapulocostal joint

Innervation
The long thoracic nerve

Arterial Supply
The dorsal scapular artery and the
lateral thoracic artery

Myofascial Meridians
Spiral line

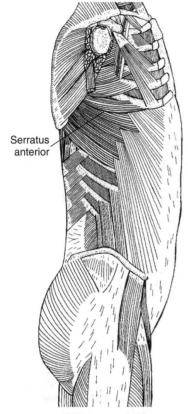

Serratus
anterior

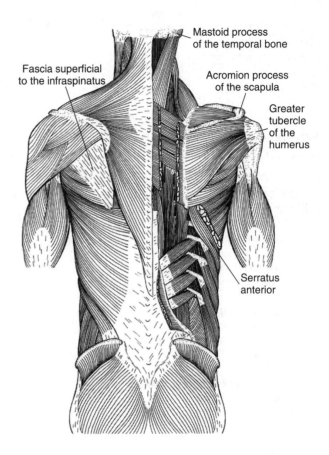

Mastoid process
of the temporal bone

Fascia superficial
to the infraspinatus

Acromion process
of the scapula

Greater
tubercle
of the
humerus

Serratus
anterior

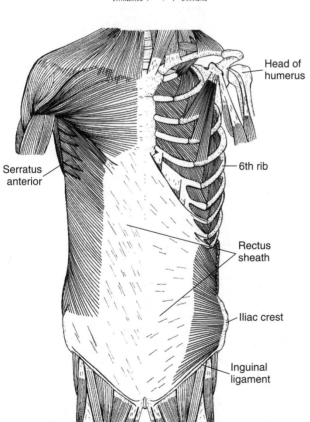

Head of
humerus

Serratus
anterior

6th rib

Rectus
sheath

Iliac crest

Inguinal
ligament

DID
YOU ?
KNOW

*In very well-developed individuals,
the serratus anterior looks like ribs
standing out in the anterolateral trunk.*

DID
YOU ?
KNOW

*The serratus anterior protracts the
scapula, but also keeps the scapula
hugged against the rib cage wall.*

SERRATUS POSTERIOR SUPERIOR

ser-**a**-tus pos-**tee**-ri-or
sue-**pee**-ri-or

Action
Elevation of ribs #2-5 at
the sternocostal and
costovertebral joints

Innervation
Intercostal nerves

Arterial Supply
The dorsal branches of
the posterior intercostal
arteries

Myofascial Meridians
Involved: Spiral line

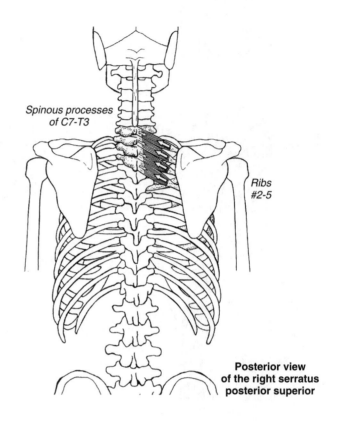

Spinous processes of C7-T3

Ribs #2-5

**Posterior view
of the right serratus
posterior superior**

SERRATUS POSTERIOR INFERIOR

ser-**a**-tus pos-**tee**-ri-or
in-**fee**-ri-or

Actions
Depression of ribs #9-12 at the
sternocostal and costovertebral
joints

Innervation
Subcostal nerve and intercostal
nerves

Arterial Supply
The dorsal branches of the posterior
intercostal arteries

Myofascial Meridians
Involved: Superficial front arm line
Involved: Superficial back line

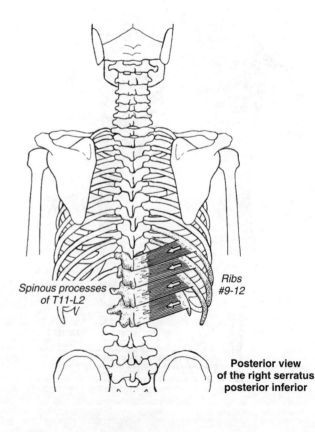

Spinous processes of T11-L2

Ribs #9-12

**Posterior view
of the right serratus
posterior inferior**

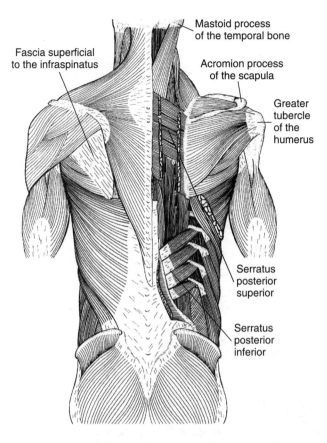

Fascia superficial
to the infraspinatus

Mastoid process
of the temporal bone

Acromion process
of the scapula

Greater
tubercle
of the
humerus

Serratus
posterior
superior

Serratus
posterior
inferior

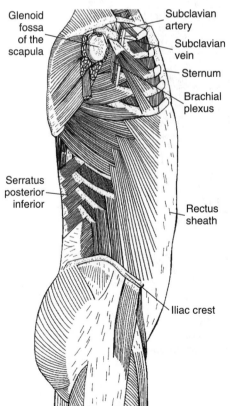

Glenoid
fossa
of the
scapula

Subclavian
artery

Subclavian
vein

Sternum

Brachial
plexus

Serratus
posterior
inferior

Rectus
sheath

Iliac crest

**DID
YOU
KNOW**

By their action of moving the ribs the serratus posterior superior and inferior muscles are primarily important as muscles of respiration.

**DID
YOU
KNOW**

The most important function of the both the serratus posterior superior and serratus posterior inferior may be to act as retinacula, acting to keep the deeper erector spinae musculature down against the trunk when they contract.

THE ERECTOR SPINAE GROUP

ee-**rek**-tor **spee**-nee

Actions
Extension of the trunk and
the neck and the head at
the spinal joints
Lateral flexion of the trunk
and the neck and the head
at the spinal joints
Ipsilateral rotation of the
trunk and the neck and the
head at the spinal joints
Anterior tilt of the pelvis at
the lumbosacral joint
Elevation of the pelvis at the
lumbosacral joint
Contralateral rotation of the
pelvis at the lumbosacral
joint

Innervation
Spinal nerves

Arterial Supply
The dorsal branches of the
posterior intercostal and
lumbar arteries

Myofascial Meridians
Superficial back line
Spiral line

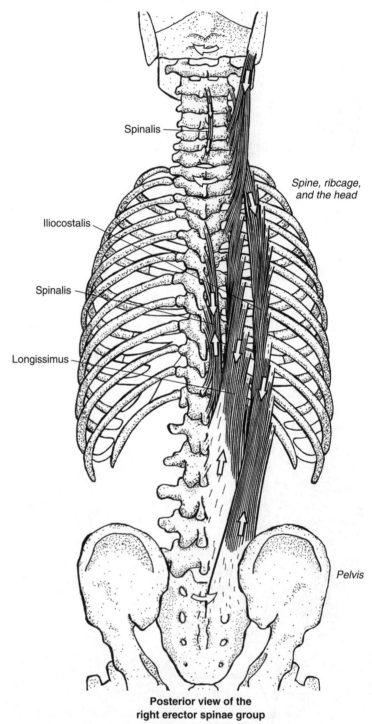

Spinalis

Iliocostalis

Spinalis

Longissimus

*Spine, ribcage,
and the head*

Pelvis

**Posterior view of the
right erector spinae group**

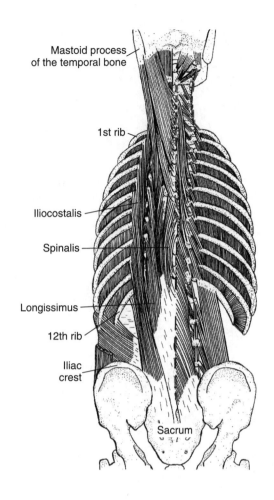

Mastoid process
of the temporal bone

1st rib

Iliocostalis

Spinalis

Longissimus

12th rib

Iliac
crest

Sacrum

DID YOU KNOW

The erector spinae group, as its name implies, makes the spine erect, i.e., it does extension of the spine.

DID YOU KNOW

The erector spinae and transversospinalis muscle groups together are often referred to as the paraspinal musculature.

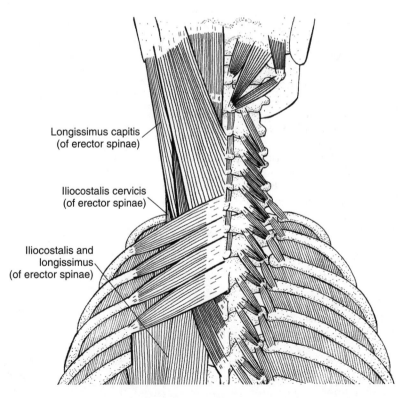

Longissimus capitis
(of erector spinae)

Iliocostalis cervicis
(of erector spinae)

Iliocostalis and
longissimus
(of erector spinae)

Actions

Extension of the trunk and the neck at the spinal joints

Lateral flexion of the trunk and the neck at the spinal joints

Ipsilateral rotation of the trunk and the neck at the spinal joints

Anterior tilt of the pelvis at the lumbosacral joint

Elevation of the pelvis at the lumbosacral joint

Contralateral rotation of the pelvis at the lumbosacral joint

Innervation

Spinal nerves

Arterial Supply

The dorsal branches of the posterior intercostal and lumbar arteries

Myofascial Meridians

Superficial back line
Spiral line

ILIOCOSTALIS
(OF THE ERECTOR SPINAE GROUP)

il-ee-o-kos-**ta**-lis

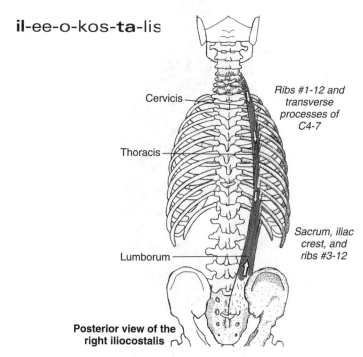

Cervicis

Ribs #1-12 and transverse processes of C4-7

Thoracis

Lumborum

Sacrum, iliac crest, and ribs #3-12

Posterior view of the right iliocostalis

Actions

Extension of the trunk and the neck and the head at the spinal joints

Lateral flexion of the trunk and the neck and the head at the spinal joints

Ipsilateral rotation of the trunk and the neck and the head at the spinal joints

Anterior tilt of the pelvis at the lumbosacral joint

Elevation of the pelvis at the lumbosacral joint

Contralateral rotation of the pelvis at the lumbosacral joint

Innervation

Spinal nerves

Arterial Supply

The dorsal branches of the posterior intercostal and lumbar arteries

Myofascial Meridians

Superficial back line
Spiral line

LONGISSIMUS
(OF THE ERECTOR SPINAE GROUP)

lon-**jis**-i-mus

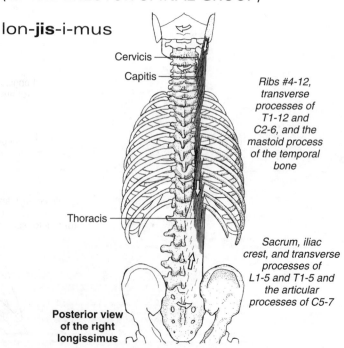

Cervicis

Capitis

Ribs #4-12, transverse processes of T1-12 and C2-6, and the mastoid process of the temporal bone

Thoracis

Sacrum, iliac crest, and transverse processes of L1-5 and T1-5 and the articular processes of C5-7

Posterior view of the right longissimus

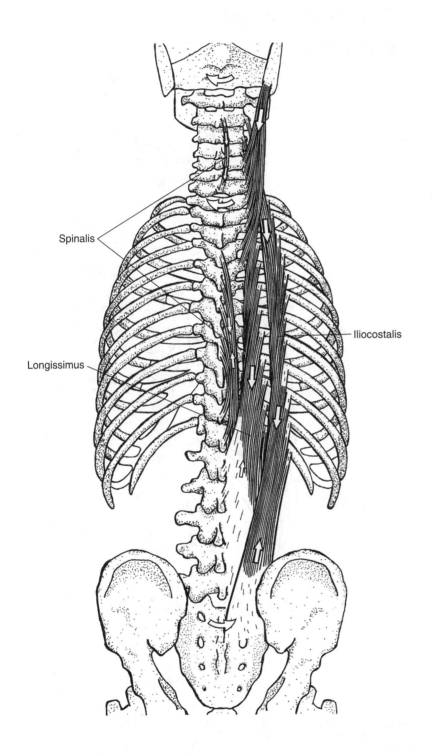

Spinalis

Longissimus

Iliocostalis

The iliocostalis, as its name implies, attaches from the ilium to the ribs.

Although not reflected in its name, the iliocostalis also has inferior attachments onto the sacrum.

The longissimus, as its name implies, is the longest of the three subgroups of the erector spinae.

The only erector spinae attachment onto the head is the longissimus capitis, attaching onto the mastoid process of the temporal bone.

SPINALIS
(OF THE ERECTOR SPINAE GROUP)

spy-**na**-lis

Actions
Extension of the trunk and the neck
   and the head at the spinal joints
Lateral flexion of the trunk and the
   neck and the head at the spinal
   joints
Ipsilateral rotation of the trunk and
   the neck and the head at the spinal
   joints

Innervation
Spinal nerves

Arterial Supply
The dorsal branches of the posterior
   intercostal and lumbar arteries

Myofascial Meridians
Superficial back line
Spiral line

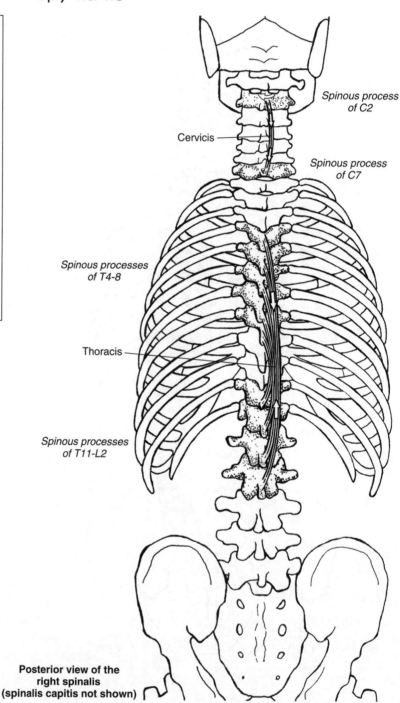

Spinous process
of C2

Cervicis

Spinous process
of C7

Spinous processes
of T4-8

Thoracis

Spinous processes
of T11-L2

**Posterior view of the
right spinalis
(spinalis capitis not shown)**

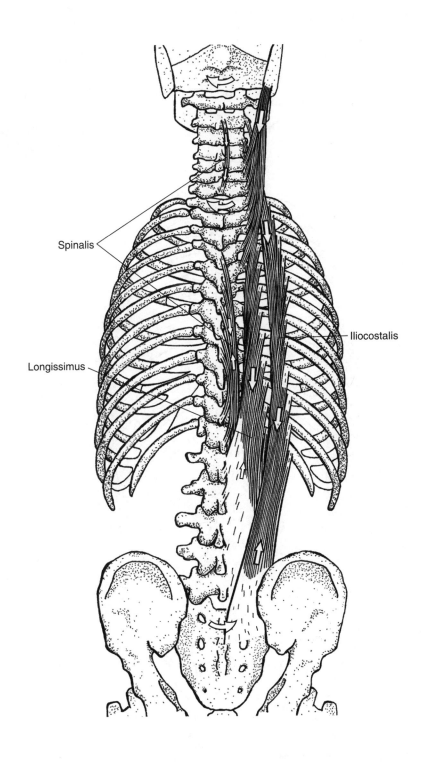

Spinalis

Longissimus

Iliocostalis

DID
YOU
KNOW ?

The spinalis, as its name implies, attaches from spinous processes to spinous processes.

DID
YOU
KNOW ?

The spinalis is, by far, the smallest subgroup of the erector spinae musculature.

THE TRANSVERSOSPINALIS GROUP

trans-**ver**-so-spy-**na**-lis

Actions

Extension of the trunk and the neck and the head at the spinal joints

Lateral flexion of the trunk and the neck and the head at the spinal joints

Contralateral rotation of the trunk and the neck at the spinal joints

Anterior tilt of the pelvis at the lumbosacral joint

Elevation of the pelvis at the lumbosacral joint

Ipsilateral rotation of the pelvis at the lumbosacral joint

Innervation

Spinal nerves

Arterial Supply

The occipital artery and the dorsal branches of the posterior intercostal and lumbar arteries

Myofascial Meridians

Superficial back line

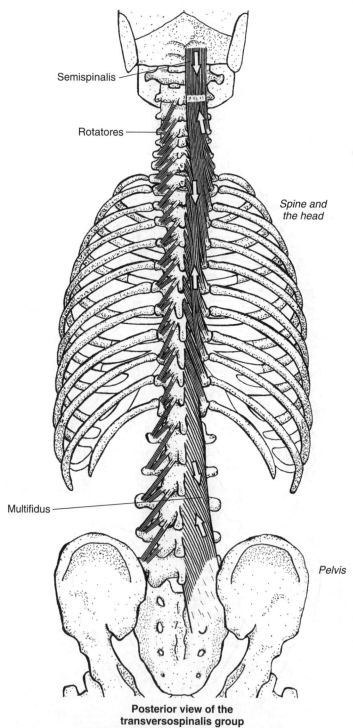

Posterior view of the transversospinalis group (semispinalis and multifidus on the right) (rotatores on the left)

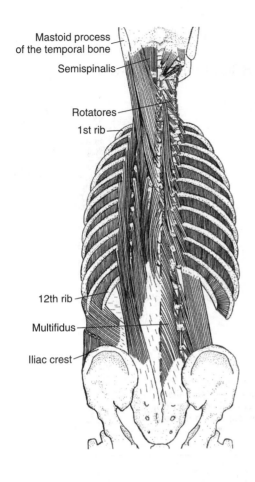

Mastoid process
of the temporal bone

Semispinalis

Rotatores

1st rib

12th rib

Multifidus

Iliac crest

**DID
YOU
KNOW ?**

*The transversospinalis group, as its
name implies, attaches from transverse
processes to spinous processes.*

**DID
YOU
KNOW ?**

*The rotatores attach 1-2 levels
above their inferior attachments,
the multifidus attach 3-4, and the
semispinalis attach 5 or more.*

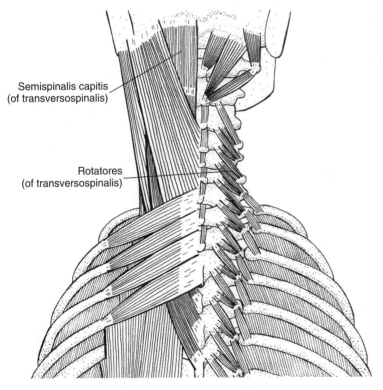

Semispinalis capitis
(of transversospinalis)

Rotatores
(of transversospinalis)

Actions

Extension of the trunk and
the neck and the head at
the spinal joints

Lateral flexion of the trunk
and the neck and the head
at the spinal joints

Contralateral rotation of the
trunk and the neck at the
spinal joints

Innervation
Spinal nerves

Arterial Supply
The occipital artery and
the dorsal branches of
the posterior intercostal
arteries

Myofascial Meridians
Superficial back line

SEMISPINALIS
(OF THE TRANSVERSOSPINALIS GROUP)

sem-ee-spy-**na**-lis

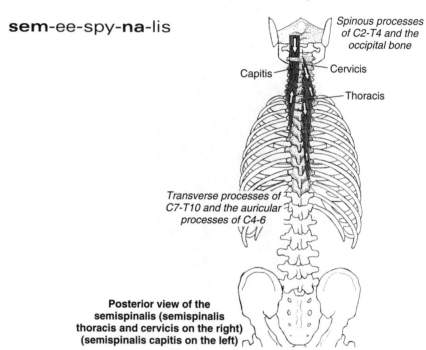

Spinous processes
of C2-T4 and the
occipital bone

Capitis   Cervicis

Thoracis

Transverse processes of
C7-T10 and the auricular
processes of C4-6

**Posterior view of the
semispinalis (semispinalis
thoracis and cervicis on the right)
(semispinalis capitis on the left)**

Actions

Extension of the trunk and the
neck at the spinal joints

Lateral flexion of the trunk
and the neck at the spinal
joints

Contralateral rotation of the
trunk and the neck at the
spinal joints

Anterior tilt of the pelvis at the
lumbosacral joint

Elevation of the pelvis at the
lumbosacral joint

Ipsilateral rotation of the
pelvis at the lumbosacral
joint

Innervation
Spinal nerves

Arterial Supply
The dorsal branches of the
posterior intercostal and
lumbar arteries

Myofascial Meridians
Superficial back line

MULTIFIDUS
(OF THE TRANSVERSOSPINALIS GROUP)

mul-**tif**-id-us

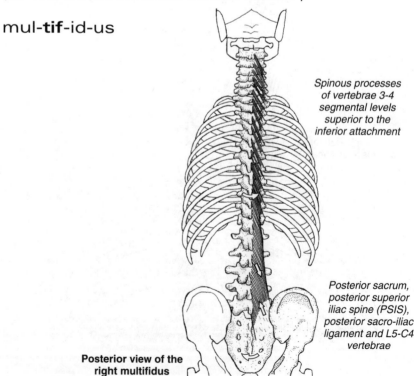

Spinous processes
of vertebrae 3-4
segmental levels
superior to the
inferior attachment

Posterior sacrum,
posterior superior
iliac spine (PSIS),
posterior sacro-iliac
ligament and L5-C4
vertebrae

**Posterior view of the
right multifidus**

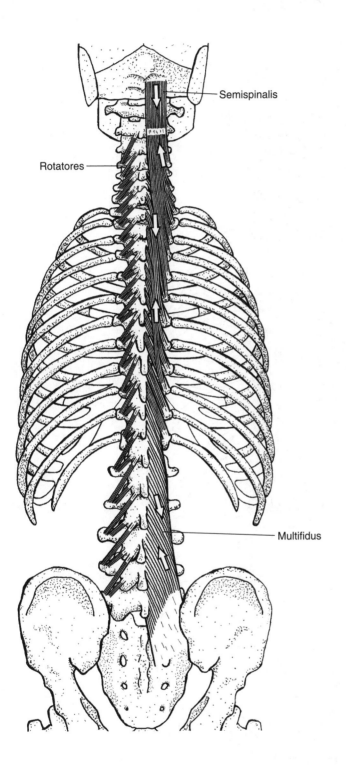

Semispinalis

Rotatores

Multifidus

DID YOU KNOW

The semispinalis capitis is the largest muscle in the posterior neck.

DID YOU KNOW

The most inferior attachment of the semispinalis is T10.

DID YOU KNOW

The multifidus is the largest muscle in the low back.

DID YOU KNOW

Where they overlap, the multifidus lies between the more superficial semispinalis and deeper rotatores.

ROTATORES
(OF THE TRANSVERSOSPINALIS GROUP)

ro-ta-**to**-reez

Actions
Contralateral rotation of the trunk
    and the neck at the spinal
    joints
Extension of the trunk and the
    neck at the spinal joints

Innervation
Spinal nerves

Arterial Supply
The dorsal branches of the
    posterior intercostal and
    lumbar arteries

Myofascial Meridians
Superficial back line

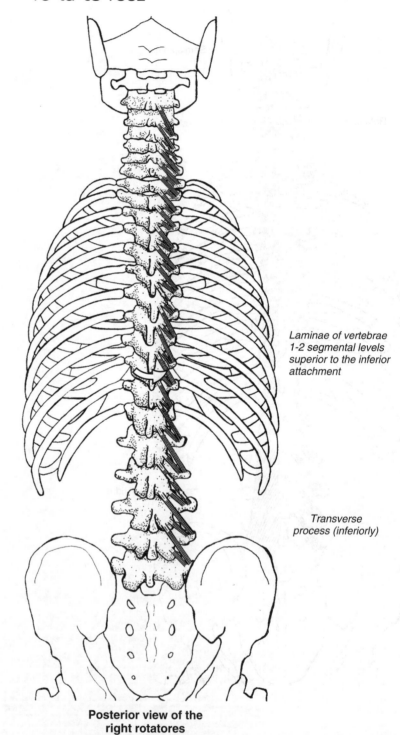

*Laminae of vertebrae
1-2 segmental levels
superior to the inferior
attachment*

*Transverse
process (inferiorly)*

**Posterior view of the
right rotatores**

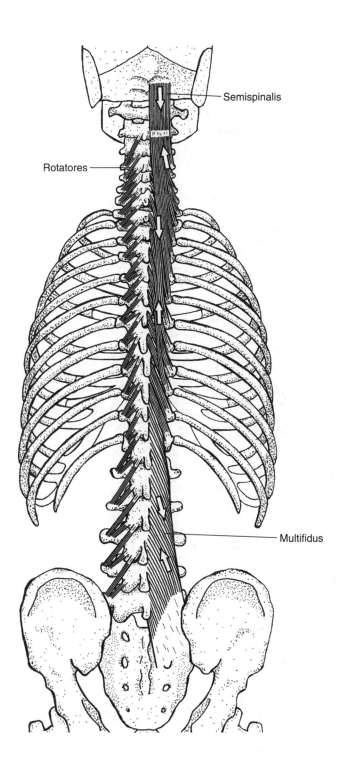

Semispinalis

Rotatores

Multifidus

DID YOU KNOW

The rotatores, as their name implies, are best at rotation (contralaterally) of the spine.

DID YOU KNOW

The rotatores are the smallest and deepest of the transversospinalis musculature.

QUADRATUS LUMBORUM ("QL")

kwod-**ray**-tus lum-**bor**-um

Actions
Elevation of the pelvis at the lumbosacral joint

Anterior tilt of the pelvis at the lumbosacral joint

Lateral flexion of the trunk at the spinal joints

Extension of the trunk at the spinal joints

Depression of the 12th rib at the costovertebral joints

Innervation
Lumbar plexus

Arterial Supply
Branches of the subcostal and lumbar arteries

Myofascial Meridians
Deep front line

Involved: Lateral line

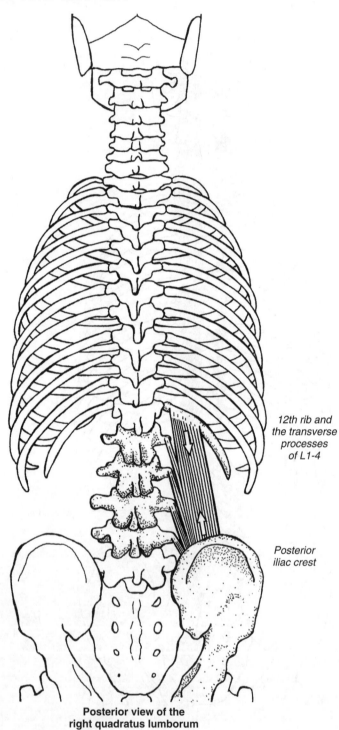

12th rib and the transverse processes of L1-4

Posterior iliac crest

Posterior view of the right quadratus lumborum

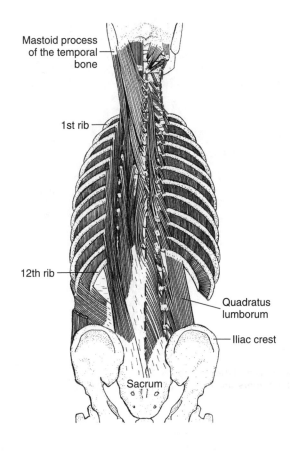

Mastoid process of the temporal bone

1st rib

12th rib

Quadratus lumborum

Iliac crest

Sacrum

DID YOU KNOW

When palpating the quadratus lumborum, it must be accessed from the side.

DID YOU KNOW

The QL attaches onto the transverse processes of L1-L4; it does not attach onto L5.

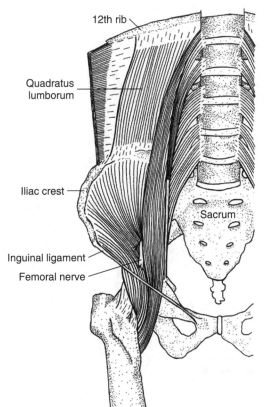

12th rib

Quadratus lumborum

Iliac crest

Inguinal ligament

Femoral nerve

Sacrum

INTERSPINALES

in-ter-spy-**na**-leez

Action
Extension of the neck and the trunk at
the spinal joints

Innervation
Spinal nerves

Arterial Supply
The dorsal branches of the posterior
intercostal arteries

Myofascial Meridians
Superficial back line

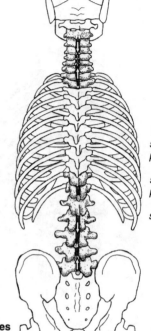

*From a
spinous
process
to the
spinous
process
directly
superior*

**Posterior view of the
right and left interspinales**

INTERTRANSVERSARII

in-ter-trans-ver-**sa**-ri-eye

Action
Lateral flexion of the neck and the
trunk at the spinal joints

Innervation
Spinal nerves

Arterial Supply
The dorsal branches of the
posterior intercostal arteries

Myofascial Meridians
Deep front line
Superficial back line

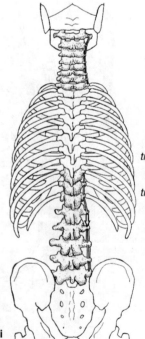

*From a
transverse
process
to the
transverse
process
directly
superior*

**Posterior view of the
right intertransversarii**

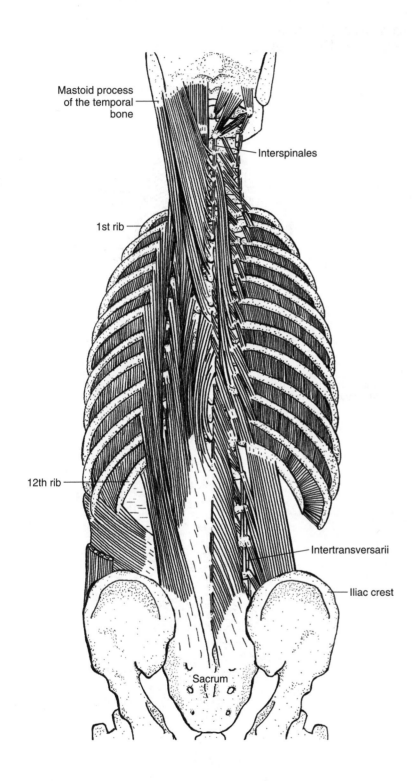

Mastoid process of the temporal bone

Interspinales

1st rib

12th rib

Intertransversarii

Iliac crest

Sacrum

DID YOU KNOW

The interspinales are small, paired muscles located between spinous processes. The intertransversarii are small muscles located between transverse processes. Both of these muscle groups are poorly developed in the thoracic region.

DID YOU KNOW

The interspinales and intertransversarii can only be stretched with very specific stretching that might be described as Grade IV joint mobilization.

LEVATORES COSTARUM

le-va-**to**-rez (singular:
le-**vay**-tor) kos-**tar**-um

Actions
Elevation of the ribs at
    the sternocostal and
    costovertebral joints
Extension of the trunk at the
    spinal joints
Lateral flexion of the trunk at
    the spinal joints
Contralateral rotation of the
    trunk at the spinal joints

Innervation
Spinal nerves

Arterial Supply
The dorsal branches of
    the posterior intercostal
    arteries

Myofascial Meridians
Superficial back line

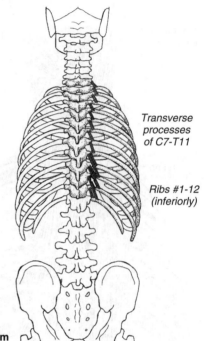

*Transverse
processes
of C7-T11*

*Ribs #1-12
(inferiorly)*

**Posterior view of the
right levatores costarum**

SUBCOSTALES

sub-kos-**tal**-eez

Action
Depression of ribs #8-10
    at the sternocostal
    and costovertebral
    joints

Innervation
Intercostal nerves

Arterial Supply
The dorsal branches of
    the posterior inter-
    costal arteries

**Myofascial
Meridians**
Lateral line

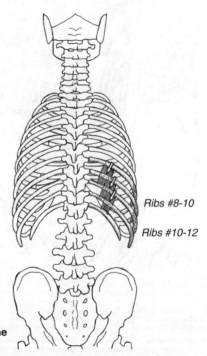

Ribs #8-10

Ribs #10-12

**Posterior view of the
right subcostales**

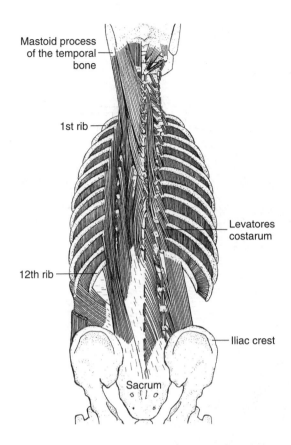

Mastoid process of the temporal bone

1st rib

Levatores costarum

12th rib

Iliac crest

Sacrum

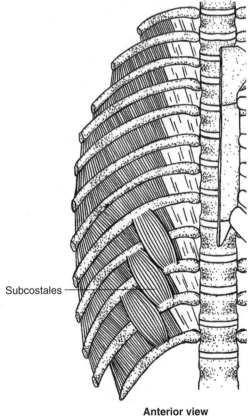

Subcostales

Anterior view

As their name implies, the levatores costarum elevate the ribs.

Given their attachment onto the rib cage, the levatores costarum are located essentially only in the thoracic region.

There are usually three subcostales muscles and they are located deep to the ribcage from the posterior perspective.

By depressing ribs 8-10, they can function synergistically with the diaphragm, acting to stabilize the lower rib cage against the upward pull of the diaphragm, allowing the diaphragm to more effectively lower its central dome for abdominal (belly) breathing.

PECTORALIS MAJOR

pek-to-ra-lis **may**-jor

Actions
Adduction of the arm at the shoulder joint

Medial rotation of the arm at the shoulder joint

Flexion of the arm at the shoulder joint (clavicular head)

Extension of the arm at the shoulder joint (sternocostal head)

Abduction of the arm at the shoulder joint (clavicular head, above 90°)

Depression of the scapula at the scapulocostal joint

Elevation of the trunk at the scapulocostal joint

Lateral deviation of the trunk at the scapulocostal joint

Ipsilateral rotation of the trunk at the scapulocostal joint

Innervation
The medial and lateral pectoral nerves

Arterial Supply
The pectoral branches of the thoracoacromial trunk

Myofascial Meridians
Superficial front arm line

Front functional line

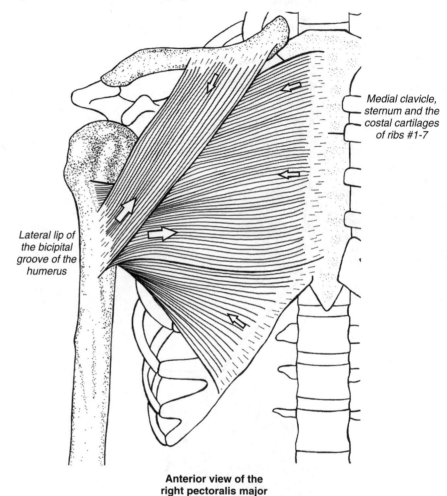

Medial clavicle, sternum and the costal cartilages of ribs #1-7

Lateral lip of the bicipital groove of the humerus

Anterior view of the right pectoralis major

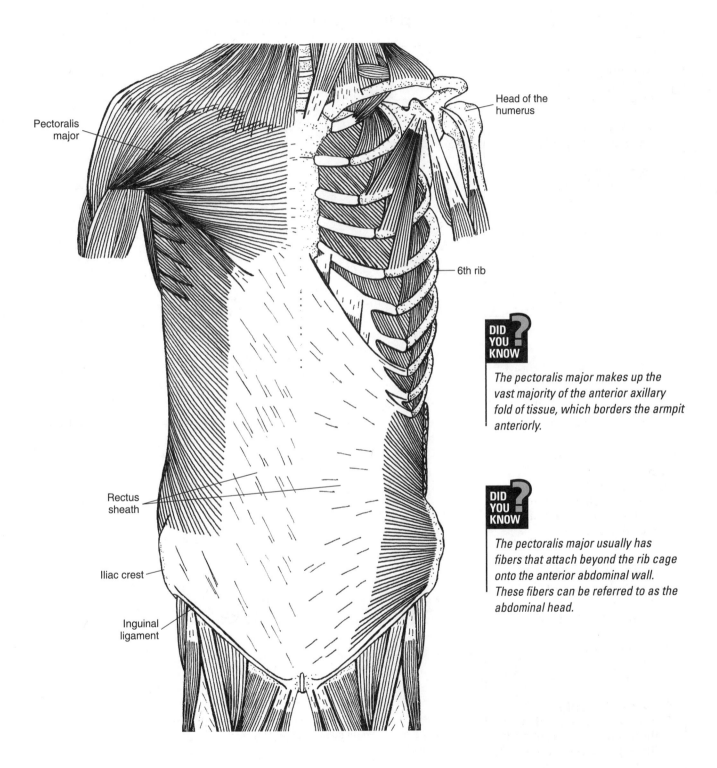

Pectoralis major

Head of the humerus

6th rib

Rectus sheath

Iliac crest

Inguinal ligament

DID YOU KNOW ?

The pectoralis major makes up the vast majority of the anterior axillary fold of tissue, which borders the armpit anteriorly.

DID YOU KNOW ?

The pectoralis major usually has fibers that attach beyond the rib cage onto the anterior abdominal wall. These fibers can be referred to as the abdominal head.

PECTORALIS MINOR

pek-to-**ra**-lis **my**-nor

Actions
Protraction (abduction)
of the scapula at the
scapulocostal joint
Depression of the scapula at
the scapulocostal joint
Downward rotation of
the scapula at the
scapulocostal joint
Elevation of ribs #3-5 at
the sternocostal and
costovertebral joints

Innervation
The medial and lateral
pectoral nerves

Arterial Supply
The pectoral branches of the
thoracoacromial trunk

Myofascial Meridians
Deep functional arm line

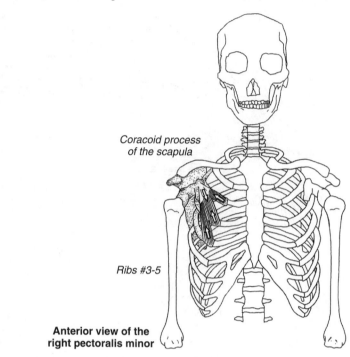

Coracoid process
of the scapula

Ribs #3-5

**Anterior view of the
right pectoralis minor**

SUBCLAVIUS

sub-**klay**-vee-us

Actions
Depression of the clavicle at
the sternoclavicular joint
Elevation of the 1st rib at
the sternocostal and
costovertebral joints
Protraction of the clavicle at
the sternoclavicular joint
Downward rotation of
the clavicle at the
sternoclavicular joint

Innervation
A nerve from the brachial
plexus

Arterial Supply
The clavicular branch of the
thoracoacromial trunk and
the suprascapular artery

Myofascial Meridians
Deep functional arm line

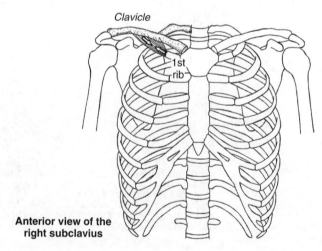

Clavicle

1st
rib

**Anterior view of the
right subclavius**

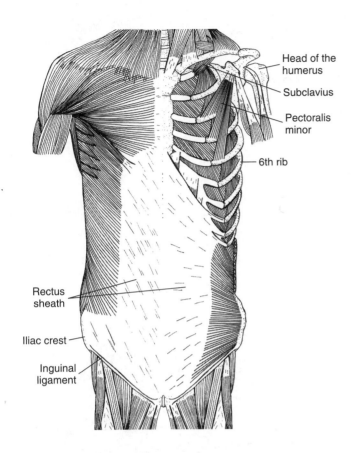

Head of the
humerus

Subclavius

Pectoralis
minor

6th rib

Rectus
sheath

Iliac crest

Inguinal
ligament

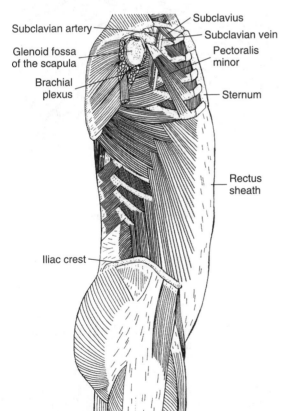

Subclavian artery

Glenoid fossa
of the scapula

Brachial
plexus

Subclavius

Subclavian vein

Pectoralis
minor

Sternum

Rectus
sheath

Iliac crest

DID YOU KNOW

If the pectoralis minor is tight, it may compress the brachial plexus of nerves and/or the subclavian artery and vein against the ribcage. This condition is called pectoralis minor syndrome, a type of thoracic outlet syndrome.

DID YOU KNOW

As the pectoralis minor contracts to protract the scapula, it also tends to pull the medial border of the scapula away from the rib cage wall, possibly causing winging of the scapula.

DID YOU KNOW

If the subclavius is tight, the brachial plexus of nerves and/or the subclavian artery and vein can be compressed between the 1st rib and the clavicle; this condition is called costoclavicular syndrome, a type of thoracic outlet syndrome.

DID YOU KNOW

The name "subclavius" literally means under the clavicle.

EXTERNAL INTERCOSTALS

eks-turn-al in-ter-**kos**-tals

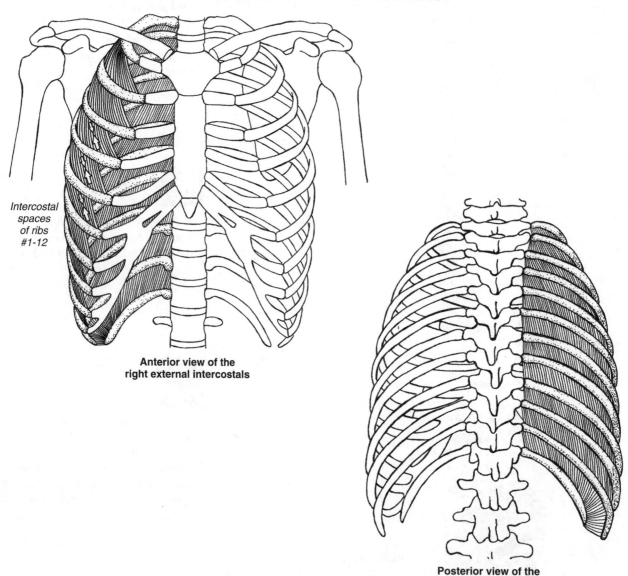

Intercostal
spaces
of ribs
#1-12

**Anterior view of the
right external intercostals**

**Posterior view of the
right external intercostals**

Actions	**Innervation**	**Myofascial Meridians**
Elevation of ribs #2-12 at the sternocostal and costoclavicular joints Depression of ribs #1-11 at the sternocostal and costoclavicular joints	Intercostal nerves **Arterial Supply** Anterior intercostal arteries and the posterior intercostal arteries	Lateral line

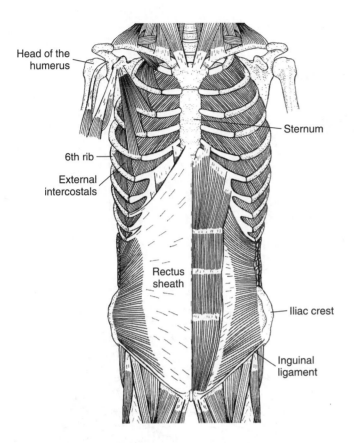

Head of the humerus

Sternum

6th rib

External intercostals

Rectus sheath

Iliac crest

Inguinal ligament

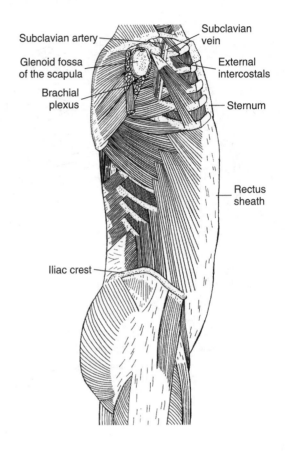

Subclavian artery

Subclavian vein

Glenoid fossa of the scapula

External intercostals

Brachial plexus

Sternum

Rectus sheath

Iliac crest

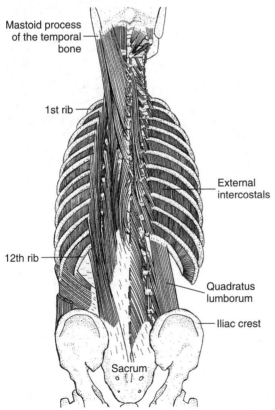

Mastoid process of the temporal bone

1st rib

External intercostals

12th rib

Quadratus lumborum

Iliac crest

Sacrum

DID YOU KNOW

Given their attachments to and movement of ribs, the external and internal intercostals are primarily muscles of respiration.

DID YOU KNOW

The external intercostals do not attach between the costal cartilages.

INTERNAL INTERCOSTALS

in-turn-al in-ter-**kos**-tals

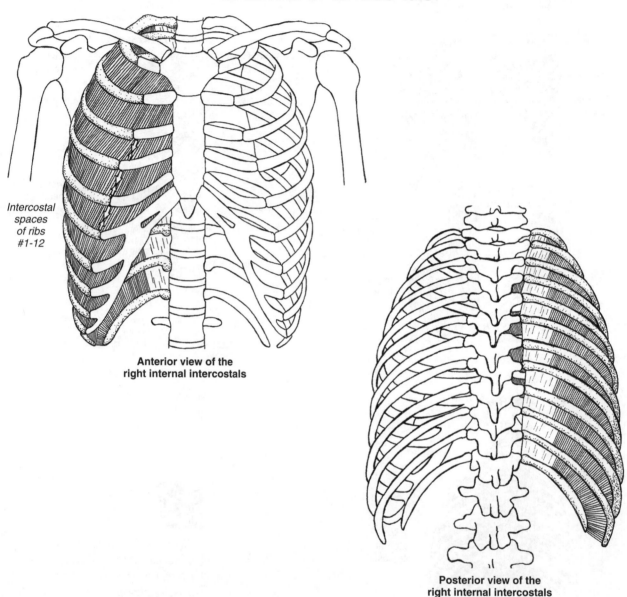

Intercostal spaces of ribs #1-12

Anterior view of the right internal intercostals

Posterior view of the right internal intercostals

Actions
Depression of ribs #1-11 at the sternocostal and costoclavicular joints
Elevation of ribs #2-12 at the sternocostal and costoclavicular joints

Innervation
Intercostal nerves

Arterial Supply
Anterior intercostal arteries and the posterior intercostal arteries

Myofascial Meridians
Lateral line

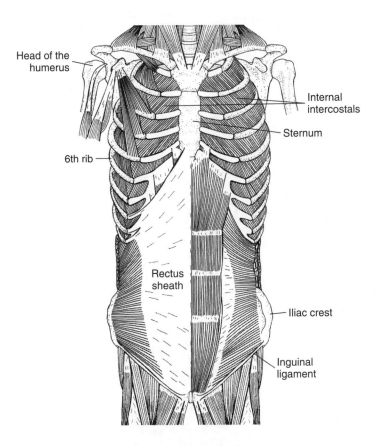

Head of the humerus

Internal intercostals

Sternum

6th rib

Rectus sheath

Iliac crest

Inguinal ligament

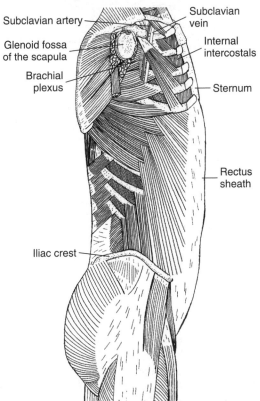

Subclavian artery

Subclavian vein

Glenoid fossa of the scapula

Internal intercostals

Brachial plexus

Sternum

Rectus sheath

Iliac crest

DID YOU KNOW ?

Given their attachments to and movement of ribs, the external and internal intercostals are primarily muscles of respiration.

DID YOU KNOW ?

As their name implies, the internal intercostals lie deep to the external intercostals.

RECTUS ABDOMINIS

rek-tus ab-dom-i-nis

Actions
Flexion of the trunk at the
    spinal joints
Posterior tilt of the pelvis at
    the lumbosacral joint
Lateral flexion of the trunk at
    the spinal joints
Compression of the abdominal
    contents

Innervation
Intercostal nerves

Arterial Supply
The superior epigastric artery
    and the inferior epigastric
    artery

Myofascial Meridians
Superficial front line
Involved: Front functional line

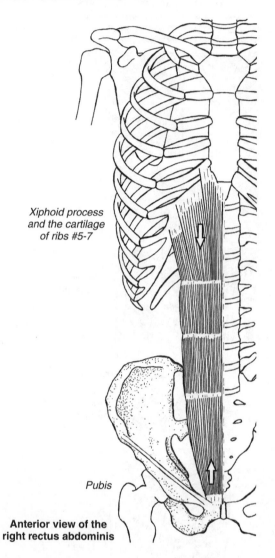

*Xiphoid process
and the cartilage
of ribs #5-7*

Pubis

**Anterior view of the
right rectus abdominis**

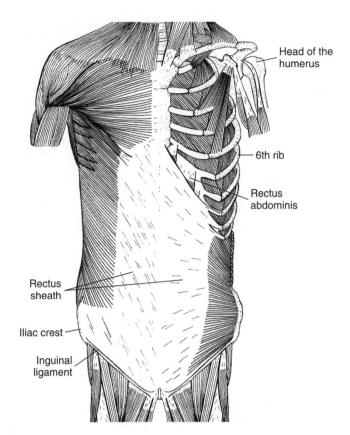

Head of the
humerus

6th rib

Rectus
abdominis

Rectus
sheath

Iliac crest

Inguinal
ligament

DID YOU KNOW

*Because of its separate compart-
ments, the rectus abdominis is often
called the 6-pack muscle. Given that
there are 8 compartments, a better
name would be the 8-pack muscle ☺.*

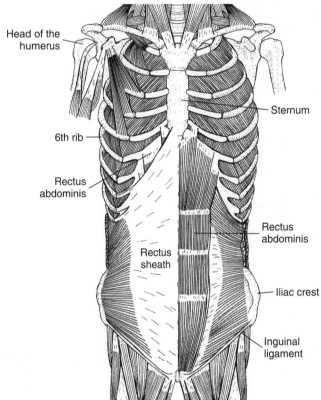

Head of the
humerus

Sternum

6th rib

Rectus
abdominis

Rectus
sheath

Rectus
abdominis

Iliac crest

Inguinal
ligament

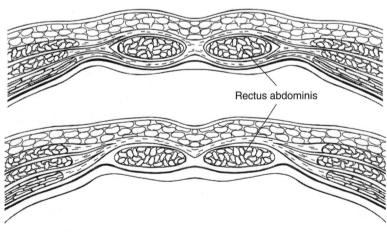

Rectus abdominis

*Anterior abdominal
wall cross section
superior to the
arcuate line*

*Anterior abdominal
wall cross section
inferior to the
arcuate line*

DID YOU KNOW

*The word "rectus" means
straight. The rectus abdominis
runs straight up and down the
anterior abdominal wall.*

EXTERNAL ABDOMINAL OBLIQUE

eks-turn-al
ab-**dom**-in-al
o-**bleek**

Actions
Flexion of the trunk at the spinal joints
Lateral flexion of the trunk at the spinal joints
Contralateral rotation of the trunk at the spinal joints
Posterior tilt of the pelvis at the lumbosacral joint
Ipsilateral rotation of the pelvis at the lumbosacral joint
Compression of the abdominal contents

Innervation
Intercostal nerves

Arterial Supply
The subcostal and posterior intercostal arteries and the deep circumflex iliac artery

Myofascial Meridians
Lateral line
Spiral line
Involved: Superficial back line
Involved: Front functional line

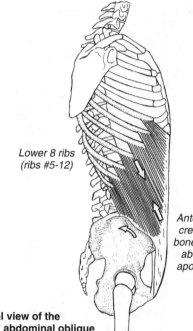

Lower 8 ribs (ribs #5-12)

Anterior iliac crest, pubic bone, and the abdominal aponeurosis

Lateral view of the right external abdominal oblique

INTERNAL ABDOMINAL OBLIQUE

in-**turn**-al
ab-**dom**-in-al
o-**bleek**

Actions
Flexion of the trunk at the spinal joints
Lateral flexion of the trunk at the spinal joints
Ipsilateral rotation of the trunk at the spinal joints
Posterior tilt of the pelvis at the lumbosacral joint
Contralateral rotation of the pelvis at the lumbosacral joint
Compression of the abdominal contents

Innervation
Intercostal nerves

Arterial Supply
The subcostal and posterior intercostal arteries and the deep circumflex iliac artery

Myofascial Meridians
Lateral line
Spiral line
Involved: Superficial back line
Involved: Front functional line

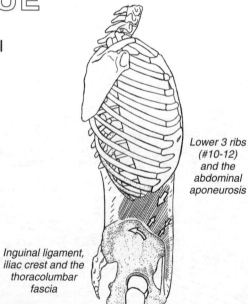

Lower 3 ribs (#10-12) and the abdominal aponeurosis

Inguinal ligament, iliac crest and the thoracolumbar fascia

Lateral view of the right internal abdominal oblique

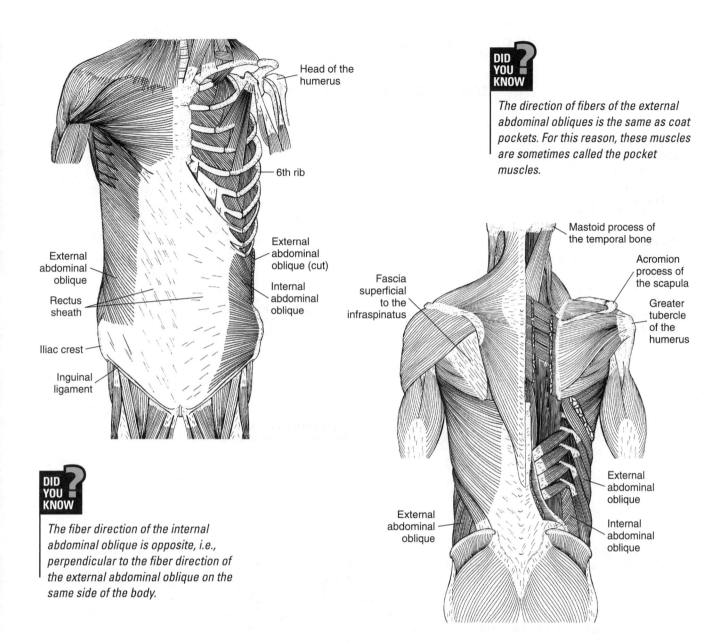

Head of the humerus

6th rib

External abdominal oblique (cut)

Internal abdominal oblique

External abdominal oblique

Rectus sheath

Iliac crest

Inguinal ligament

DID YOU KNOW?

The direction of fibers of the external abdominal obliques is the same as coat pockets. For this reason, these muscles are sometimes called the pocket muscles.

Mastoid process of the temporal bone

Acromion process of the scapula

Greater tubercle of the humerus

Fascia superficial to the infraspinatus

External abdominal oblique

Internal abdominal oblique

External abdominal oblique

DID YOU KNOW?

The fiber direction of the internal abdominal oblique is opposite, i.e., perpendicular to the fiber direction of the external abdominal oblique on the same side of the body.

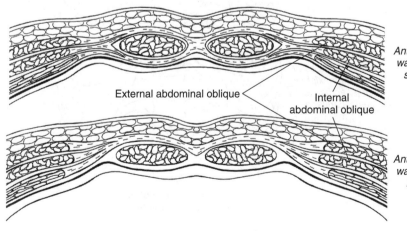

External abdominal oblique

Internal abdominal oblique

Anterior abdominal wall cross section superior to the arcuate line

Anterior abdominal wall cross section inferior to the arcuate line

DID YOU KNOW?

With respect to rotation (and flexion), the external abdominal oblique on one side of the body is synergistic with the internal abdominal oblique on the other side of the body.

TRANSVERSUS ABDOMINIS

trans-**ver**-sus ab-**dom**-i-nis

Action
Compression of the abdominal
contents

Innervation
Intercostal nerves

Arterial Supply
The subcostal and posterior
intercostal arteries and the deep
circumflex iliac artery

Myofascial Meridians
Deep front line

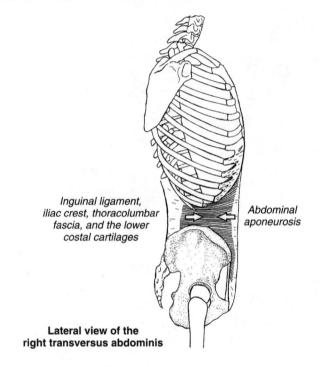

*Inguinal ligament,
iliac crest, thoracolumbar
fascia, and the lower
costal cartilages*

*Abdominal
aponeurosis*

**Lateral view of the
right transversus abdominis**

TRANSVERSUS THORACIS

trans-**ver**-sus thor-**as**-is

Action
Depression of ribs #2-6 at the
sternocostal and costovertebral
joints

Innervation
Intercostal nerves

Arterial Supply
The anterior intercostal arteries

Myofascial Meridians
Deep front line

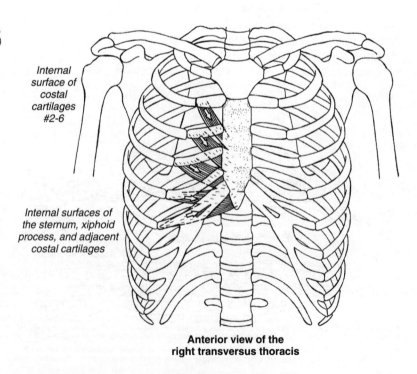

*Internal
surface of
costal
cartilages
#2-6*

*Internal surfaces of
the sternum, xiphoid
process, and adjacent
costal cartilages*

**Anterior view of the
right transversus thoracis**

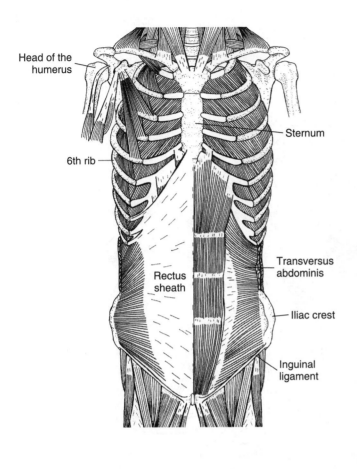

Head of the
humerus

Sternum

6th rib

Transversus
abdominis

Rectus
sheath

Iliac crest

Inguinal
ligament

DID
YOU
KNOW

*The transversus abdominis is sometimes called
the corset muscle because it wraps around the
abdomen like a corset, and like a corset, it functions
to hold in the abdomen.*

DID
YOU
KNOW

*The transversus is considered to be one of the most
important muscles for core (Powerhouse) stability.*

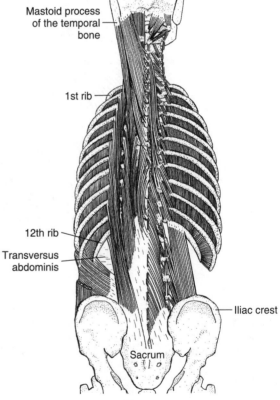

Mastoid process
of the temporal
bone

1st rib

12th rib

Transversus
abdominis

Iliac crest

Sacrum

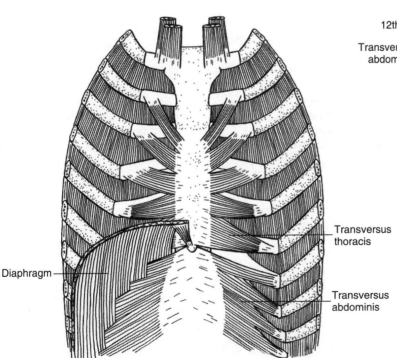

Transversus
thoracis

Diaphragm

Transversus
abdominis

**Posterior view of
the anterior ribcage**

DID
YOU
KNOW

*The transversus thoracis is located
deep to the ribcage.*

DID
YOU
KNOW

*The transversus thoracis (as with all
muscles of the rib cage) functions as a
muscle of respiration.*

DIAPHRAGM

di-a-fram

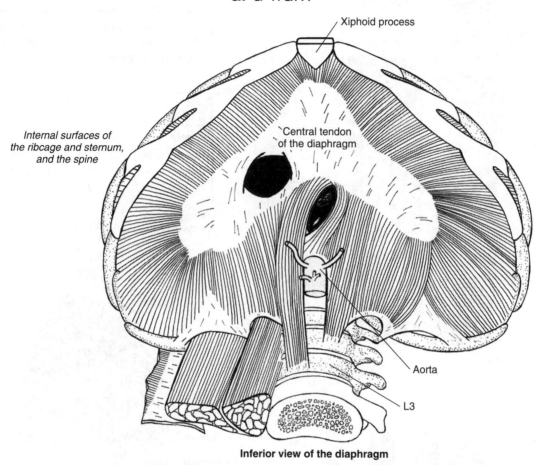

Xiphoid process

Internal surfaces of
the ribcage and sternum,
and the spine

Central tendon
of the diaphragm

Aorta

L3

Inferior view of the diaphragm

Action	**Arterial Supply**	**Myofascial Meridians**
Increases the volume of the thoracic cavity	Branches of the aorta and the internal thoracic artery	Deep front line
Innervation		
The phrenic nerve		

The diaphragm is an unusual muscle in that it is under both conscious and unconscious control by the nervous system.

The diaphragm can contract to drop its central dome for abdominal (belly) breathing and/or elevate the lower rib cage for thoracic (chest) breathing.

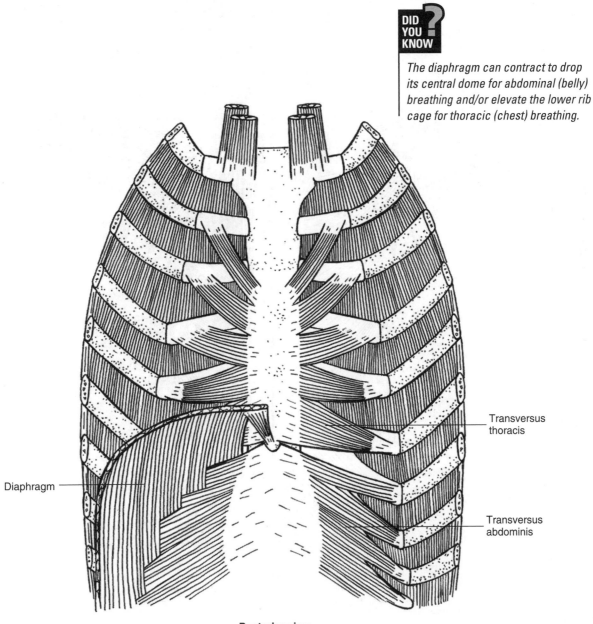

Transversus thoracis

Transversus abdominis

Diaphragm

Posterior view

POSTERIOR VIEW OF THE TRUNK (SUPERFICIAL AND INTERMEDIATE)

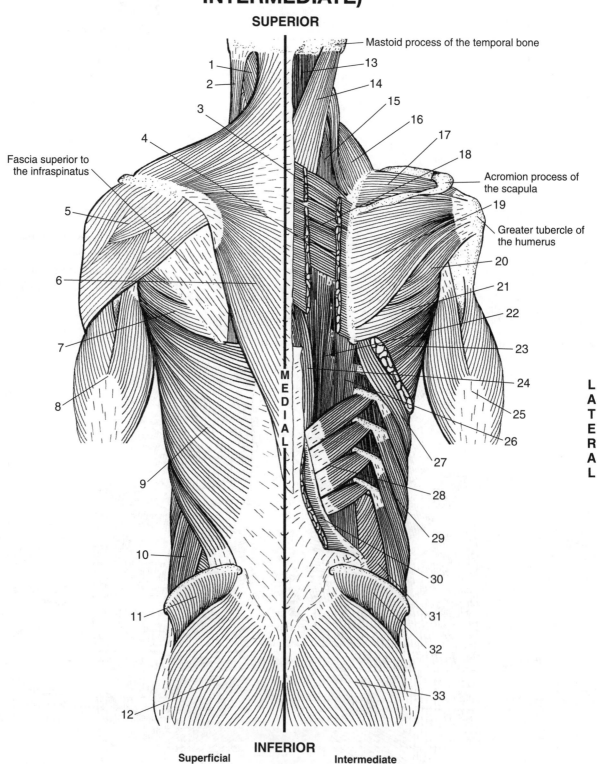

SUPERIOR

Mastoid process of the temporal bone

1
2
3
4
Fascia superior to the infraspinatus
5
6
7
8
9
10
11
12

13
14
15
16
17
18
Acromion process of the scapula
19
Greater tubercle of the humerus
20
21
22
23
24
25
26
27
28
29
30
31
32
33

LATERAL

MEDIAL

LATERAL

INFERIOR

Superficial   Intermediate

Answers to labeling exercises are on p. 484.

POSTERIOR VIEW OF THE TRUNK (DEEP LAYERS)

SUPERIOR

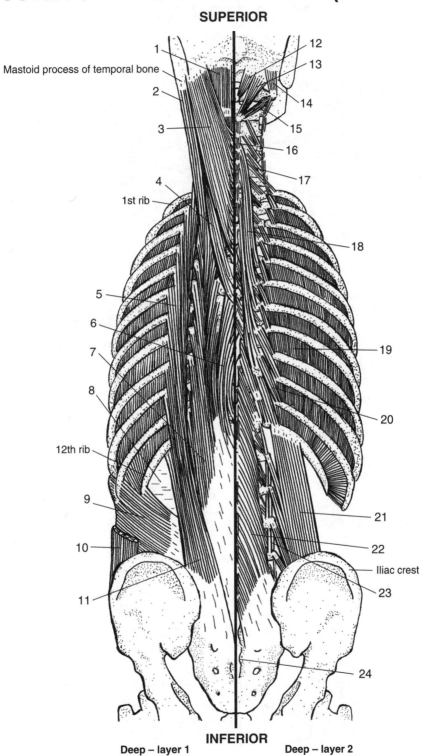

Mastoid process of temporal bone

1st rib

12th rib

Iliac crest

LATERAL

LATERAL

INFERIOR

Deep – layer 1   Deep – layer 2

ANTERIOR VIEW OF THE TRUNK (SUPERFICIAL AND INTERMEDIATE)

SUPERIOR

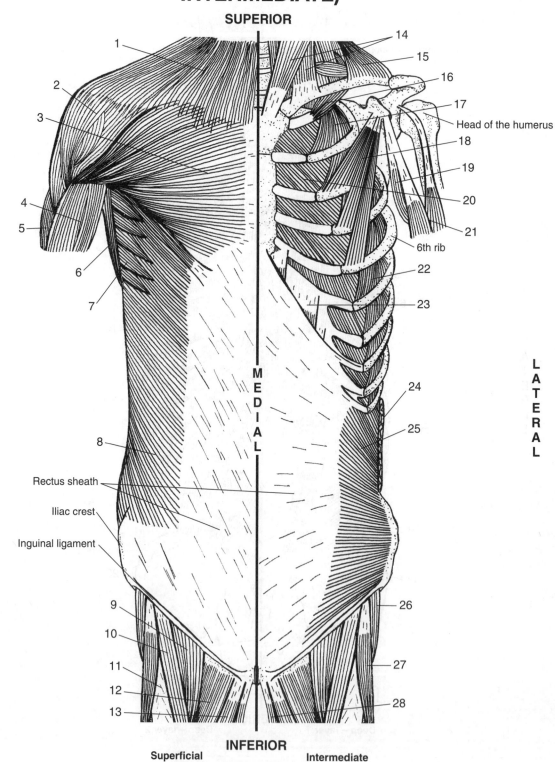

LATERAL

MEDIAL

LATERAL

Head of the humerus

6th rib

Rectus sheath

Iliac crest

Inguinal ligament

INFERIOR

Superficial   Intermediate

ANTERIOR VIEW OF THE TRUNK (INTERMEDIATE AND DEEP)

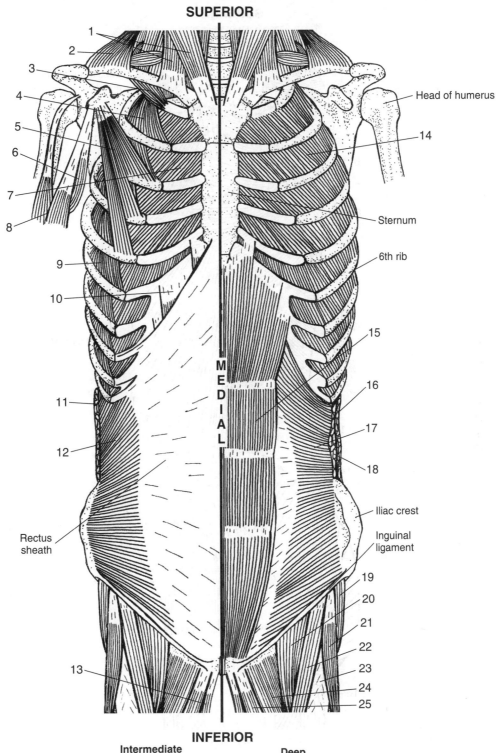

SUPERIOR

Head of humerus

14

Sternum

6th rib

15

16

17

18

Iliac crest

Inguinal
ligament

19

20

21

22

23

24

25

LATERAL

MEDIAL

LATERAL

1
2
3
4
5
6
7
8
9
10
11
12
13

Rectus
sheath

INFERIOR

Intermediate

Deep

LATERAL VIEW OF THE TRUNK

SUPERIOR

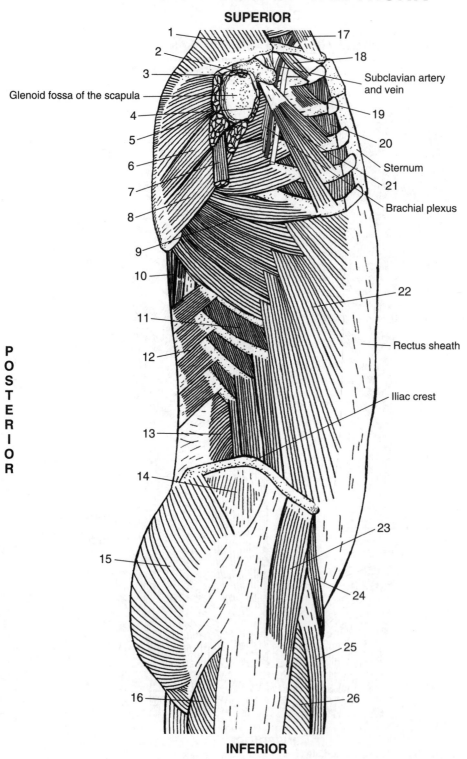

Glenoid fossa of the scapula

Subclavian artery and vein

Sternum

Brachial plexus

Rectus sheath

Iliac crest

POSTERIOR

ANTERIOR

INFERIOR

CROSS SECTION VIEWS OF THE TRUNK

ANTERIOR

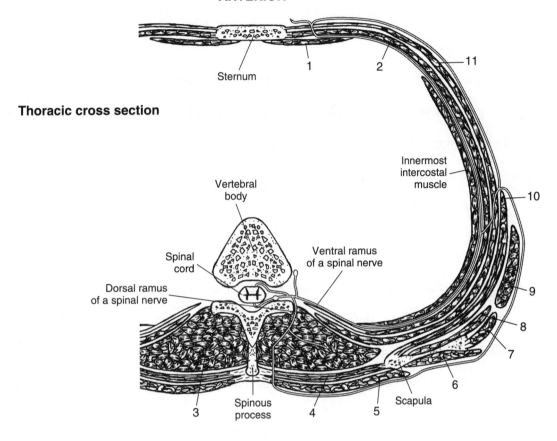

Thoracic cross section

Sternum

1 · 2 · 11

Innermost intercostal muscle

Vertebral body

Spinal cord

Dorsal ramus of a spinal nerve

Ventral ramus of a spinal nerve

10

9

8

7

6

Spinous process

Scapula

3 · 4 · 5

L A T E R A L

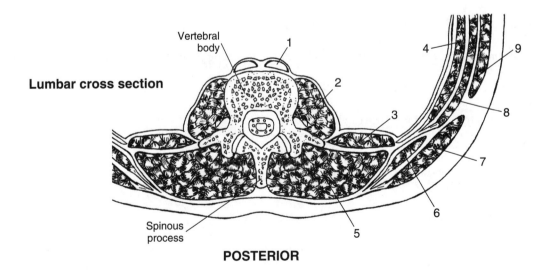

Vertebral body

1

Lumbar cross section

2

4 · 9

8

3

7

Spinous process

6

5

POSTERIOR

Review Questions

Muscles of the Trunk

Answers to these questions are found on page 485.

1. What subgroup of the transversospinalis is immediately superficial to the rotatores?

2. What muscle makes up the vast majority of the anterior axillary fold of tissue?

3. What muscles sit the deepest in the laminar groove of the spine?

4. What are the two heads of the pectoralis major?

5. With regard to flexion of the trunk at the spinal joints, what two abdominal wall muscles are synergistic with the rectus abdominis?

6. What joint action is occurring when the right-sided intertransversarii are eccentrically contracting?

7. Name two actions of the serratus anterior that are synergistic with actions of the pectoralis minor.

8. What muscle is immediately superficial to the pectoralis minor?

9. True or false: The diaphragm is under both conscious and unconscious control.

10. What is the direction of fibers of the external abdominal oblique compared to the internal abdominal oblique on the same side?

11. What two muscles make up the vast majority of the posterior axillary fold of tissue?

12. What structures can the pectoralis minor compress against the ribcage?

13. What joint action is occurring when the interspinales are lengthening?

14. If the pelvis is anteriorly tilting at the lumbosacral joint, what is happening to the length of the erector spinae group?

15. What two muscles pierce the diaphragm posteriorly?

16. What muscle attaches to the underside of the clavicle?

17. Would left lateral flexion of the trunk at the spinal joints lengthen or shorten the right-sided levatores costarum?

18. Which subgroup of the erector spinae goes from spinous processes to spinous processes?

19. The serratus anterior interdigitates (blends) with what muscle anteriorly?

20. What muscle group is immediately superficial to the levatores costarum?

21. The upper fibers on the ribcage of the serratus anterior are deep to what two muscles?

22. If the superior rib attachment of an external intercostal muscle is fixed, what action will occur?

23. What muscles are often called the coat pocket muscles?

24. What is happening to the length of the left quadratus lumborum when the pelvis is posteriorly tilting at the lumbosacral joint?

25. What two abdominal wall muscles attach into the thoracolumbar fascia?

26. What happens to the length of the rhomboids as the scapula protracts (abducts) at the scapulocostal joint?

27. What muscles are known as the "Christmas Tree" muscles?

28. What muscle is located deep (posterior) to the anterior ribcage and is analogous to the transversus abdominis?

29. If the inferior rib attachment of an external intercostal muscle is fixed, what action will occur?

30. What two muscles can upwardly rotate the scapula at the scapulocostal joint?

31. How are the serratus posterior inferior and quadratus lumborum synergistic with each other?

32. Where the latissimus dorsi and trapezius overlap, which muscle is superficial?

33. What happens to the length of the rectus abdominis as the pelvis anteriorly tilts at the lumbosacral joint?

34. The serratus posterior inferior is immediately deep to what muscle?

35. If the right-sided rotatores are concentrically contracting, what type of rotation of the spine is occurring?

36. Where are intercostal muscles not deep to external intercostals?

37. If the pectoralis minor is eccentrically contracting, is the scapula protracting or retracting at the scapulocostal joint?

38. Which subgroup of the erector spinae is the most lateral?

39. What is the only subgroup of the transversospinalis that attaches to the pelvis?

40. The direction of fibers of the external intercostals is similar to what muscle?

41. How is the right external abdominal oblique synergistic with and also antagonistic to the right internal abdominal oblique?

42. Which subgroup of the erector spinae is the longest?

43. What happens to the length of the left rectus abdominis as the trunk is passively left laterally flexed at the spinal joints?

44. If the latissimus dorsi eccentrically contracts as the pelvis moves, how is the pelvis moving?

45. What three muscles are located lateral to the rectus abdominis?

46. If the arm medially rotates at the shoulder joint, what happens to the length of the latissimus dorsi?

47. What happens to the length of the right-sided rotatores if the spine is rotated to the right?

48. Name a muscle that is antagonistic to the elevation of the 12th rib action of the internal intercostals.

49. Which subgroup of the transversospinalis is the deepest?

50. If the right-sided rotatores are eccentrically contracting, what type of rotation of the spine is occurring?

51. Which subgroup of the erector spinae is the most medial?

52. Which subgroup of the erector spinae goes from the pelvis to ribs?

53. Which subgroup of the transversospinalis is the most superficial?

54. What is happening to the length of the left quadratus lumborum when the spine is laterally flexing to the left?

55. What muscle is superficial to the rhomboids?

56. As a rule, transversospinalis musculature attaches from where to where?

57. Which muscle attaches farther posteriorly, the external or internal abdominal oblique?

58. How are the serratus posterior superior and scalenes synergistic with each other?

59. What muscle is immediately deep to the internal abdominal oblique?

60. What happens to the length of the transversus abdominis as a person breathes in and their belly rises?

61. When the diaphragm concentrically contracts, what happens to its dome (central tendon)?

62. In what region is the multifidus of the transversospinalis group the largest?

63. What muscle is deep to the rhomboids and has the same direction of fibers?

64. What muscle attaches from the pelvis to the lumbar spine and 12th rib and is deep to the erector spinae group?

65. What is the name of the connective tissue that envelops the rectus abdominis?

66. In the thoracic region, the transversospinalis musculature is deep to which muscle of the erector spinae group.?

67. Name a synergist to the pectoralis minor's action of protraction of the scapula at the scapulocostal joint.

68. What happens to the length of the pectoralis major if the arm laterally rotates at the shoulder joint?

69. What muscle is immediately superficial to the transversus abdominis?

70. What muscle group is immediately superficial to the quadratus lumborum?

71. If the subclavius is tight, what condition might be caused?

72. Which subgroup of the transversospinalis is best suited for rotation of the spine and why?

73. What is the superior attachment of the rotatores?

74. From a posterior perspective, which is deeper, the intercostals or the subcostales?

75. What muscle is immediately deep to the external intercostals?

76. How are the rhomboids synergistic with the middle trapezius?

77. What muscle is immediately superficial to the semispinalis in the suboccipital region?

78. If the serratus posterior inferior is eccentrically contracting, what joint motion is occurring?

79. What spinal rotation is created by the transversospinalis musculature on the right side of the body?

80. In what region is the semispinalis of the transversospinalis group the largest?

81. If the trunk is passively flexing at the spinal joints, what is happening to the length of the erector spinae group?

82. What muscle group is deep to the rhomboids and has a vertical direction to its fibers?

83. What is the superior attachment of the diaphragm?

84. Which head of the pectoralis major is better suited to create flexion of the arm at the shoulder joint?

85. Are the right and left side intertransversarii synergistic with or antagonistic to each other?

86. What muscle has the same humeral actions as the latissimus dorsi?

87. Where they overlap, which is deeper, the erector spinae group or the transversospinalis group?

88. What muscle is known as the corset muscle?

89. What muscle is immediately deep to the distal attachment of the pectoralis major?

90. If a person's trunk is actively rotated to the right, what happens to the length of the transversospinalis musculature on the right?

91. The direction of fibers of the internal intercostals is similar to what muscle?

92. What region of the spine is mostly missing interspinales?

93. What is the action upon the spine if both quadratus lumborum muscles contract together?

94. What muscle is immediately superficial to the internal intercostals?

95. Why are the levatores costarum and subcostales antagonistic to each other?

Muscles of the Pelvis 6

Note: Throughout this chapter, muscle attachments are indicated by italics.

⊖ More review activities on Evolve at: http://evolve.elsevier.com/Muscolino/anatomycoloring/

PSOAS MAJOR
(OF THE ILIOPSOAS)

so-as **may**-jor

Actions
Flexion of the thigh at the
hip joint
Lateral rotation of the thigh
at the hip joint
Flexion of the trunk at the
spinal joints
Lateral flexion of the trunk
at the spinal joints
Anterior tilt of the pelvis at
the hip joint
Contralateral rotation of the
trunk at the spinal joints
Contralateral rotation of the
pelvis at the hip joint

Innervation
Lumbar plexus

Arterial Supply
The lumbar arteries

**Myofascial
Meridians**
Deep front line

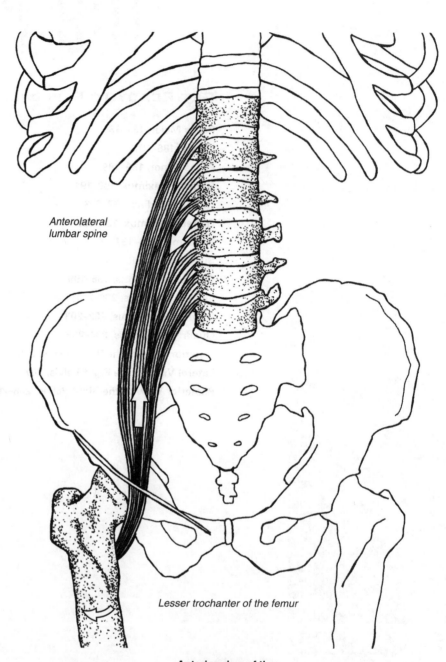

*Anterolateral
lumbar spine*

Lesser trochanter of the femur

**Anterior view of the
right psoas major**

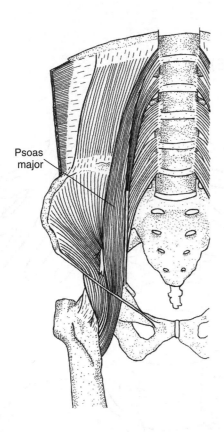

Psoas
major

DID
YOU
KNOW

The reason that old-fashioned sit-ups
have been replaced by abdominal curl-
ups or crunches is to avoid creating
an overly strengthened and perhaps
overly tight psoas major.

DID
YOU
KNOW

The psoas major is the only hip flexor
that also crosses the spinal joints.

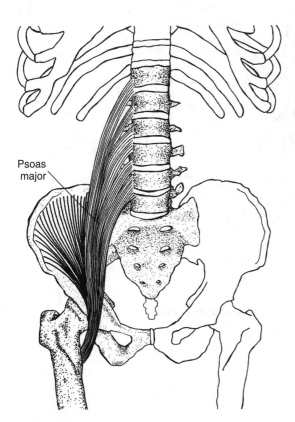

Psoas
major

ILIACUS
(OF THE ILIOPSOAS)

i-lee-**ak**-us

Actions
Flexion of the thigh at the hip
joint
Lateral rotation of the thigh at
the hip joint
Anterior tilt of the pelvis at
the hip joint
Contralateral rotation of the
pelvis at the hip joint

Innervation
The femoral nerve

Arterial Supply
The iliolumbar artery

Myofascial Meridians
Deep front line

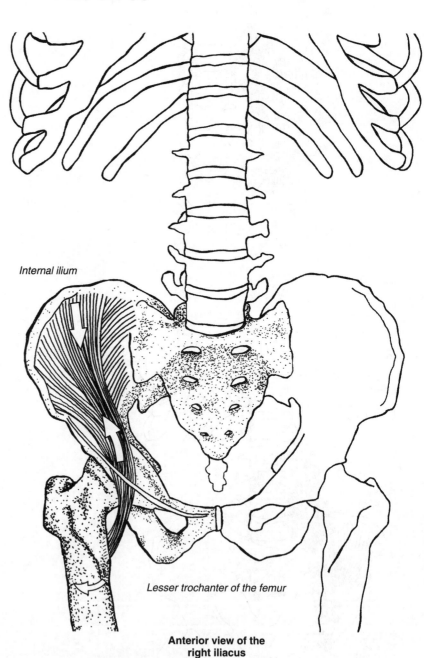

Internal ilium

Lesser trochanter of the femur

**Anterior view of the
right iliacus**

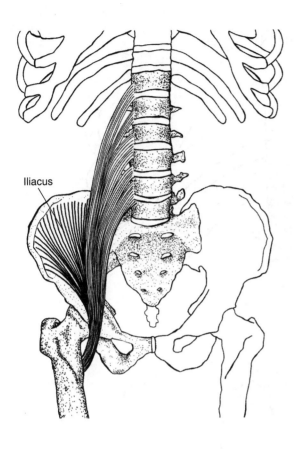

Iliacus

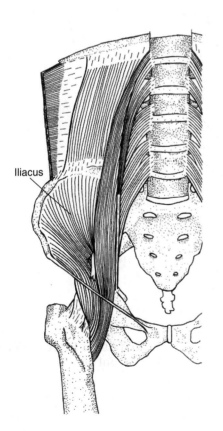

Iliacus

DID
YOU
KNOW

The distal tendon of the iliacus joins into the distal tendon of the psoas major; together, these two muscles are often called the iliopsoas muscle.

DID
YOU
KNOW

In the anterior proximal thigh, the iliacus is usually wider than the adjacent psoas major.

PSOAS MINOR

so-as my-nor

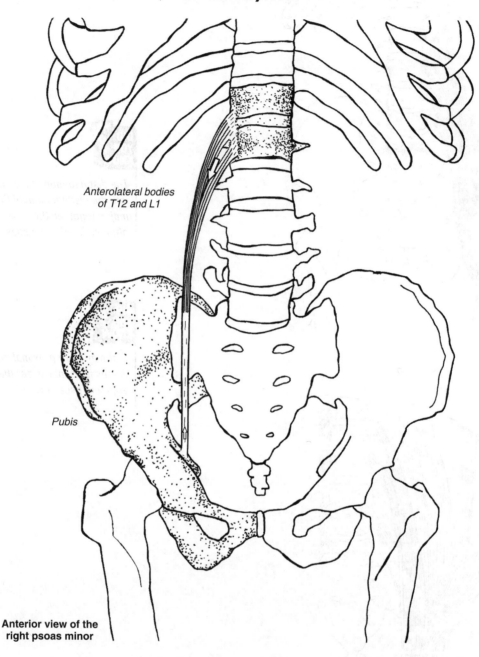

Anterolateral bodies
of T12 and L1

Pubis

**Anterior view of the
right psoas minor**

Actions	**Innervation**	**Myofascial Meridians**
Flexion of the trunk at the spinal joints	L1 spinal nerve	Deep front line
Posterior tilt of the pelvis at the lumbosacral joint	**Arterial Supply**	
	Lumbar arteries	

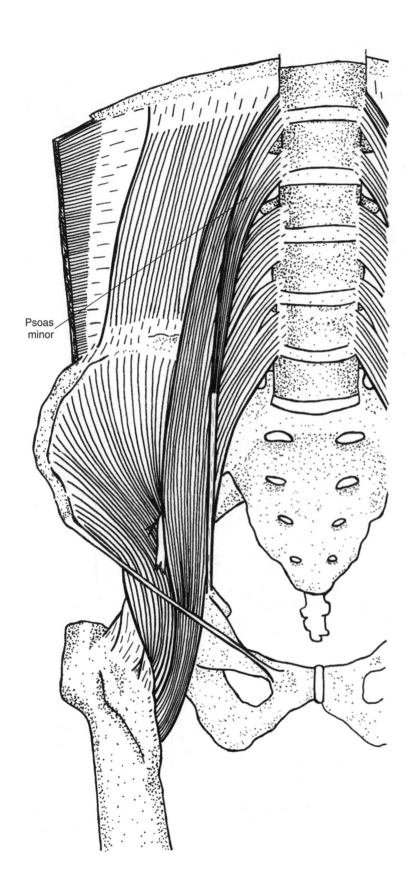

Psoas
minor

The psoas minor is absent in up to 40% of individuals.

The psoas minor, unlike the psoas major, does not cross the hip joint.

GLUTEUS MAXIMUS

gloo-tee-us **max**-i-mus

Actions
Extension of the thigh at the hip joint

Lateral rotation of the thigh at the hip joint

Abduction of the thigh at the hip joint (upper ⅓)

Adduction of the thigh at the hip joint (lower ⅔)

Posterior tilt of the pelvis at the hip joint

Contralateral rotation of the pelvis at the hip joint

Extension of the leg at the knee joint

Innervation
The inferior gluteal nerve (L5, S1, 2)

Arterial Supply
The superior gluteal artery and the inferior gluteal artery

Myofascial Meridians
Lateral line

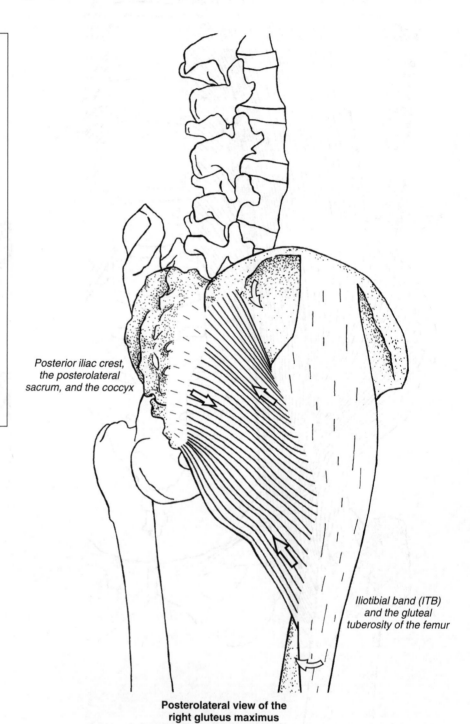

Posterior iliac crest, the posterolateral sacrum, and the coccyx

Iliotibial band (ITB) and the gluteal tuberosity of the femur

Posterolateral view of the right gluteus maximus

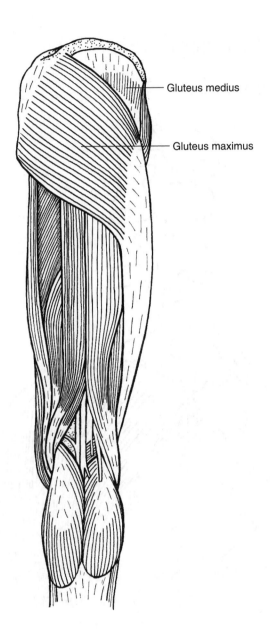

Gluteus medius

Gluteus maximus

The gluteus maximus is the largest muscle in the human body.

Because of its ability to extend and laterally rotate (and the upper fibers' ability to abduct), the gluteus maximus is often known as the "speedskater's muscle."

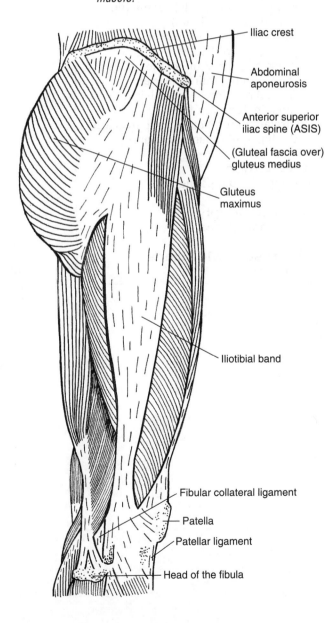

Iliac crest

Abdominal aponeurosis

Anterior superior iliac spine (ASIS)

(Gluteal fascia over) gluteus medius

Gluteus maximus

Iliotibial band

Fibular collateral ligament

Patella

Patellar ligament

Head of the fibula

GLUTEUS MEDIUS

gloo-tee-us **meed**-ee-us

Actions

Abduction of the thigh at the hip joint (entire muscle)

Flexion of the thigh at the hip joint (anterior fibers)

Medial rotation of the thigh at the hip joint (anterior fibers)

Extension of the thigh at the hip joint (posterior fibers)

Lateral rotation of the thigh at the hip joint (posterior fibers)

Posterior tilt of the pelvis at the hip joint (posterior fibers)

Anterior tilt of the pelvis at the hip joint (anterior fibers)

Depression (lateral tilt) of the pelvis at the hip joint (entire muscle)

Ipsilateral rotation of the pelvis at the hip joint (anterior fibers)

Contralateral rotation of the pelvis at the hip joint (posterior fibers)

Innervation
The superior gluteal nerve

Arterial Supply
The superior gluteal artery

Myofascial Meridians
Lateral line

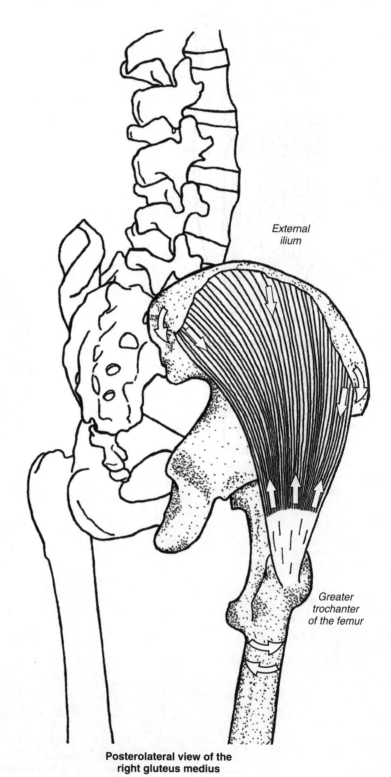

External ilium

Greater trochanter of the femur

Posterolateral view of the right gluteus medius

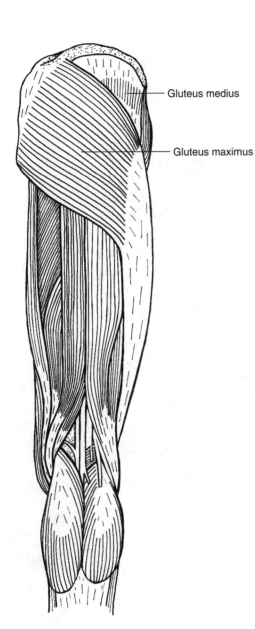

Gluteus medius

Gluteus maximus

Depression of the pelvis at the hip joint during walking is actually the most important action of the gluteus medius.

Because of its joint actions, the gluteus medius is often described as the "deltoid of the hip joint."

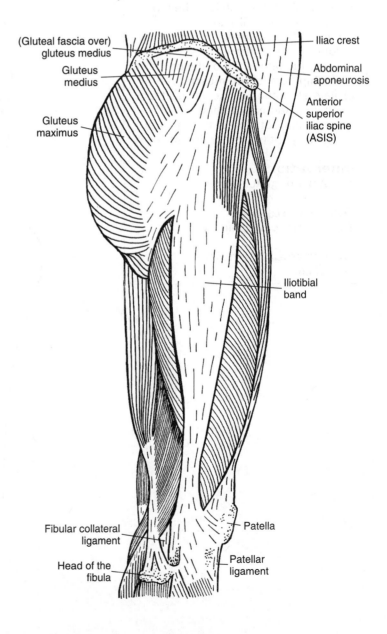

(Gluteal fascia over) gluteus medius

Gluteus medius

Gluteus maximus

Iliac crest

Abdominal aponeurosis

Anterior superior iliac spine (ASIS)

Iliotibial band

Fibular collateral ligament

Head of the fibula

Patella

Patellar ligament

GLUTEUS MINIMUS

gloo-tee-us **min-i-mus**

Actions
Abduction of the thigh at the hip joint
  (entire muscle)
Flexion of the thigh at the hip joint
  (anterior fibers)
Medial rotation of the thigh at the hip
  joint (anterior fibers)
Extension of the thigh at the hip joint
  (posterior fibers)
Lateral rotation of the thigh at the hip
  joint (posterior fibers)
Posterior tilt of the pelvis at the hip
  joint (posterior fibers)
Anterior tilt of the pelvis at the hip
  joint (anterior fibers)
Depression (lateral tilt) of the pelvis at
  the hip joint (entire muscle)
Ipsilateral rotation of the pelvis at the
  hip joint (anterior fibers)
Contralateral rotation of the pelvis at
  the hip joint (posterior fibers)

Innervation
The superior gluteal nerve

Arterial Supply
The superior gluteal artery

Myofascial Meridians
Lateral line

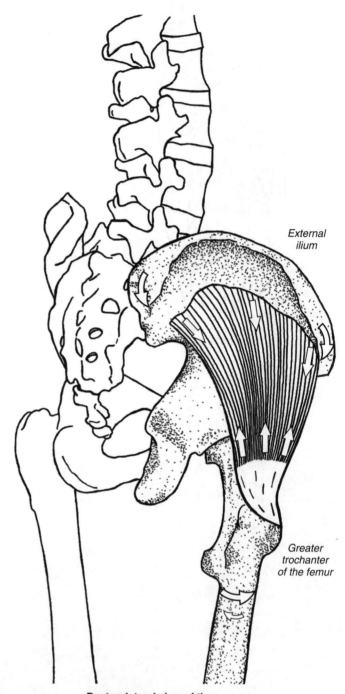

External
ilium

Greater
trochanter
of the femur

**Posterolateral view of the
right gluteus minimus**

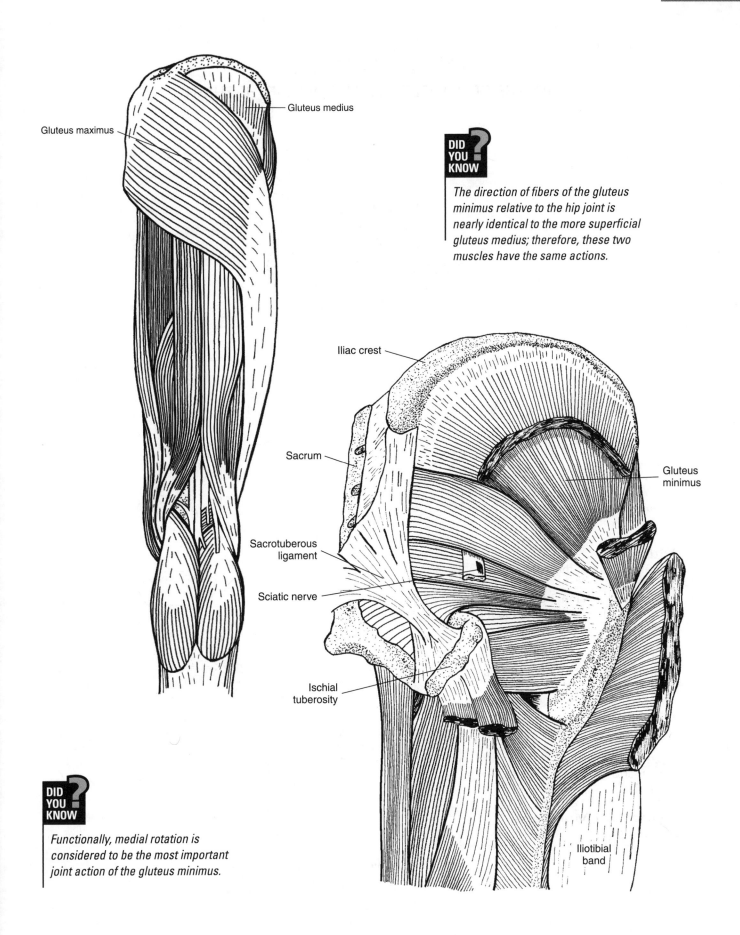

Gluteus maximus

Gluteus medius

Iliac crest

Sacrum

Gluteus minimus

Sacrotuberous ligament

Sciatic nerve

Ischial tuberosity

Iliotibial band

PIRIFORMIS

(OF THE DEEP LATERAL ROTATORS OF THE THIGH)

pi-ri-**for**-mis

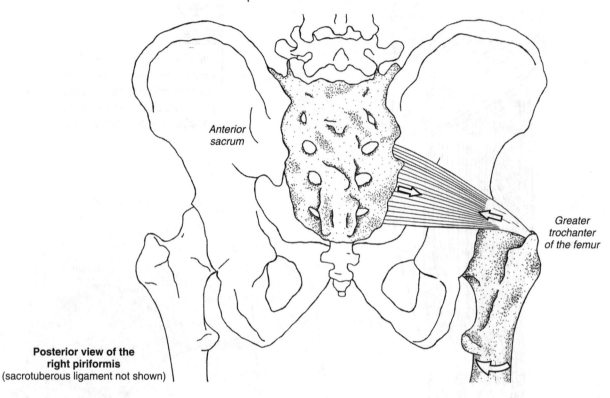

Anterior sacrum

Greater trochanter of the femur

Posterior view of the right piriformis
(sacrotuberous ligament not shown)

Actions
Lateral rotation of the thigh at the
hip joint
Horizontal extension (horizontal
abduction) of the thigh at the hip
joint (if the thigh is flexed)
Medial rotation of the thigh at the
hip joint (if the thigh is flexed)
Contralateral rotation of the pelvis
at the hip joint

Innervation
The lumbosacral plexus

Arterial Supply
The superior and inferior gluteal
arteries

Myofascial Meridians
Deep front line

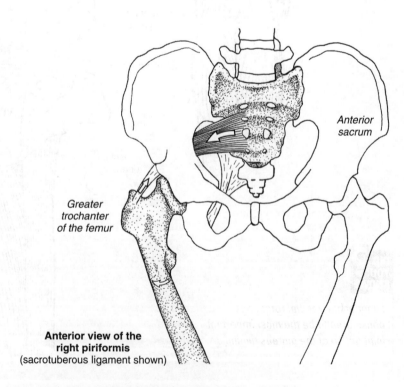

Anterior sacrum

Greater trochanter of the femur

Anterior view of the right piriformis
(sacrotuberous ligament shown)

A tight piriformis can compress the sciatic nerve causing symptoms of sciatica. This condition is called piriformis syndrome.

The piriformis is the only member of the deep lateral rotator group that attaches onto the sacrum and therefore has a function at the sacroiliac joint.

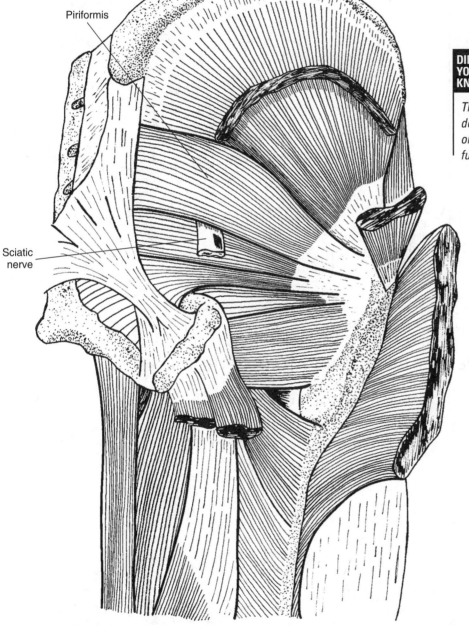

Piriformis

Sciatic nerve

SUPERIOR GEMELLUS
(OF THE DEEP LATERAL ROTATORS OF THE THIGH)

su-**pee**-ree-or jee-**mel**-us

Actions
Lateral rotation of the thigh at
    the hip joint
Horizontal extension
    (horizontal abduction) of the
    thigh at the hip joint (if the
    thigh is flexed)
Contralateral rotation of the
    pelvis at the hip joint

Innervation
The lumbosacral plexus

Arterial Supply
The inferior gluteal artery

Myofascial Meridians
Deep front line

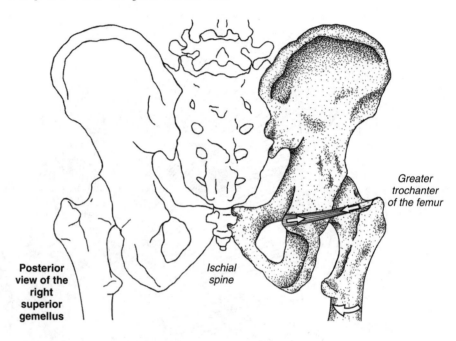

Greater
trochanter
of the femur

Posterior
view of the
right
superior
gemellus

Ischial
spine

OBTURATOR INTERNUS
(OF THE DEEP LATERAL ROTATORS OF THE THIGH)

ob-too-**ray**-tor in-**ter**-nus

Actions
Lateral rotation of the thigh at
    the hip joint
Horizontal extension
    (horizontal abduction) of
    the thigh at the hip joint (if
    the thigh is flexed)
Contralateral rotation of the
    pelvis at the hip joint

Innervation
The lumbosacral plexus

Arterial Supply
The superior and inferior
    gluteal arteries

Myofascial Meridians
Deep front line

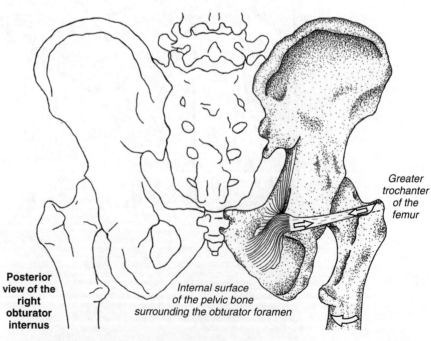

Greater
trochanter
of the
femur

Posterior
view of the
right
obturator
internus

Internal surface
of the pelvic bone
surrounding the obturator foramen

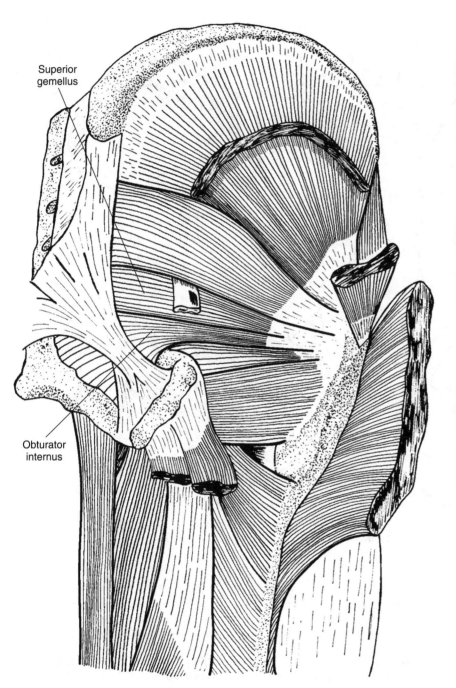

Superior gemellus

Obturator internus

The distal tendons of the superior gemellus, obturator internus, and inferior gemellus usually blend together.

The word "gemellus" means twin. The superior and inferior gemellus muscles can be thought of as twin muscles of the deep lateral rotator group.

The obturator internus turns 90 degrees around the pelvic bone to then attach onto the greater trochanter of the femur.

INFERIOR GEMELLUS
(OF THE DEEP LATERAL ROTATORS OF THE THIGH)
in-**fee**-ree-or jee-**mel**-us

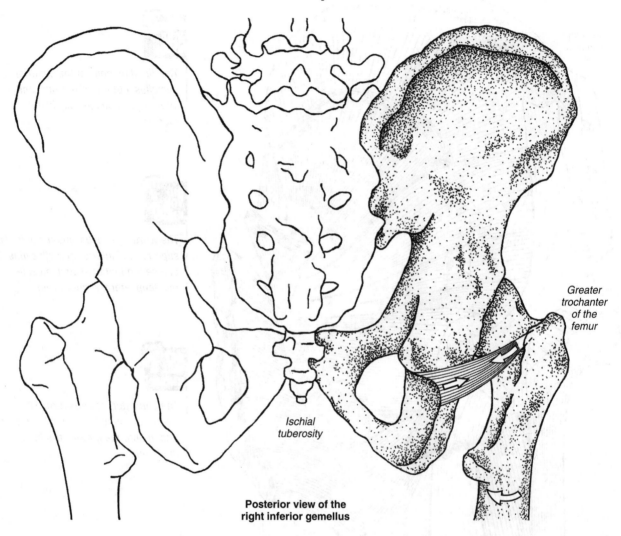

Greater
trochanter
of the
femur

Ischial
tuberosity

**Posterior view of the
right inferior gemellus**

Actions
Lateral rotation of the thigh at
    the hip joint
Horizontal extension (horizontal
    abduction) of the thigh at the
    hip joint (if the thigh is flexed)

Contralateral rotation of the
    pelvis at the hip joint

Innervation
The lumbosacral plexus

Arterial Supply
The inferior gluteal artery

Myofascial Meridians
Deep front line

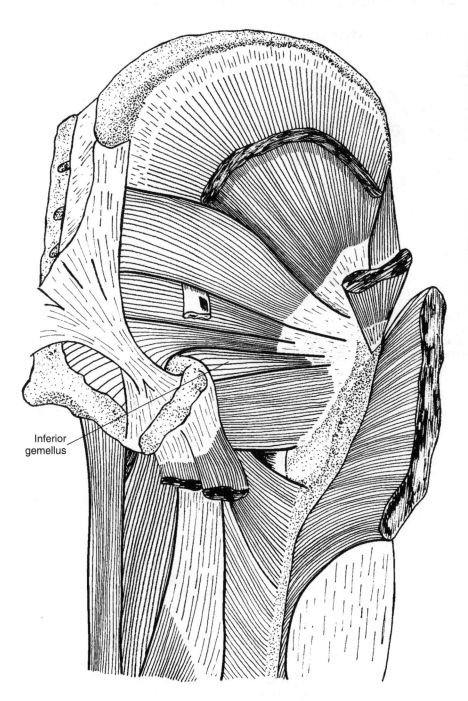

Inferior
gemellus

DID
YOU
KNOW

The distal tendons of the superior gemellus, obturator internus, and inferior gemellus usually blend together.

DID
YOU
KNOW

The inferior and superior gemellus muscles are "twin" muscles of the deep lateral rotator group. "Gemellus" means twin (think "Gemini").

OBTURATOR EXTERNUS
(OF THE DEEP LATERAL ROTATORS OF THE THIGH)

ob-too-**ray**-tor ex-**ter**-nus

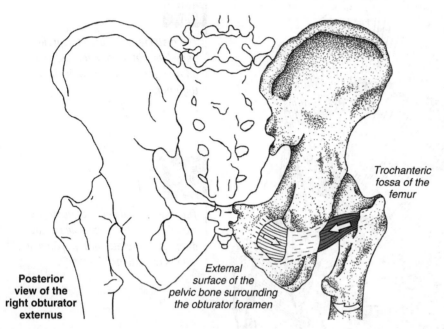

Posterior
view of the
right obturator
externus

External
surface of the
pelvic bone surrounding
the obturator foramen

Trochanteric
fossa of the
femur

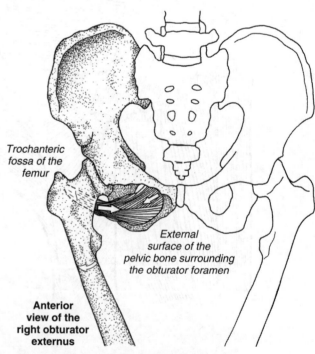

Trochanteric
fossa of the
femur

External
surface of the
pelvic bone surrounding
the obturator foramen

Anterior
view of the
right obturator
externus

Actions
Lateral rotation of the thigh at
   the hip joint
Contralateral rotation of the
   pelvis at the hip joint

Innervation
The obturator nerve

Arterial Supply
The obturator artery

Myofascial Meridians
Deep front line

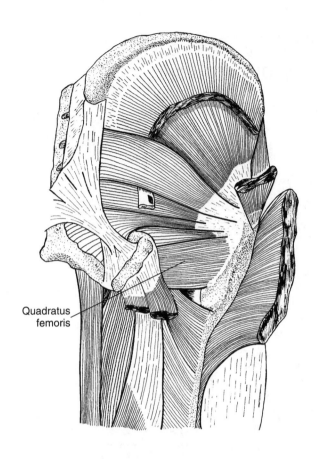

Quadratus femoris

DID YOU KNOW

The obturator externus is located deeper and has a different innervation than the other deep lateral rotators of the thigh.

DID YOU KNOW

If there is an obturator externus muscle, there must be an obturator internus muscle.

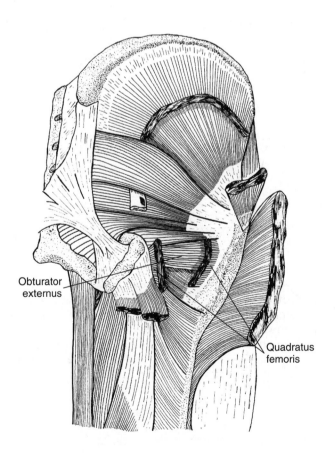

Obturator externus

Quadratus femoris

QUADRATUS FEMORIS
(OF THE DEEP LATERAL ROTATORS OF THE THIGH)

kwod-**rate**-us **fem**-o-ris

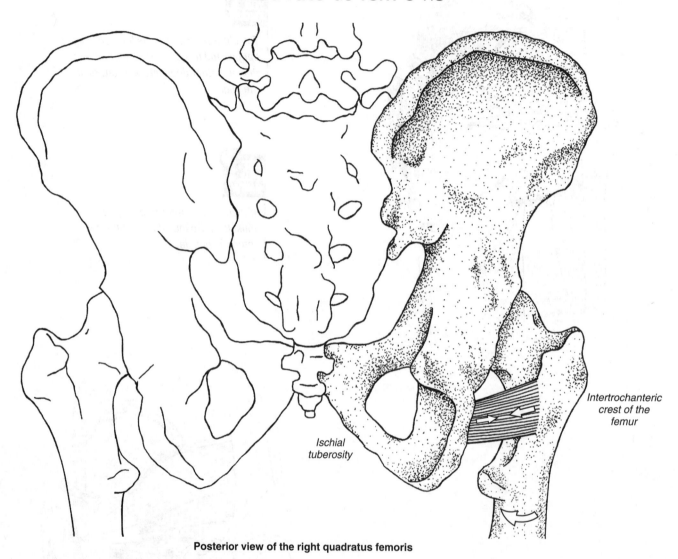

Ischial
tuberosity

Intertrochanteric
crest of the
femur

Posterior view of the right quadratus femoris

Actions	Contralateral rotation of the	**Arterial Supply**
Lateral rotation of the thigh at the hip joint	pelvis at the hip joint	The inferior gluteal artery
Adduction of the thigh at the hip joint	**Innervation**	**Myofascial Meridians**
	The lumbosacral plexus	Deep front line

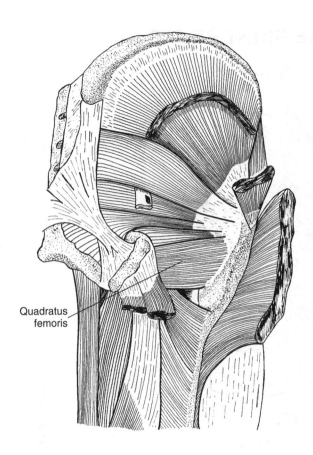

Quadratus
femoris

DID
YOU
KNOW

The quadratus femoris attaches
sufficiently distal on the femur to be
able to do adduction of the thigh at the
hip joint.

DID
YOU
KNOW

The quadratus femoris is often the
largest of the six muscles of the deep
lateral rotator group.

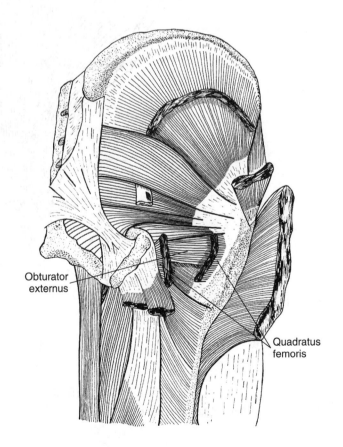

Obturator
externus

Quadratus
femoris

ANTERIOR VIEW OF THE RIGHT PELVIS

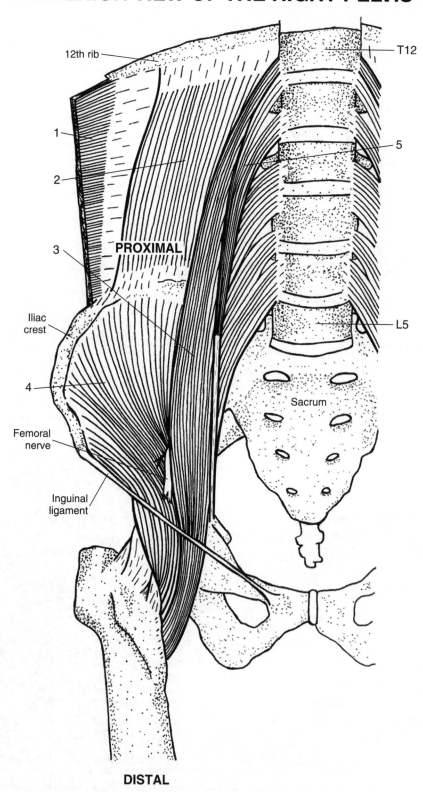

12th rib

T12

1

2

5

PROXIMAL

3

Iliac
crest

L5

4

Sacrum

Femoral
nerve

Inguinal
ligament

LATERAL

MEDIAL

DISTAL

Answers to labeling exercises are on p. 486.

LATERAL VIEW OF THE RIGHT PELVIS

PROXIMAL

P
O
S
T
E
R
I
O
R

A
N
T
E
R
I
O
R

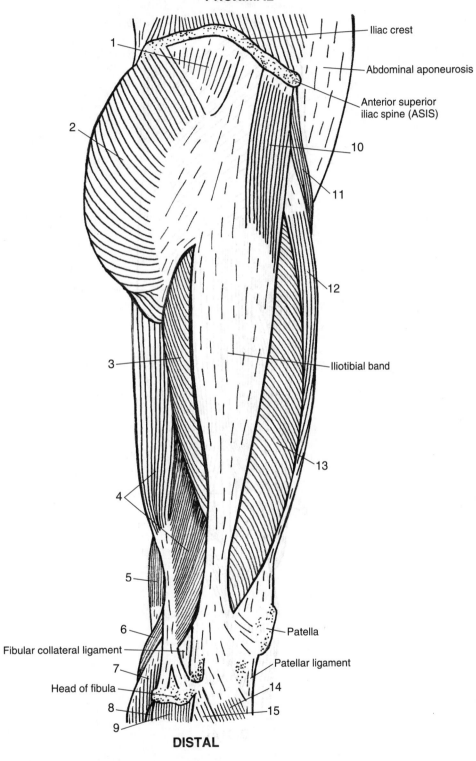

Iliac crest

Abdominal aponeurosis

Anterior superior
iliac spine (ASIS)

Iliotibial band

Patella

Fibular collateral ligament

Patellar ligament

Head of fibula

DISTAL

POSTERIOR VIEW OF THE RIGHT PELVIS (SUPERFICIAL)

PROXIMAL

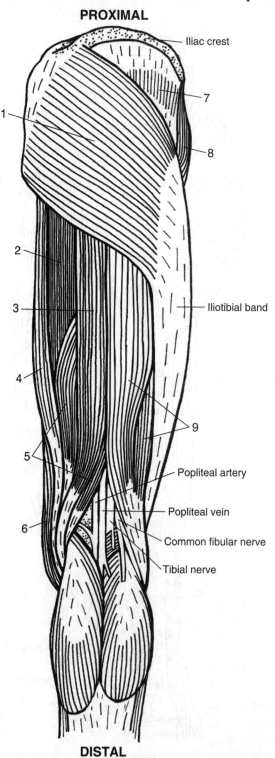

Iliac crest

7

1

8

MEDIAL

LATERAL

2

3

Iliotibial band

4

9

5

Popliteal artery

Popliteal vein

6

Common fibular nerve

Tibial nerve

DISTAL

POSTERIOR VIEW OF THE RIGHT PELVIS (DEEP)

PROXIMAL

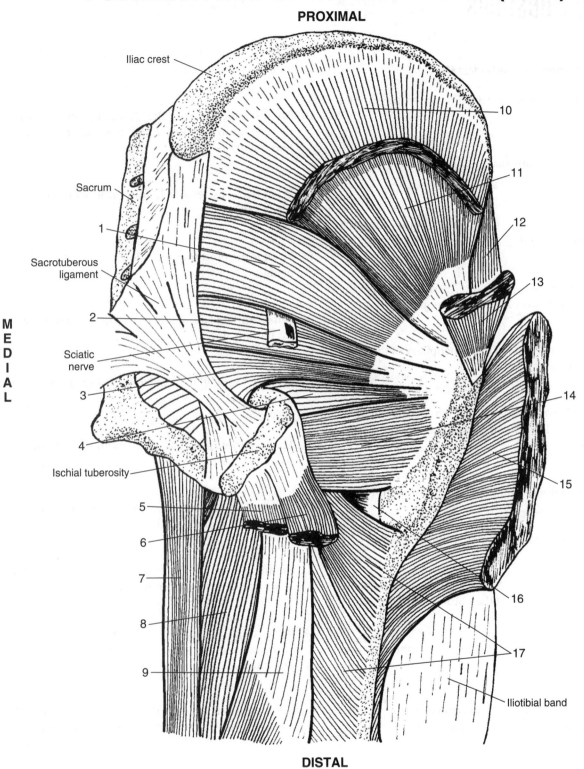

Iliac crest

Sacrum

Sacrotuberous
ligament

Sciatic
nerve

Ischial tuberosity

MEDIAL

LATERAL

Iliotibial band

DISTAL

Review Questions

Muscles of the Pelvis
Answers to these questions are found on page 486.

1. What muscle is immediately superior to the inferior gemellus?

2. What muscle is immediately superior to the superior gemellus?

3. If the quadratus femoris is being lengthened, what joint action of the thigh is occurring?

4. What are the most superior and inferior muscles of the deep lateral rotators of the thigh group?

5. What two muscles attach to the periphery of the obturator foramen?

6. What effect would passive flexion of the thigh at the hip joint have upon the length of the gluteus maximus?

7. What three muscles comprise the gluteal group?

8. What is the largest muscle in the human body?

9. The distal tendons of what two muscles usually blend with the distal tendon of the obturator internus?

10. Name an antagonist to the obturator externus' action upon the thigh.

11. Are the superior gemellus and obturator internus synergistic with or antagonistic to each other?

12. What muscle is immediately deep to the psoas minor?

13. Passive extension of the trunk at the spinal joints results in what change in length to the psoas minor?

14. What rotation of the pelvis at the hip joint does the right piriformis create?

15. Besides the gluteus maximus, what other muscle attaches into the iliotibial band?

16. Are the upper fibers of the gluteus maximus synergistic with or antagonistic to the lower fibers of the gluteus maximus?

17. What two muscles attach onto the lesser trochanter of the femur?

18. What is the most important joint action of the gluteus medius?

19. What frontal plane action of the thigh can the quadratus femoris do?

20. Relative to the gluteus maximus, where is the piriformis located?

21. The superior gemellus and obturator internus are members of what group?

22. Where does the sciatic nerve usually exit the pelvis relative to the piriformis?

23. Are the gluteus medius and minimus synergistic with or antagonistic to each other?

24. If the thigh is passively laterally rotated at the hip joint, what happens to the length of the obturator externus?

25. What joint action of the thigh is occurring if there is a concentric contraction of the superior gemellus?

26. What muscle is superficial to the inferior gemellus?

27. What muscle is directly inferior to the piriformis?

28. How are the psoas major and psoas minor synergistic with each other?

29. How is the gluteus medius antagonistic to itself?

30. How can the two quadratus femoris muscles be antagonistic to each other?

31. What muscle is superficial to the piriformis?

32. If the right psoas major is eccentrically contracting, what sagittal plane joint motion of the thigh is occurring?

33. If the thigh is first flexed, what joint actions of the thigh could be done to stretch the piriformis?

34. Are the psoas major and iliacus synergistic with or antagonistic to the sartorius? Why?

35. What two muscles are superficial to the gluteus medius?

36. Would passive medial rotation of the thigh at the hip joint shorten or lengthen the psoas major and iliacus?

37. What joint action of the thigh occurs when the superior gemellus eccentrically contracts?

38. What other muscles share the quadratus femoris' proximal attachment?

39. If the thigh is medially rotated at the hip joint, what happens to the length of the inferior gemellus?

40. What effect would active flexion of the thigh at the hip joint have upon the length of the gluteus maximus?

41. What joint action is occurring if the left psoas minor is concentrically contracting?

42. What muscle is immediately superficial to the obturator externus?

43. What two muscles of the lower extremity attach to the anterolateral lumbar spine?

44. If the thigh is actively extended and laterally rotated, what happens to the length of the piriformis?

45. What muscle is immediately superior to the obturator externus?

46. What six muscles comprise the deep lateral rotators of the thigh group?

47. What muscle is immediately inferior to the obturator internus?

48. What muscle of the abdomen and pelvis is absent in approximately 40% of individuals?

49. What pelvic action is created by the right inferior gemellus?

50. Old-fashioned straight-leg sit-ups are no longer recommended because they overly strengthen what muscle?

51. What muscle's tendon is located directly lateral to the distal tendon of the iliacus?

52. Which muscle is deeper, the gluteus medius or the gluteus minimus?

53. If the thigh is moving and the obturator externus is eccentrically contracting, what joint action is occurring?

54. What muscle is immediately deep to the quadratus femoris?

Muscles of the Thigh 7

Note: Throughout this chapter, muscle attachments are indicated by italics.

⊝ More review activities on Evolve at: http://evolve.elsevier.com/Muscolino/anatomycoloring/

213

ANTERIOR VIEW OF THE RIGHT THIGH (SUPERFICIAL)

PROXIMAL

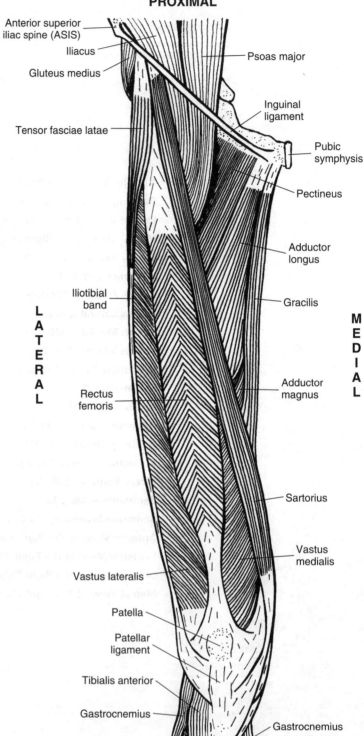

Anterior superior iliac spine (ASIS)

Iliacus

Gluteus medius

Tensor fasciae latae

Psoas major

Inguinal ligament

Pubic symphysis

Pectineus

Adductor longus

Gracilis

Iliotibial band

Adductor magnus

Rectus femoris

Sartorius

Vastus medialis

Vastus lateralis

Patella

Patellar ligament

Tibialis anterior

Gastrocnemius

Fibularis longus

Gastrocnemius

Tibial tuberosity

L A T E R A L

M E D I A L

DISTAL

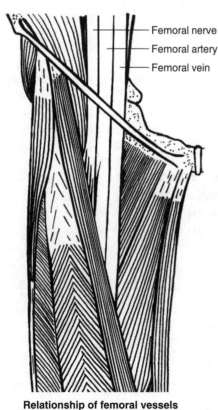

Femoral nerve

Femoral artery

Femoral vein

Relationship of femoral vessels to anterior thigh

ANTERIOR VIEW OF THE RIGHT THIGH (DEEP)

PROXIMAL

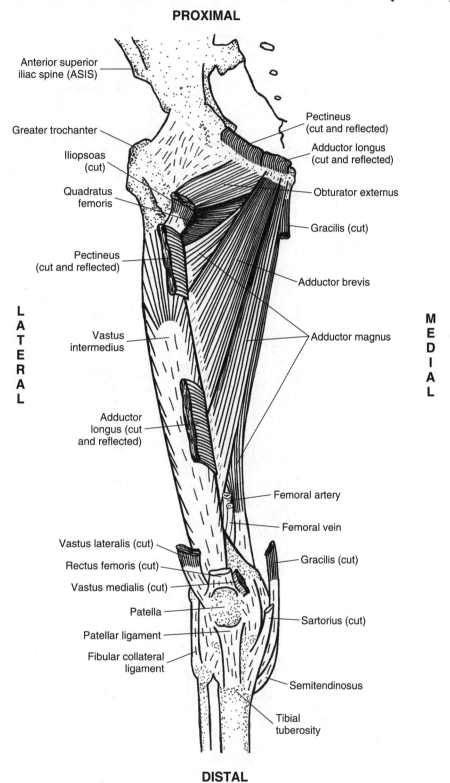

Anterior superior
iliac spine (ASIS)

Greater trochanter

Iliopsoas
(cut)

Quadratus
femoris

Pectineus
(cut and reflected)

Vastus
intermedius

Adductor
longus (cut
and reflected)

Vastus lateralis (cut)

Rectus femoris (cut)

Vastus medialis (cut)

Patella

Patellar ligament

Fibular collateral
ligament

Pectineus
(cut and reflected)

Adductor longus
(cut and reflected)

Obturator externus

Gracilis (cut)

Adductor brevis

Adductor magnus

Femoral artery

Femoral vein

Gracilis (cut)

Sartorius (cut)

Semitendinosus

Tibial
tuberosity

LATERAL

MEDIAL

DISTAL

POSTERIOR VIEW OF THE RIGHT THIGH (SUPERFICIAL)

PROXIMAL

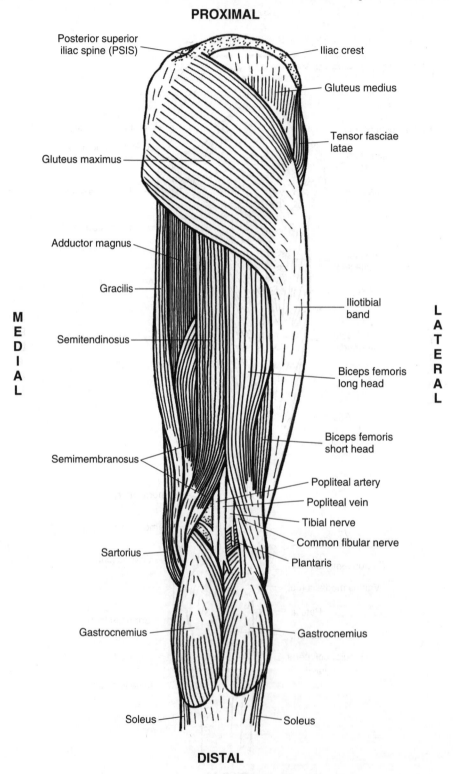

Posterior superior iliac spine (PSIS)

Iliac crest

Gluteus medius

Tensor fasciae latae

Gluteus maximus

Adductor magnus

Gracilis

Iliotibial band

Semitendinosus

Biceps femoris long head

MEDIAL

LATERAL

Biceps femoris short head

Semimembranosus

Popliteal artery

Popliteal vein

Tibial nerve

Common fibular nerve

Sartorius

Plantaris

Gastrocnemius

Gastrocnemius

Soleus

Soleus

DISTAL

POSTERIOR VIEW OF THE RIGHT THIGH (DEEP)

PROXIMAL

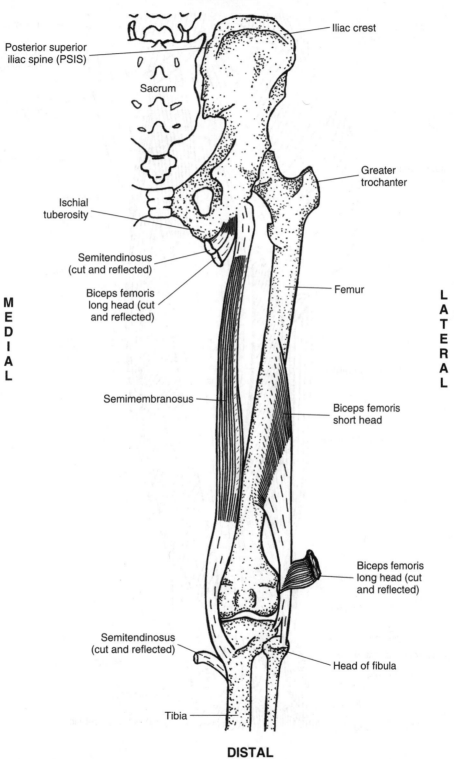

Posterior superior
iliac spine (PSIS)

Iliac crest

Sacrum

Greater
trochanter

Ischial
tuberosity

Semitendinosus
(cut and reflected)

Biceps femoris
long head (cut
and reflected)

Femur

**M
E
D
I
A
L**

**L
A
T
E
R
A
L**

Semimembranosus

Biceps femoris
short head

Biceps femoris
long head (cut
and reflected)

Semitendinosus
(cut and reflected)

Head of fibula

Tibia

DISTAL

LATERAL VIEW OF THE RIGHT THIGH

PROXIMAL

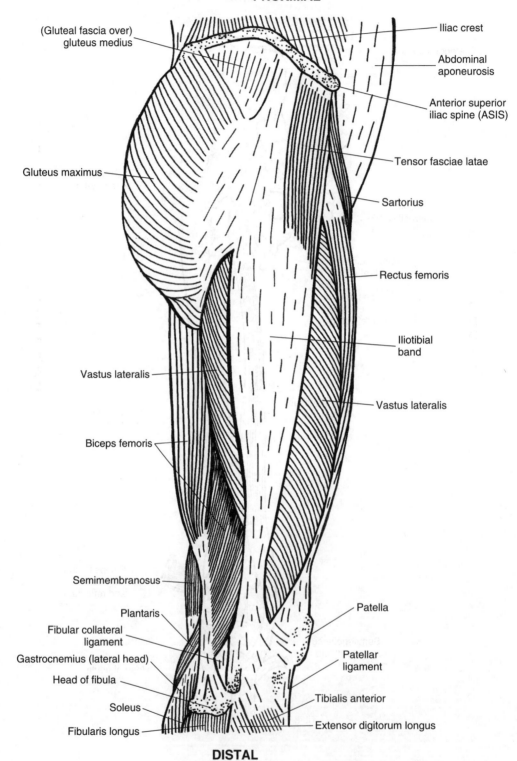

(Gluteal fascia over) gluteus medius

Iliac crest

Abdominal aponeurosis

Anterior superior iliac spine (ASIS)

Gluteus maximus

Tensor fasciae latae

Sartorius

Rectus femoris

POSTERIOR

ANTERIOR

Iliotibial band

Vastus lateralis

Vastus lateralis

Biceps femoris

Semimembranosus

Patella

Plantaris

Fibular collateral ligament

Patellar ligament

Gastrocnemius (lateral head)

Head of fibula

Tibialis anterior

Soleus

Extensor digitorum longus

Fibularis longus

DISTAL

MEDIAL VIEW OF THE RIGHT THIGH

PROXIMAL

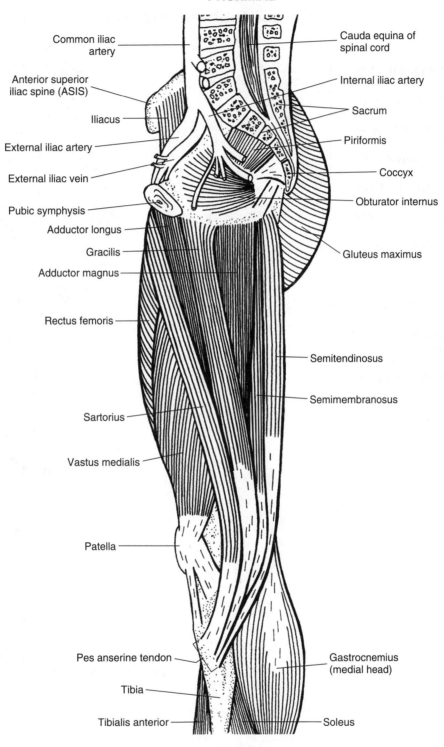

Common iliac artery

Anterior superior iliac spine (ASIS)

Iliacus

External iliac artery

External iliac vein

Pubic symphysis

Adductor longus

Gracilis

Adductor magnus

Rectus femoris

Sartorius

Vastus medialis

Patella

Pes anserine tendon

Tibia

Tibialis anterior

Cauda equina of spinal cord

Internal iliac artery

Sacrum

Piriformis

Coccyx

Obturator internus

Gluteus maximus

Semitendinosus

Semimembranosus

Gastrocnemius (medial head)

Soleus

ANTERIOR

POSTERIOR

DISTAL

TENSOR FASCIAE LATAE ("TFL")

ten-sor **fash**-ee-a **la**-tee

Actions
Flexion of the thigh at the hip joint

Abduction of the thigh at the hip joint

Medial rotation of the thigh at the hip joint

Anterior tilt of the pelvis at the hip joint

Depression (lateral tilt) of the pelvis at the hip joint

Ipsilateral rotation of the pelvis at the hip joint

Extension of the leg at the knee joint

Innervation
The superior gluteal nerve

Arterial Supply
The superior gluteal artery

Myofascial Meridians
Lateral line
Spiral line

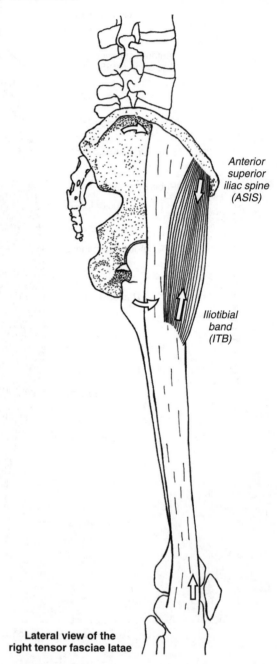

Anterior superior iliac spine (ASIS)

Iliotibial band (ITB)

Lateral view of the right tensor fasciae latae

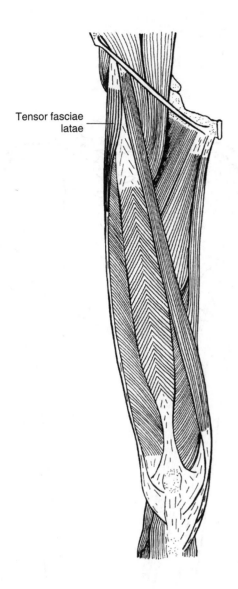

Tensor fasciae latae

The tensor fasciae latae is one of two muscles that attach into the iliotibial band.

The TFL is a transitional muscle between and anterior flexor compartment and lateral abductor compartment of the thigh.

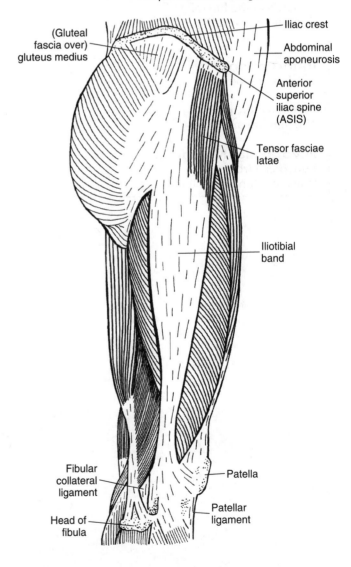

(Gluteal fascia over) gluteus medius

Iliac crest

Abdominal aponeurosis

Anterior superior iliac spine (ASIS)

Tensor fasciae latae

Iliotibial band

Fibular collateral ligament

Patella

Head of fibula

Patellar ligament

SARTORIUS

sar-**tor**-ee-us

Actions
Flexion of the thigh at the hip
   joint
Abduction of the thigh at the hip
   joint
Lateral rotation of the thigh at the
   hip joint
Flexion of the leg at the knee joint
Anterior tilt of the pelvis at the
   hip joint
Medial rotation of the leg at the
   knee joint
Depression (lateral tilt) of the
   pelvis at the hip joint
Contralateral rotation of the
   pelvis at the hip joint

Innervation
The femoral nerve

Arterial Supply
The femoral artery

Myofascial Meridians
Superficial front line
Ipsilateral functional line

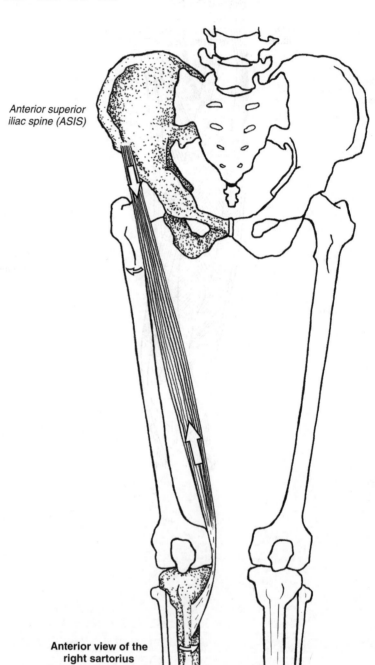

Anterior superior
iliac spine (ASIS)

**Anterior view of the
right sartorius**

Pes anserine tendon

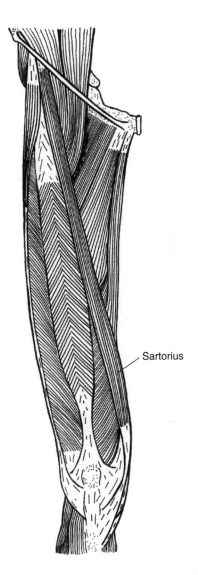

Sartorius

The sartorius is the longest muscle in the human body. It is also one of three muscles that attach into the pes anserine tendon.

The sartorius crosses the hip joint anteriorly but crosses the knee joint posteriorly.

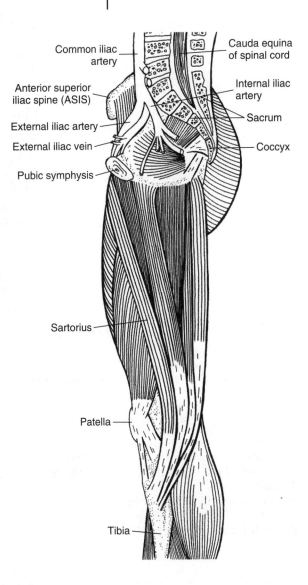

Common iliac artery

Cauda equina of spinal cord

Anterior superior iliac spine (ASIS)

Internal iliac artery

External iliac artery

Sacrum

External iliac vein

Coccyx

Pubic symphysis

Sartorius

Patella

Tibia

RECTUS FEMORIS
(OF THE QUADRICEPS FEMORIS GROUP)

rek-tus fem-o-ris

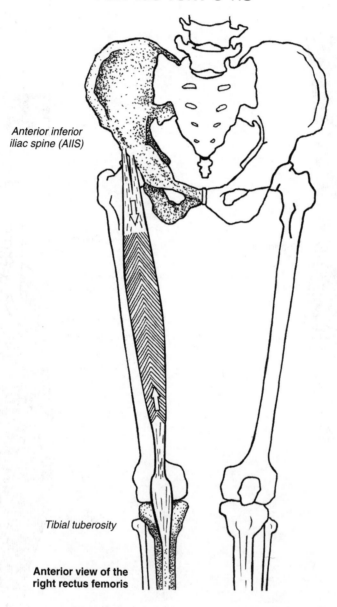

Anterior inferior
iliac spine (AIIS)

Tibial tuberosity

**Anterior view of the
right rectus femoris**

Actions	**Innervation**	**Arterial Supply**
Extension of the leg at the knee joint	The femoral nerve	The femoral artery and the deep femoral artery
Flexion of the thigh at the hip joint		
Anterior tilt of the pelvis at the hip joint		**Myofascial Meridians**
		Superficial front line

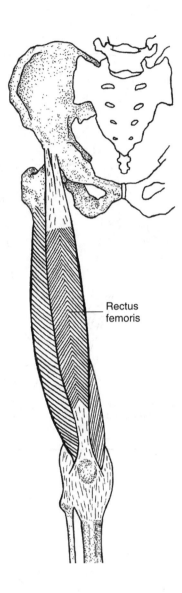

Rectus
femoris

The rectus femoris is the only quadriceps femoris muscle that can create movement of the thigh or pelvis at the hip joint because it is the only one that crosses the hip joint.

The rectus femoris runs straight up and down the femur; "rectus" means straight and "femoris" refers to the femur.

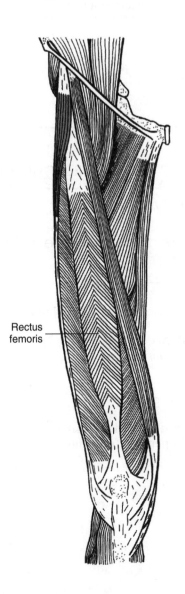

Rectus
femoris

VASTUS LATERALIS
(OF THE QUADRICEPS FEMORIS GROUP)

vas-tus lat-er-**a**-lis

Action
Extension of the leg at the knee joint

Innervation
The femoral nerve

Arterial Supply
The femoral artery and the deep femoral artery

Myofascial Meridians
Back functional line
Involved: Superficial front line

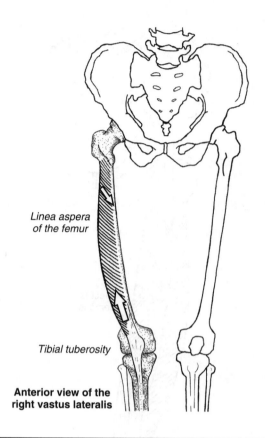

*Linea aspera
of the femur*

Tibial tuberosity

**Anterior view of the
right vastus lateralis**

VASTUS MEDIALIS
(OF THE QUADRICEPS FEMORIS GROUP)

vas-tus mee-dee-**a**-lis

Action
Extension of the leg at the knee joint

Innervation
The femoral nerve

Arterial Supply
The femoral artery

Myofascial Meridians
Involved: Superficial front line

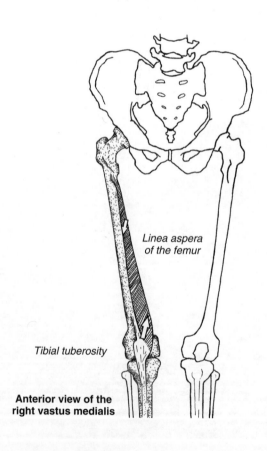

*Linea aspera
of the femur*

Tibial tuberosity

**Anterior view of the
right vastus medialis**

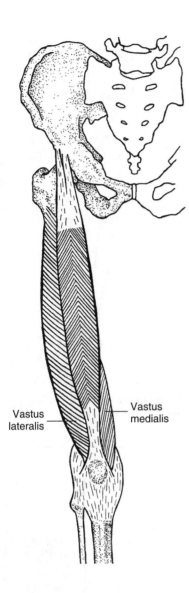

Vastus
lateralis

Vastus
medialis

DID YOU KNOW

The vastus lateralis is the largest of the four quadriceps femoris muscles. Pain attributed to the iliotibial band is often due to this large muscle that lies deep to it.

DID YOU KNOW

The vastus lateralis tracks the patella laterally along the femur.

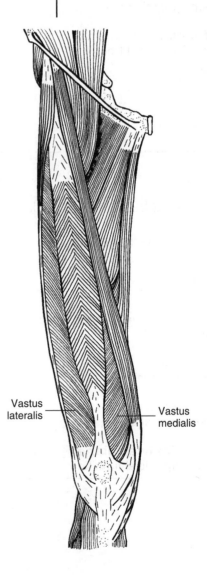

Vastus
lateralis

Vastus
medialis

DID YOU KNOW

The most distal aspect of the vastus medialis is bulky and may form a bulge in well-toned individuals.

DID YOU KNOW

The vastus medialis tracts the patella medially along the femur.

VASTUS INTERMEDIUS
(OF THE QUADRICEPS FEMORIS GROUP)

vas-tus in-ter-**mee**-dee-us

Action
Extension of the leg at the knee joint

Innervation
The femoral nerve

Arterial Supply
The deep femoral artery

Myofascial Meridians
Involved: Superficial front line

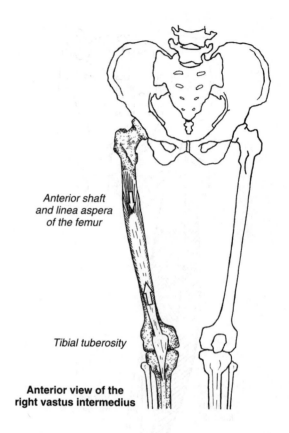

Anterior shaft and linea aspera of the femur

Tibial tuberosity

Anterior view of the right vastus intermedius

ARTICULARIS GENUS

ar-**tik**-you-**la**-ris **je**-new

Action
Tenses and pulls the joint capsule of the knee joint proximally

Innervation
The femoral nerve

Arterial Supply
The deep femoral artery

Myofascial Meridians
Involved: Superficial front line

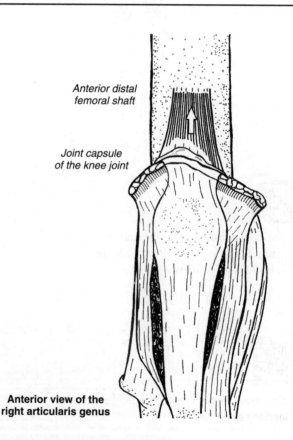

Anterior distal femoral shaft

Joint capsule of the knee joint

Anterior view of the right articularis genus

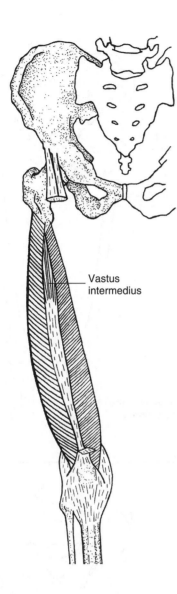

Vastus
intermedius

From most perspectives, the vastus intermedius is the deepest of the four quadriceps femoris muscles.

The vastus intermedius blends into the adjacent vastus medialis.

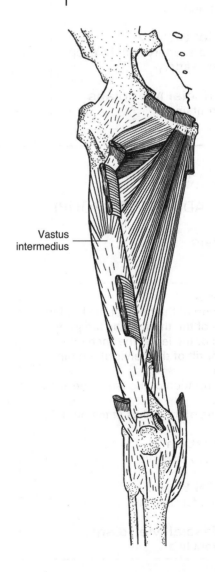

Vastus
intermedius

The articularis genus has no skeletal function to move bones. It acts to move the joint capsule of the knee so that it doesn't get pinched between the femur and tibia when the knee joint moves.

The word "genu" means knee.

PECTINEUS
(OF THE ADDUCTOR GROUP)

pek-**tin**-ee-us

Actions
Adduction of the thigh at the hip
   joint
Flexion of the thigh at the hip
   joint
Anterior tilt of the pelvis at the
   hip joint
Elevation of the pelvis at the hip
   joint

Innervation
The femoral nerve

Arterial Supply
The femoral artery and the deep
   femoral artery

Myofascial Meridians
Deep front line

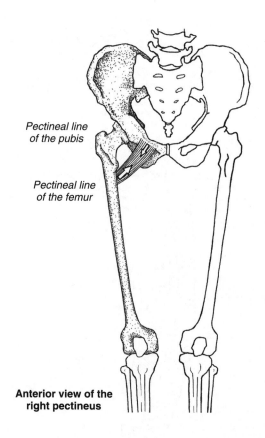

*Pectineal line
of the pubis*

*Pectineal line
of the femur*

**Anterior view of the
right pectineus**

GRACILIS
(OF THE ADDUCTOR GROUP)

gra-**sil**-is

Actions
Adduction of the thigh at the hip joint
Flexion of the thigh at the hip joint
Flexion of the leg at the knee joint
Anterior tilt of the pelvis at the hip
   joint
Medial rotation of the leg at the knee
   joint
Elevation of the pelvis at the hip joint

Innervation
The obturator nerve

Arterial Supply
The deep femoral artery

Myofascial Meridians
Deep front line

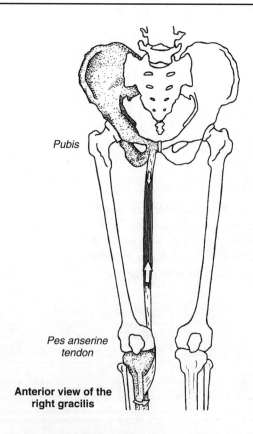

Pubis

*Pes anserine
tendon*

**Anterior view of the
right gracilis**

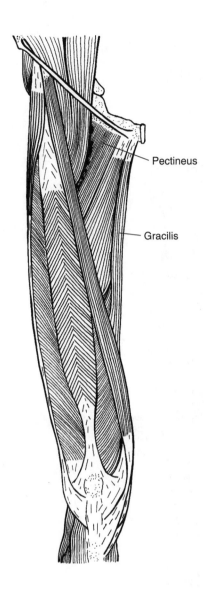

Pectineus

Gracilis

The pectineus attaches from the pectineal line of the pubis to the pectineal line of the femur.

The pectineus is a transitional muscle between the anterior flexor compartment and the medial adductor compartment of the thigh.

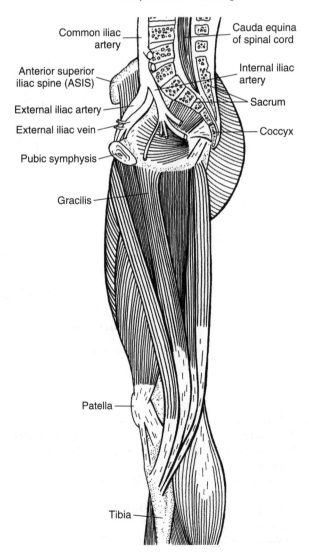

Common iliac artery

Anterior superior iliac spine (ASIS)

External iliac artery

External iliac vein

Pubic symphysis

Gracilis

Cauda equina of spinal cord

Internal iliac artery

Sacrum

Coccyx

Patella

Tibia

The gracilis muscle is the second longest muscle in the human body. It is also one of three muscles that attach into the pes anserine tendon.

The gracilis is often described as the adductor gracilis.

ADDUCTOR LONGUS
(OF THE ADDUCTOR GROUP)

ad-**duk**-tor **long**-us

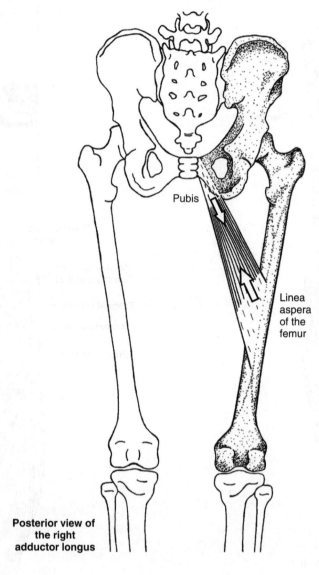

Pubis

Linea
aspera
of the
femur

**Posterior view of
the right
adductor longus**

Actions
Adduction of the thigh at the hip
   joint
Flexion of the thigh at the hip
   joint
Anterior tilt of the pelvis at the hip
   joint
Elevation of the pelvis at the hip
   joint

Innervation
The obturator nerve

Arterial Supply
The femoral artery and the deep
   femoral artery

Myofascial Meridians
Deep front line
Front functional line

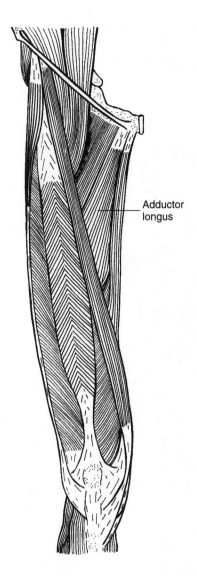

Adductor
longus

DID
YOU
KNOW

*The adductor longus is easy to locate
because it has the most prominent
tendon in the groin region. Its
proximal tendon can also be useful
as a landmark for palpating other
muscles of the region (the more
lateral pectineus and the more medial
gracilis).*

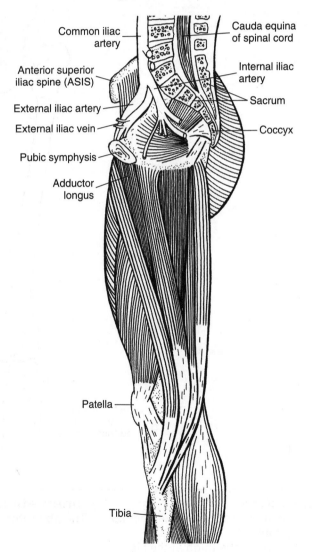

Common iliac
artery

Anterior superior
iliac spine (ASIS)

External iliac artery

External iliac vein

Pubic symphysis

Adductor
longus

Cauda equina
of spinal cord

Internal iliac
artery

Sacrum

Coccyx

Patella

Tibia

ADDUCTOR BREVIS
(OF THE ADDUCTOR GROUP)

ad-**duk**-tor **bre**-vis

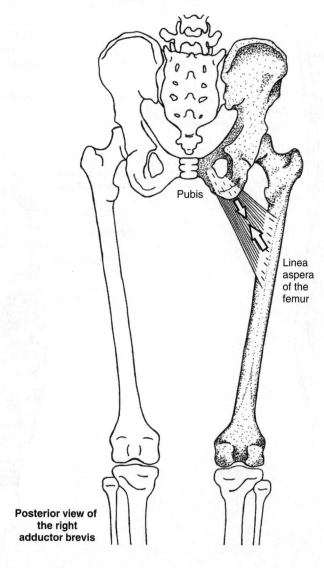

Pubis

Linea
aspera
of the
femur

**Posterior view of
the right
adductor brevis**

Actions
Adduction of the thigh at the hip
joint
Flexion of the thigh at the hip
joint
Anterior tilt of the pelvis at the hip
joint
Elevation of the pelvis at the hip
joint

Innervation
The obturator nerve

Arterial Supply
The femoral artery and the deep
femoral artery

Myofascial Meridians
Deep front line
Front functional line

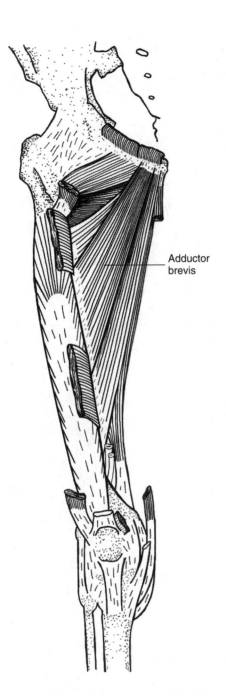

Adductor
brevis

*The adductor brevis is located
between the adductor longus and
adductor magnus.*

*All three "adductor" muscles attach
onto the linea aspera of the femur.*

ADDUCTOR MAGNUS

(OF THE ADDUCTOR GROUP)

ad-**duk**-tor **mag**-nus

Actions
Adduction of the thigh at the
  hip joint
Extension of the thigh at the
  hip joint
Posterior tilt of the pelvis at
  the hip joint
Elevation of the pelvis at the
  hip joint

Innervation
The obturator nerve and the
  sciatic nerve

Arterial Supply
Anterior head: the femoral
  artery and the deep
  femoral artery
Posterior head: the deep
  femoral artery and the
  inferior gluteal artery

**Myofascial
Meridians**
Involved with spiral line

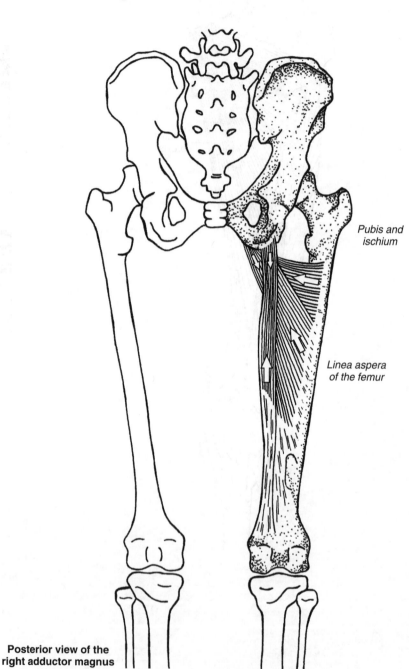

Pubis and
ischium

Linea aspera
of the femur

**Posterior view of the
right adductor magnus**

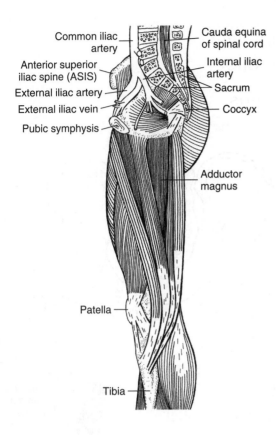

Common iliac artery

Anterior superior iliac spine (ASIS)

External iliac artery

External iliac vein

Pubic symphysis

Cauda equina of spinal cord

Internal iliac artery

Sacrum

Coccyx

Adductor magnus

Patella

Tibia

Because the adductor magnus is so far posterior, attaches to the ischial tuberosity, and can extend the thigh at the hip joint, it is sometimes called the 4th hamstring.

The adductor magnus has an anterior head and a posterior head. There is a gap between the two heads called the adductor hiatus.

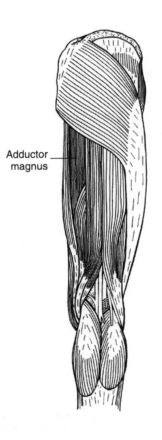

Adductor magnus

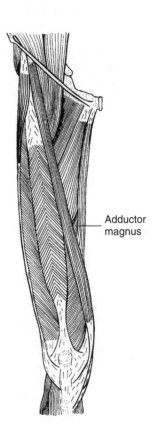

Adductor magnus

BICEPS FEMORIS
(OF THE HAMSTRING GROUP)
by-seps fem-o-ris

Actions
Flexion of the leg at the knee
    joint (entire muscle)
Extension of the thigh at the hip
    joint (long head)
Posterior tilt of the pelvis at the
    hip joint (long head)
Lateral rotation of the leg at the
    knee joint (entire muscle)
Adduction of the thigh at the hip
    joint (long head)
Lateral rotation of the thigh at
    the hip joint (long head)

Innervation
The sciatic nerve

Arterial Supply
Long head: the inferior gluteal
    artery and perforating
    branches of the deep femoral
    artery
Short head: perforating branches
    of the deep femoral artery

Myofascial Meridians
Superficial back line
Spiral line

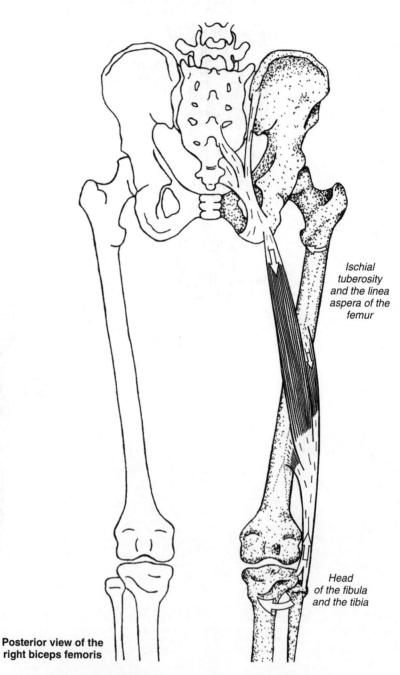

Ischial
tuberosity
and the linea
aspera of the
femur

Head
of the fibula
and the tibia

**Posterior view of the
right biceps femoris**

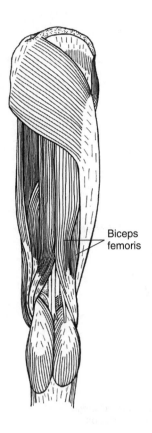

Biceps
femoris

DID
YOU **?**
KNOW

*The biceps femoris is a lateral
hamstring muscle. As its name implies,
it has two heads. Its short head is the
only part of the hamstring group that
does not cross the hip joint.*

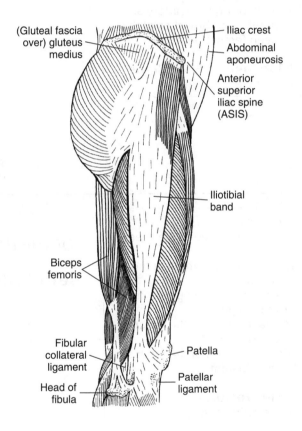

(Gluteal fascia
over) gluteus
medius

Iliac crest

Abdominal
aponeurosis

Anterior
superior
iliac spine
(ASIS)

Iliotibial
band

Biceps
femoris

Fibular
collateral
ligament

Patella

Head of
fibula

Patellar
ligament

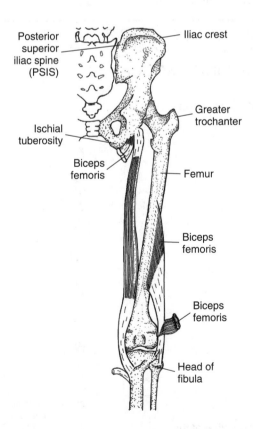

Posterior
superior
iliac spine
(PSIS)

Iliac crest

Greater
trochanter

Ischial
tuberosity

Biceps
femoris

Femur

Biceps
femoris

Biceps
femoris

Head of
fibula

Actions
Flexion of the leg at the knee
joint
Extension of the thigh at the
hip joint
Posterior tilt of the pelvis at
the hip joint
Medial rotation of the leg at
the knee joint
Medial rotation of the thigh at
the hip joint

Innervation
The sciatic nerve

Arterial Supply
The inferior gluteal artery and
perforating branches of the
deep femoral artery

Myofascial Meridians
Superficial back line

SEMITENDINOSUS
(OF THE HAMSTRING GROUP)

sem-i-**ten**-di-**no**-sus

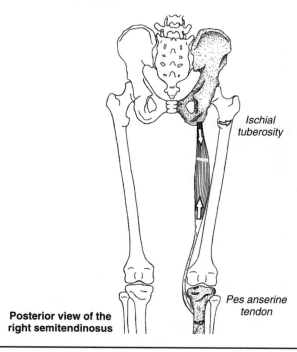

Ischial
tuberosity

Pes anserine
tendon

**Posterior view of the
right semitendinosus**

Actions
Flexion of the leg at the knee
joint
Extension of the thigh at the
hip joint
Posterior tilt of the pelvis at
the hip joint
Medial rotation of the leg at
the knee joint
Medial rotation of the thigh at
the hip joint

Innervation
The sciatic nerve

Arterial Supply
The inferior gluteal artery and
perforating branches of the
deep femoral artery

Myofascial Meridians
Superficial back line

SEMIMEMBRANOSUS
(OF THE HAMSTRING GROUP)

sem-i-**mem**-bra-**no**-sus

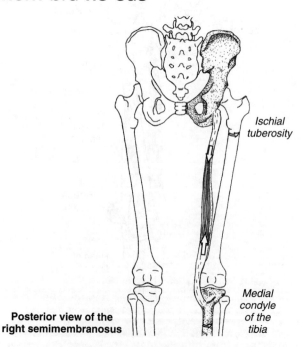

Ischial
tuberosity

Medial
condyle
of the
tibia

**Posterior view of the
right semimembranosus**

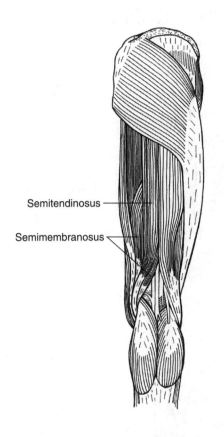

Semitendinosus

Semimembranosus

The semitendinosus and semimembranosus are the medial hamstrings. The semitendinosus is named for its long distal tendon. It is also one of three muscles that attach into the pes anserine tendon.

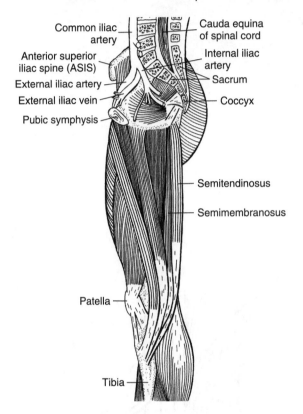

Common iliac artery
Anterior superior iliac spine (ASIS)
External iliac artery
External iliac vein
Pubic symphysis

Cauda equina of spinal cord
Internal iliac artery
Sacrum
Coccyx

Semitendinosus

Semimembranosus

Patella

Tibia

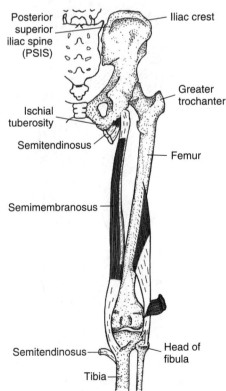

Posterior superior iliac spine (PSIS)
Ischial tuberosity
Semitendinosus
Semimembranosus
Semitendinosus
Tibia

Iliac crest
Greater trochanter
Femur
Head of fibula

The semimembranosus is named for its long membranous proximal tendon.

The semimembranosus lies deep to the semitendinosus.

ANTERIOR VIEW OF THE RIGHT THIGH (SUPERFICIAL)

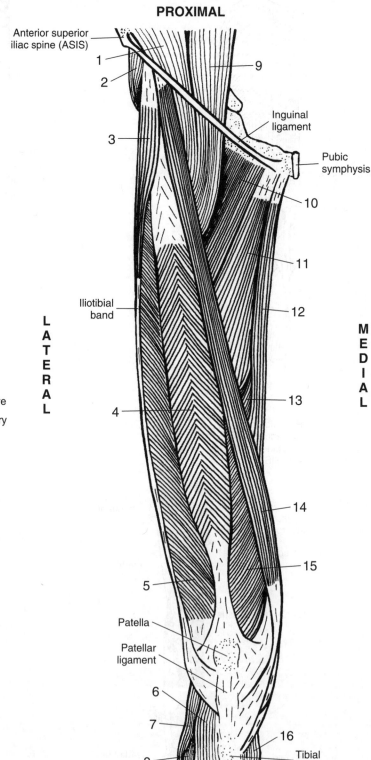

PROXIMAL

Anterior superior
iliac spine (ASIS)

1

2

3

4

5

6

7

8

9

Inguinal
ligament

Pubic
symphysis

10

11

12

13

14

15

Iliotibial
band

Patella

Patellar
ligament

16

Tibial
tuberosity

LATERAL

MEDIAL

DISTAL

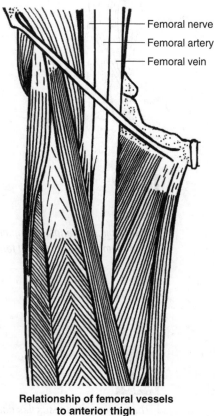

Femoral nerve

Femoral artery

Femoral vein

**Relationship of femoral vessels
to anterior thigh**

Answers to labeling exercises are on p. 486.

ANTERIOR VIEW OF THE RIGHT THIGH (DEEP)

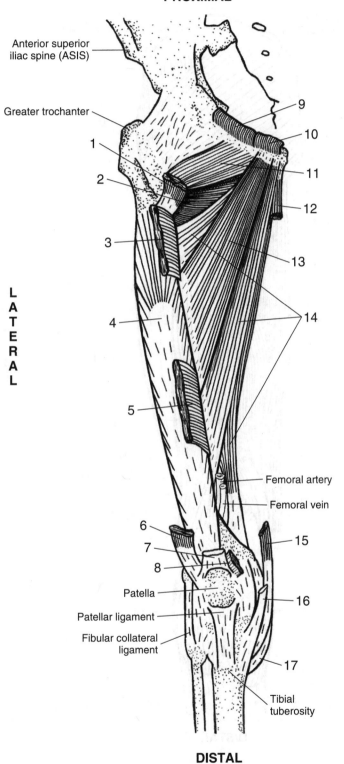

PROXIMAL

Anterior superior
iliac spine (ASIS)

Greater trochanter

9

10

1

11

2

12

3

13

L
A
T
E
R
A
L

4

14

M
E
D
I
A
L

5

Femoral artery

Femoral vein

6

15

7

8

16

Patella

Patellar ligament

Fibular collateral
ligament

17

Tibial
tuberosity

DISTAL

POSTERIOR VIEW OF THE RIGHT THIGH (SUPERFICIAL)

PROXIMAL

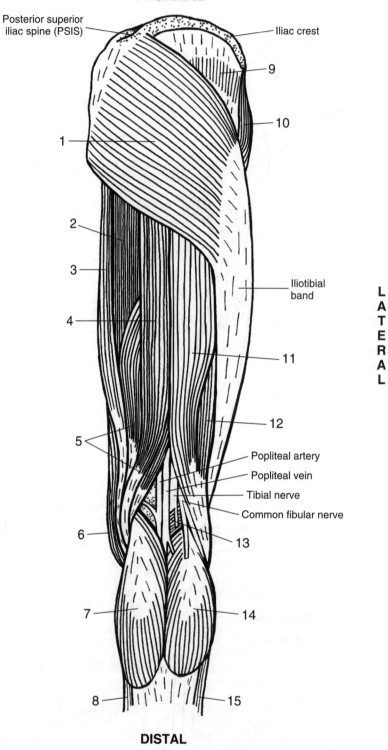

Posterior superior
iliac spine (PSIS)

Iliac crest

9

10

1

2

3

4

Iliotibial
band

11

M
E
D
I
A
L

L
A
T
E
R
A
L

12

5

Popliteal artery

Popliteal vein

Tibial nerve

Common fibular nerve

6

13

7

14

8

15

DISTAL

POSTERIOR VIEW OF THE RIGHT THIGH (DEEP)

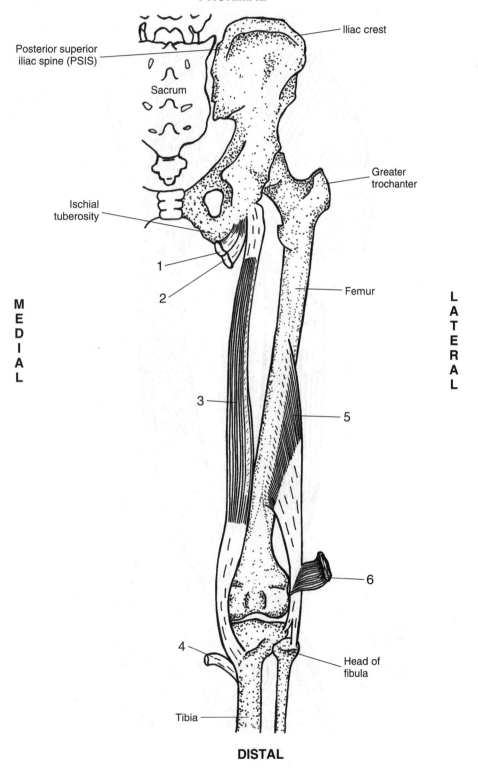

PROXIMAL

Posterior superior
iliac spine (PSIS)

Iliac crest

Sacrum

Ischial
tuberosity

Greater
trochanter

Femur

**M
E
D
I
A
L**

**L
A
T
E
R
A
L**

1

2

3

5

6

4

Head of
fibula

Tibia

DISTAL

LATERAL VIEW OF THE RIGHT THIGH

PROXIMAL

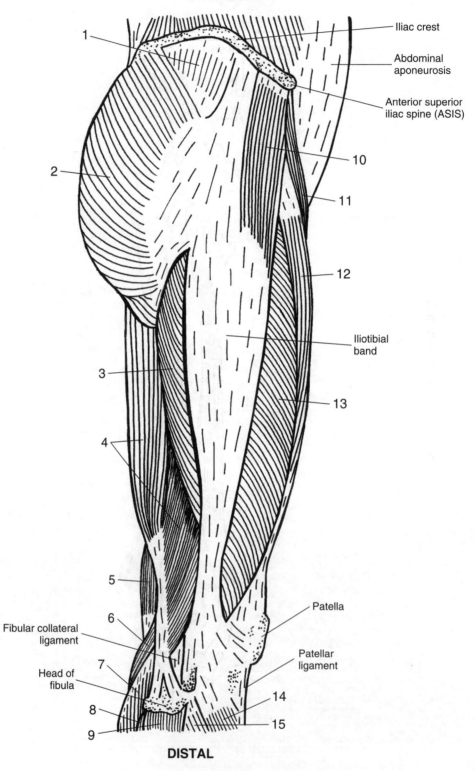

Iliac crest

Abdominal
aponeurosis

Anterior superior
iliac spine (ASIS)

10

11

12

Iliotibial
band

13

1

2

**P
O
S
T
E
R
I
O
R**

**A
N
T
E
R
I
O
R**

3

4

5

6

Fibular collateral
ligament

7

Head of
fibula

8

9

Patella

Patellar
ligament

14

15

DISTAL

MEDIAL VIEW OF THE RIGHT THIGH

PROXIMAL

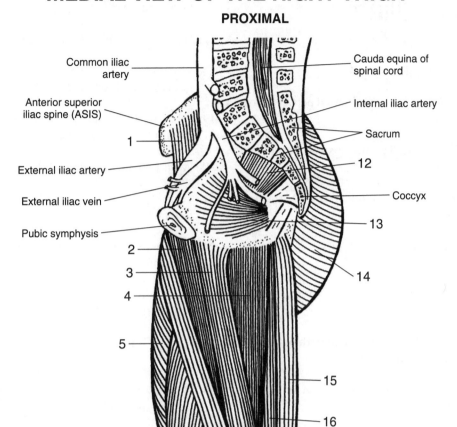

Common iliac artery

Anterior superior iliac spine (ASIS)

1

External iliac artery

External iliac vein

Pubic symphysis

2

3

4

5

6

7

Patella

8, 9, 10

Tibia

11

Cauda equina of spinal cord

Internal iliac artery

Sacrum

12

Coccyx

13

14

15

16

17

18

ANTERIOR

POSTERIOR

DISTAL

Review Questions

Muscles of the Thigh
Answers to these questions are found on page 487.

1. Proximally, the rectus femoris is located between what two muscles?

2. What muscle is superficial to the proximal attachment of the biceps femoris?

3. How many muscles of the adductor group attach to the linea aspera?

4. Which thigh muscle is named for its long distal tendon?

5. What joint action is occurring if the vastus lateralis is eccentrically contracting?

6. Name a muscle that is antagonistic to both of the pectineus' joint actions of the thigh?

7. What muscle is located immediately medial to the medial hamstrings?

8. What happens to the length of the semitendinosus if the pelvis is anteriorly tilted?

9. What is the only part of the hamstring group that cannot extend the thigh at the hip joint?

10. Besides the TFL, what muscle attaches to the anterior superior iliac spine of the pelvis?

11. What muscle acts to move the joint capsule of the knee?

12. Which of the following joint actions of the pelvis at the hip joint is occurring if the semimembranosus concentrically contracts? anterior tilt / posterior tilt

13. Name three synergists to the rectus femoris at the knee joint.

14. How many of the muscles of the adductor group can flex the thigh at the hip joint?

15. How are the biceps femoris and the semitendinosus antagonistic to each other?

16. How are all four quadriceps femoris muscles synergistic with each other?

17. Why are the hamstrings antagonistic to the TFL?

18. What is the only part of the hamstring group that does not cross the hip joint?

19. What is the common distal attachment of all four quadriceps femoris muscles?

20. What two muscles attach into the iliotibial band?

21. What three muscles attach into the pes anserine tendon?

22. What happens to the length of the sartorius when the knee joint extends?

23. What muscle's tendon is located directly medial to the distal tendon of the sartorius?

24. How is the pectineus synergistic with the rectus femoris?

25. During what joint actions of the pelvis does the adductor longus lengthen?

26. What joint action of the knee lengthens the biceps femoris?

27. What joint actions are antagonistic to the pelvic actions of the adductor longus?

28. What three muscles attach into the pes anserine tendon?

29. What muscle is sometimes known as the 4th hamstring?

30. What muscle is deep to the vastus intermedius?

31. Which muscle of the adductor group is the most posterior?

32. What three muscles comprise the hamstring group?

33. What happens to the length of the adductor magnus if the thigh is actively extended at the hip joint?

34. Which of the following joint actions of the thigh at the hip joint occurs if the adductor magnus eccentrically contracts? extension / flexion

35. Which quadriceps femoris muscle is the largest?

36. If the thigh is passively flexed at the hip joint, what happens to the length of the TFL?

37. What is the only muscle of the adductor group that crosses the knee joint?

38. Which hamstring muscle is located the most laterally?

39. What happens to the length of the vastus intermedius if the leg is passively extended at the knee joint?

40. Why is the semitendinosus antagonistic to the sartorius?

41. What muscle is immediately deep to the TFL?

42. If the sartorius is eccentrically contracting, what action is occurring at the hip joint?

43. What muscle is immediately medial to the pectineus?

44. What muscle is deep to the iliotibial band for most of its length?

45. What muscle is immediately lateral to the pectineus?

46. What muscle is immediately deep to the adductor longus?

47. How can the rectus abdominis be considered to be synergistic with the adductor magnus?

48. How many of the quadriceps femoris muscles attach to the linea aspera of the femur?

49. What is the longest muscle in the human body?

50. Which muscle of the adductor group has the most prominent proximal tendon?

51. What muscle is located directly deep to the rectus femoris?

52. If the thigh is passively laterally rotated at the hip joint, what happens to the length of the TFL?

53. What seven muscles attach to the linea aspera of the femur?

54. What happens to the length of the rectus femoris if the hip joint flexes?

55. What five muscles comprise the adductors of the thigh group?

56. What happens to the length of the gracilis if the pelvis is posteriorly tilted at the hip joint?

57. What is the only quadriceps femoris muscle that crosses the hip joint?

58. What four muscles comprise the quadriceps femoris group?

59. Name a synergist to the vastus intermedius.

Muscles of the Leg

8

GET READY TO EXPLORE:

Note: Throughout this chapter, muscle attachments are indicated by italics.

⊖ More review activities on Evolve at: http://evolve.elsevier.com/Muscolino/anatomycoloring/

ANTERIOR VIEW OF THE RIGHT LEG

PROXIMAL

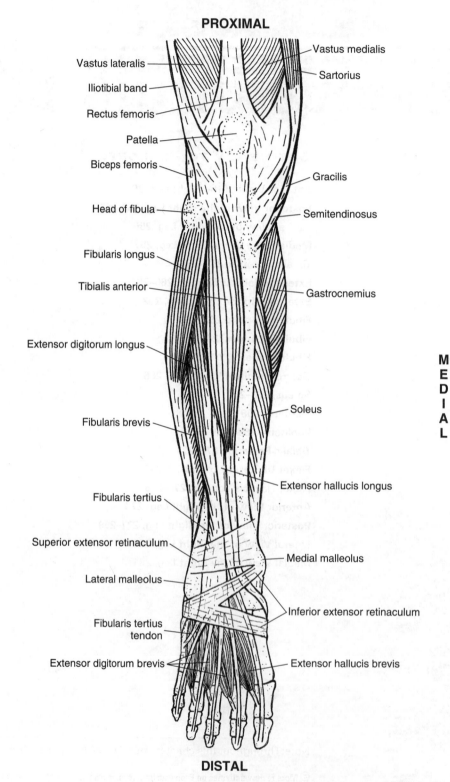

Vastus lateralis

Iliotibial band

Rectus femoris

Patella

Biceps femoris

Head of fibula

Fibularis longus

Tibialis anterior

Extensor digitorum longus

Fibularis brevis

Fibularis tertius

Superior extensor retinaculum

Lateral malleolus

Fibularis tertius tendon

Extensor digitorum brevis

Vastus medialis

Sartorius

Gracilis

Semitendinosus

Gastrocnemius

Soleus

Extensor hallucis longus

Medial malleolus

Inferior extensor retinaculum

Extensor hallucis brevis

L A T E R A L

M E D I A L

DISTAL

POSTERIOR VIEW OF THE RIGHT LEG (SUPERFICIAL)

PROXIMAL

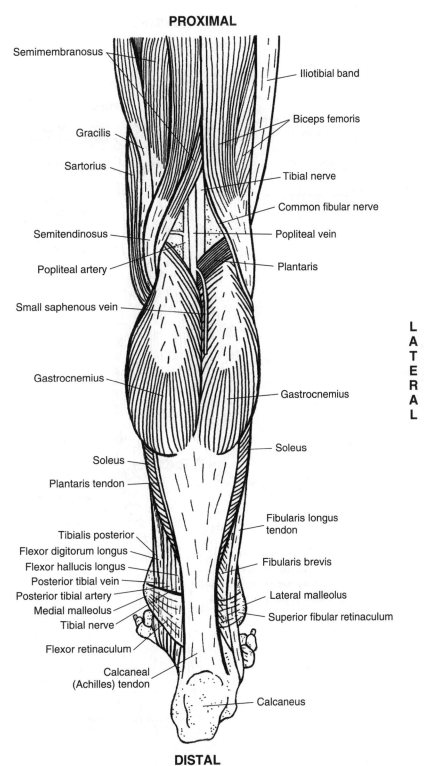

Semimembranosus

Gracilis

Sartorius

Semitendinosus

Popliteal artery

Small saphenous vein

M E D I A L

Gastrocnemius

Soleus

Plantaris tendon

Tibialis posterior
Flexor digitorum longus
Flexor hallucis longus
Posterior tibial vein
Posterior tibial artery
Medial malleolus
Tibial nerve

Flexor retinaculum

Calcaneal
(Achilles) tendon

Iliotibial band

Biceps femoris

Tibial nerve

Common fibular nerve

Popliteal vein

Plantaris

L A T E R A L

Gastrocnemius

Soleus

Fibularis longus
tendon

Fibularis brevis

Lateral malleolus

Superior fibular retinaculum

Calcaneus

DISTAL

POSTERIOR VIEW OF THE RIGHT LEG (INTERMEDIATE)

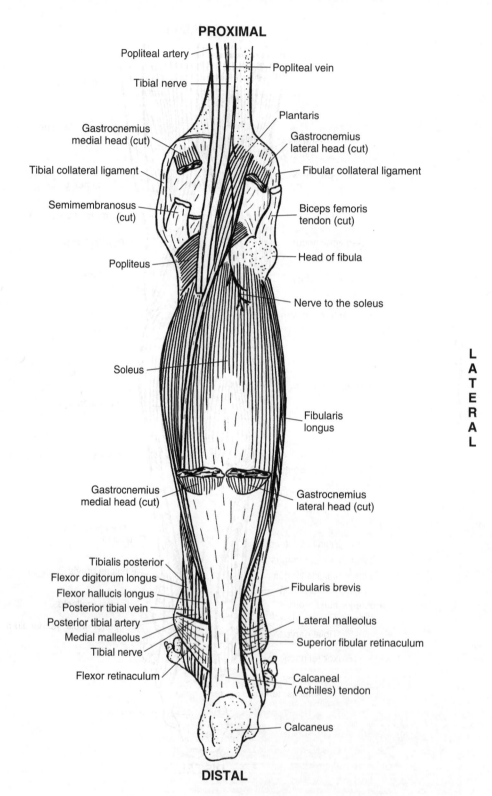

PROXIMAL

Popliteal artery

Tibial nerve

Gastrocnemius
medial head (cut)

Tibial collateral ligament

Semimembranosus
(cut)

Popliteus

Soleus

Gastrocnemius
medial head (cut)

Tibialis posterior
Flexor digitorum longus
Flexor hallucis longus
Posterior tibial vein
Posterior tibial artery
Medial malleolus
Tibial nerve
Flexor retinaculum

Popliteal vein

Plantaris

Gastrocnemius
lateral head (cut)

Fibular collateral ligament

Biceps femoris
tendon (cut)

Head of fibula

Nerve to the soleus

Fibularis
longus

Gastrocnemius
lateral head (cut)

Fibularis brevis

Lateral malleolus

Superior fibular retinaculum

Calcaneal
(Achilles) tendon

Calcaneus

MEDIAL

LATERAL

DISTAL

POSTERIOR VIEW OF THE RIGHT LEG (DEEP)

PROXIMAL

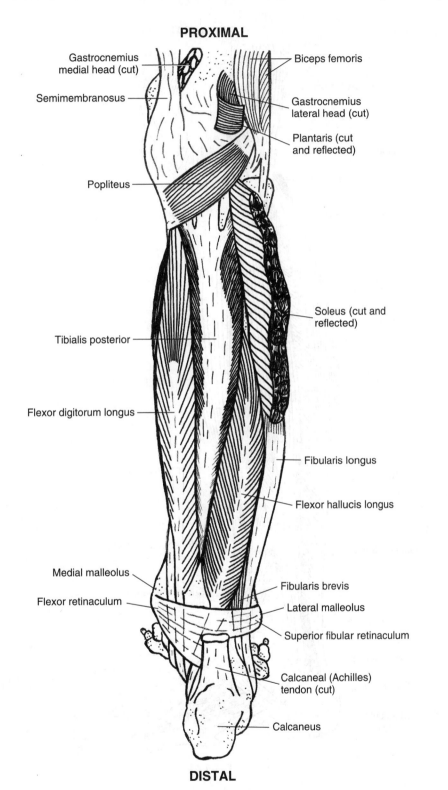

Gastrocnemius medial head (cut)

Semimembranosus

Popliteus

Tibialis posterior

Flexor digitorum longus

Biceps femoris

Gastrocnemius lateral head (cut)

Plantaris (cut and reflected)

Soleus (cut and reflected)

Fibularis longus

Flexor hallucis longus

MEDIAL

LATERAL

Medial malleolus

Flexor retinaculum

Fibularis brevis

Lateral malleolus

Superior fibular retinaculum

Calcaneal (Achilles) tendon (cut)

Calcaneus

DISTAL

LATERAL VIEW OF THE RIGHT LEG

PROXIMAL

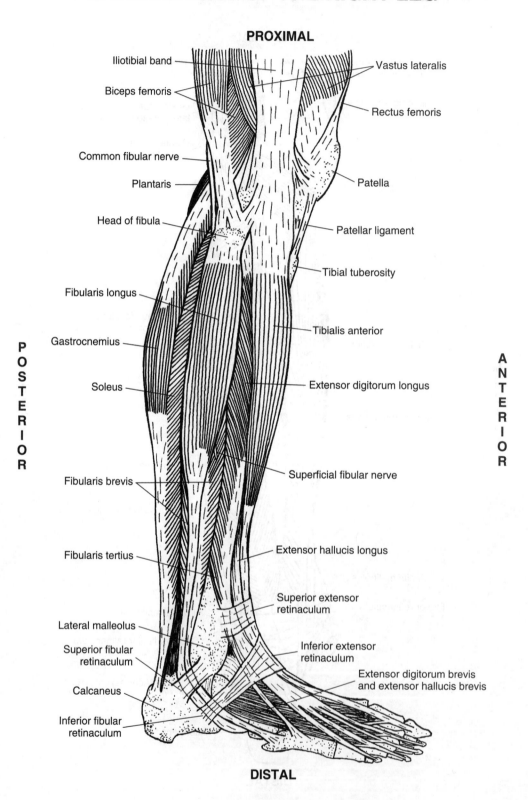

Iliotibial band

Biceps femoris

Common fibular nerve

Plantaris

Head of fibula

Fibularis longus

Gastrocnemius

Soleus

Fibularis brevis

Fibularis tertius

Lateral malleolus

Superior fibular
retinaculum

Calcaneus

Inferior fibular
retinaculum

Vastus lateralis

Rectus femoris

Patella

Patellar ligament

Tibial tuberosity

Tibialis anterior

Extensor digitorum longus

Superficial fibular nerve

Extensor hallucis longus

Superior extensor
retinaculum

Inferior extensor
retinaculum

Extensor digitorum brevis
and extensor hallucis brevis

P O S T E R I O R

A N T E R I O R

DISTAL

MEDIAL VIEW OF THE RIGHT LEG

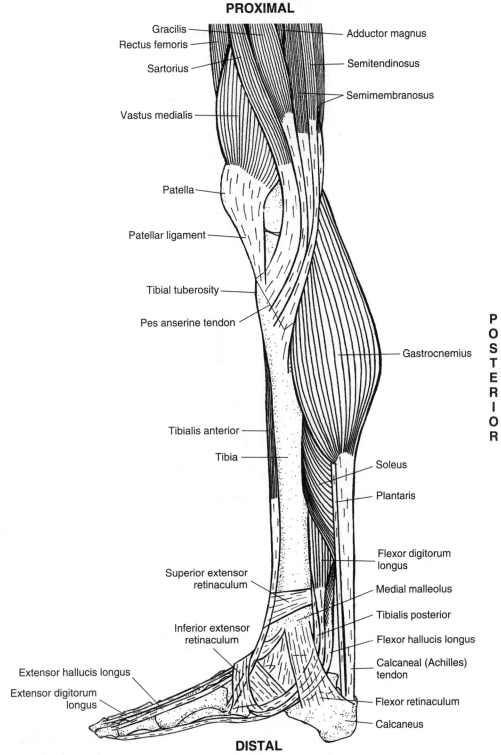

PROXIMAL

Gracilis

Rectus femoris

Sartorius

Vastus medialis

Patella

Patellar ligament

Tibial tuberosity

Pes anserine tendon

Tibialis anterior

Tibia

Superior extensor
retinaculum

Inferior extensor
retinaculum

Extensor hallucis longus

Extensor digitorum
longus

Adductor magnus

Semitendinosus

Semimembranosus

Gastrocnemius

Soleus

Plantaris

Flexor digitorum
longus

Medial malleolus

Tibialis posterior

Flexor hallucis longus

Calcaneal (Achilles)
tendon

Flexor retinaculum

Calcaneus

ANTERIOR

POSTERIOR

DISTAL

TIBIALIS ANTERIOR
(IN THE ANTERIOR COMPARTMENT)

tib-ee-**a**-lis an-**tee**-ri-or

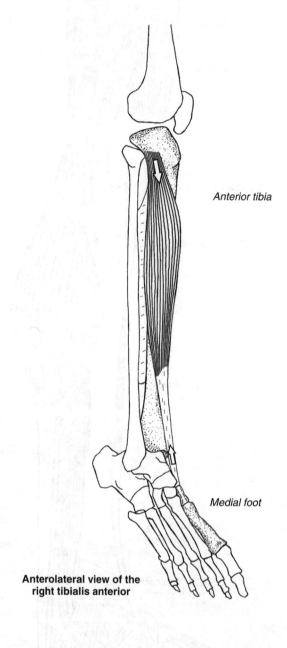

Anterior tibia

Medial foot

**Anterolateral view of the
right tibialis anterior**

Actions	**Innervation**	**Myofascial Meridians**
Dorsiflexion of the foot at the ankle joint	The deep fibular nerve	Superficial front line
Inversion of the foot at the subtalar joint	**Arterial Supply**	Spiral line
	The anterior tibial artery	

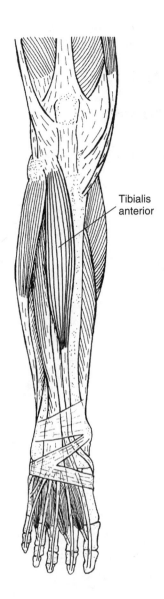

Tibialis anterior

DID YOU KNOW

The tibialis anterior is the most commonly affected muscle when a person has shin splints. The tibialis anterior is also one of the two "stirrup muscles."

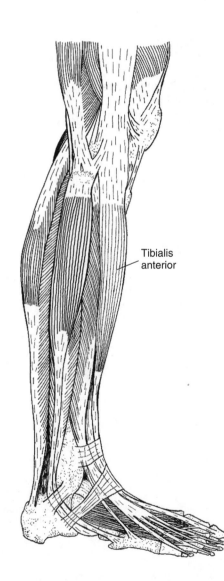

Tibialis anterior

DID YOU KNOW

The other stirrup muscle is the fibularis longus.

EXTENSOR HALLUCIS LONGUS
(IN THE ANTERIOR COMPARTMENT)

eks-**ten**-sor hal-**oo**-sis **long**-us

Actions
Extension of the big toe
(toe #1) at the meta-
tarsophalangeal joint and
the interphalan-geal joint
Dorsiflexion of the foot at
the ankle joint
Inversion of the foot at the
subtalar joint

Innervation
The deep fibular nerve

Arterial Supply
The anterior tibial artery

Myofascial Meridians
Superficial front line

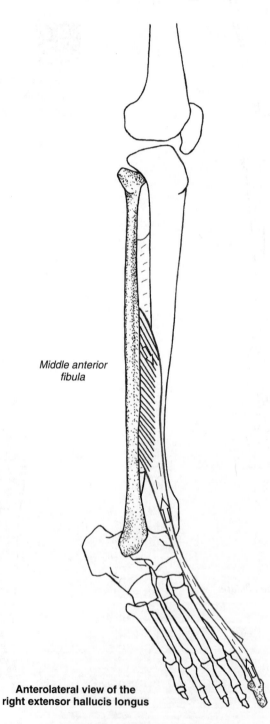

*Middle anterior
fibula*

**Anterolateral view of the
right extensor hallucis longus**

*Dorsal surface of the
big toe (toe #1)*

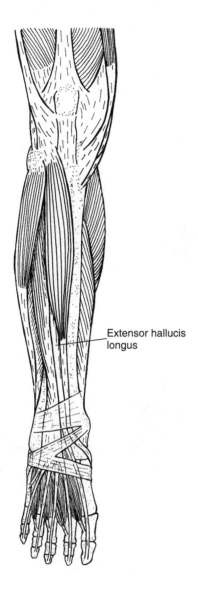

Extensor hallucis longus

DID YOU KNOW

The extensor hallucis longus is in the anterior compartment of the leg, along with the tibialis anterior, extensor digitorum longus, and fibularis tertius.

DID YOU KNOW

The extensor hallucis longus is the only muscle that can extend the distal phalanx of the big toe.

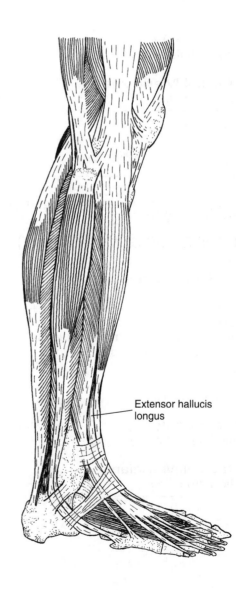

Extensor hallucis longus

EXTENSOR DIGITORUM LONGUS

(IN THE ANTERIOR COMPARTMENT)

eks-**ten**-sor dij-i-**toe**-rum **long**-us

Actions
Extension of toes #2-5 at the metatarsophalan-geal joint and the proximal and distal interphalangeal joints
Dorsiflexion of the foot at the ankle joint
Eversion of the foot at the subtalar joint

Innervation
The deep fibular nerve

Arterial Supply
The anterior tibial artery

Myofascial Meridians
Superficial front line

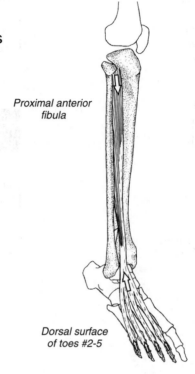

Proximal anterior fibula

Dorsal surface of toes #2-5

Anterolateral view of the right extensor digitorum longus

FIBULARIS TERTIUS

(IN THE ANTERIOR COMPARTMENT)

fib-you **la**-ris **ter**-she-us

Actions
Dorsiflexion of the foot at the ankle joint
Eversion of the foot at the subtalar joint

Innervation
The deep fibular nerve

Arterial Supply
The anterior tibial artery

Myofascial Meridians
Superficial front line

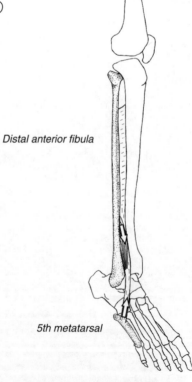

Distal anterior fibula

5th metatarsal

Anterolateral view of the right fibularis tertius

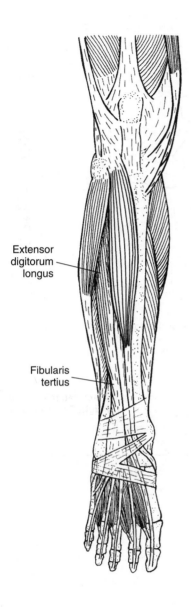

Extensor
digitorum
longus

Fibularis
tertius

DID
YOU
KNOW

The most distal and lateral part of the
extensor digitorum longus does not attach
onto "digits," therefore it is given another
name, the fibularis tertius. Therefore, the
fibularis tertius is actually the most distal
and lateral part of the extensor digitorum
longus. It is given a separate name
because it does not attach onto "digits."

DID
YOU
KNOW

The fibularis tertius used to be named
the peroneus tertius.

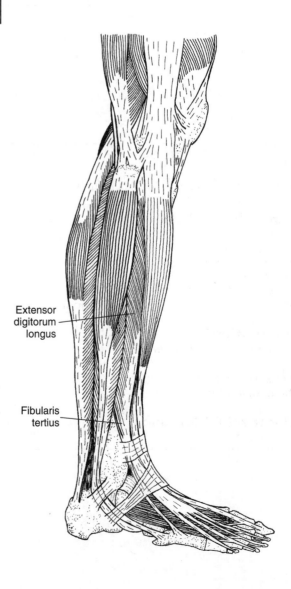

Extensor
digitorum
longus

Fibularis
tertius

FIBULARIS LONGUS
(IN THE LATERAL COMPARTMENT)

fib-you-**la**-ris **long**-us

Actions
Eversion of the foot at the subtalar joint
Plantarflexion of the foot at the ankle joint

Innervation
The superficial fibular nerve

Arterial Supply
The fibular artery

Myofascial Meridians
Lateral line
Spiral line

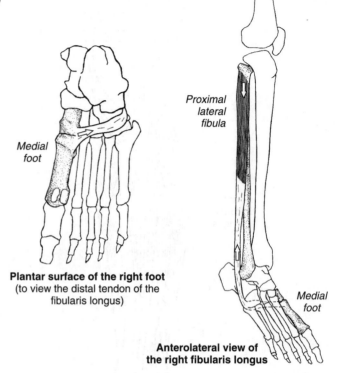

Medial foot

Proximal lateral fibula

Medial foot

Plantar surface of the right foot
(to view the distal tendon of the
fibularis longus)

**Anterolateral view of
the right fibularis longus**

FIBULARIS BREVIS
(IN THE LATERAL COMPARTMENT)

fib-you-**la**-ris **bre**-vis

Actions
Eversion of the foot at the subtalar joint
Plantarflexion of the foot at the ankle joint

Innervation
The superficial fibular nerve

Arterial Supply
The fibular artery

Myofascial Meridians
Lateral line

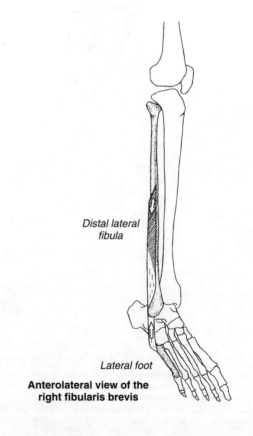

Distal lateral fibula

Lateral foot

**Anterolateral view of the
right fibularis brevis**

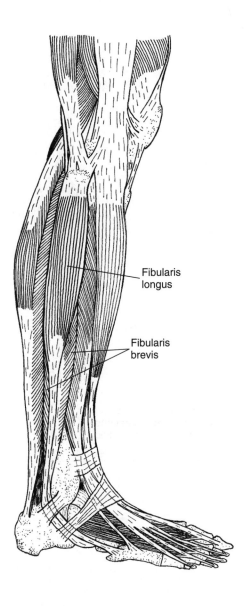

Fibularis
longus

Fibularis
brevis

The fibularis longus, along with the tibialis anterior, are often called the "stirrup muscles" because their distal tendons form a stirrup around the foot.

The fibularis longus used to be named the peroneus longus.

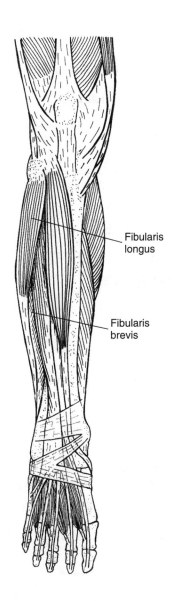

Fibularis
longus

Fibularis
brevis

The fibularis brevis is located deep to the fibularis longus and has the same actions as the fibularis longus.

The fibularis brevis used to be named the peroneus brevis.

GASTROCNEMIUS ("GASTROC")

(OF THE TRICEPS SURAE AND IN
THE SUPERFICIAL POSTERIOR
COMPARTMENT)

gas-trok-**nee**-me-us

Actions
Plantarflexion of the foot at the ankle joint
Flexion of the leg at the knee joint
Inversion of the foot at the subtalar joint

Innervation
The tibial nerve

Arterial Supply
Sural branches of the popliteal artery

Myofascial Meridians
Superficial back line

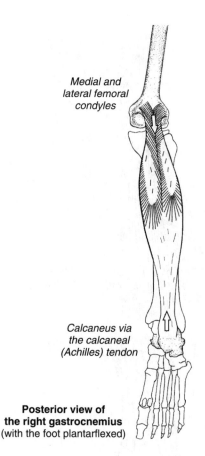

*Medial and
lateral femoral
condyles*

*Calcaneus via
the calcaneal
(Achilles) tendon*

**Posterior view of
the right gastrocnemius**
(with the foot plantarflexed)

SOLEUS

(OF THE TRICEPS SURAE AND IN
THE SUPERFICIAL POSTERIOR
COMPARTMENT)

so-lee-us

Actions
Plantarflexion of the foot at the ankle joint
Inversion of the foot at the subtalar joint

Innervation
The tibial nerve

Arterial Supply
Sural branches of the popliteal artery

Myofascial Meridians
Superficial back line

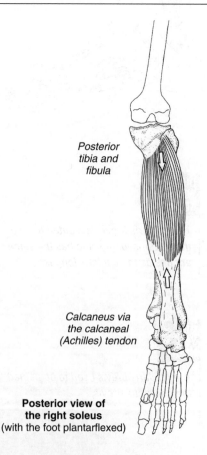

*Posterior
tibia and
fibula*

*Calcaneus via
the calcaneal
(Achilles) tendon*

**Posterior view of
the right soleus**
(with the foot plantarflexed)

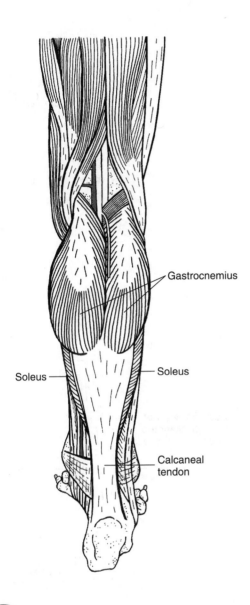

Gastrocnemius

Soleus

Soleus

Calcaneal tendon

DID YOU KNOW

The gastrocnemius (and soleus) attaches into the calcaneus via the calcaneal tendon, which is more well known as the Achilles tendon.

DID YOU KNOW

The gastrocnemius has two heads, a lateral head and a medial head.

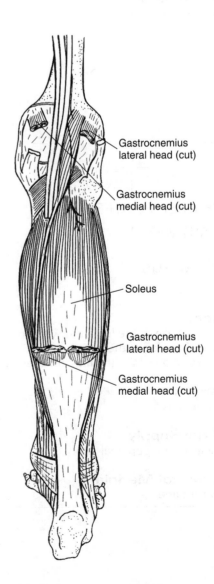

Gastrocnemius lateral head (cut)

Gastrocnemius medial head (cut)

Soleus

Gastrocnemius lateral head (cut)

Gastrocnemius medial head (cut)

DID YOU KNOW

The soleus is actually quite large and massive, accounting for the contours of the gastrocnemius being so visible. "Behind every great gastrocnemius is a great soleus ☺."

DID YOU KNOW

The soleus and two heads of the gastrocnemius are often referred to as the "triceps surae."

PLANTARIS

(IN THE SUPERFICIAL POSTERIOR COMPARTMENT)

plan-**ta**-ris

Actions
Plantarflexion of the foot at the ankle joint
Flexion of the leg at the knee joint

Innervation
The tibial nerve

Arterial Supply
Sural branches of the popliteal artery

Myofascial Meridians
Superficial back line

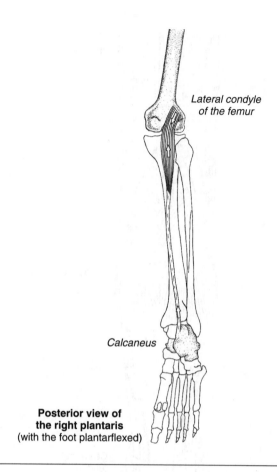

Lateral condyle
of the femur

Calcaneus

**Posterior view of
the right plantaris**
(with the foot plantarflexed)

POPLITEUS

(IN THE DEEP POSTERIOR COMPARTMENT)

pop-**lit**-ee-us

Actions
Medial rotation of the leg at the knee joint
Flexion of the leg at the knee joint
Lateral rotation of the thigh at the knee joint

Innervation
The tibial nerve

Arterial Supply
Branches of the popliteal artery

Myofascial Meridians
Deep front line

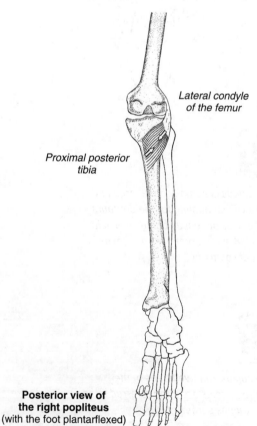

Lateral condyle
of the femur

Proximal posterior
tibia

**Posterior view of
the right popliteus**
(with the foot plantarflexed)

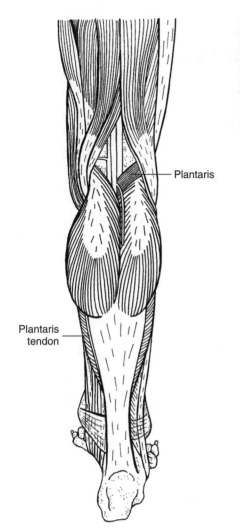

Plantaris

Plantaris
tendon

Sometimes the plantaris joints the gastrocnemius and soleus, attaching into the Achilles tendon.

The vast majority of the length of the plantaris is its long, slender, distal tendon.

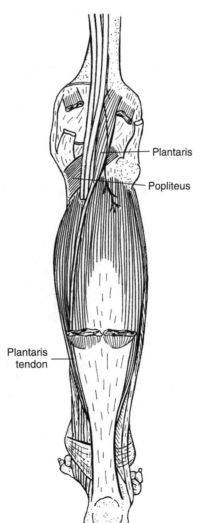

Plantaris

Popliteus

Plantaris
tendon

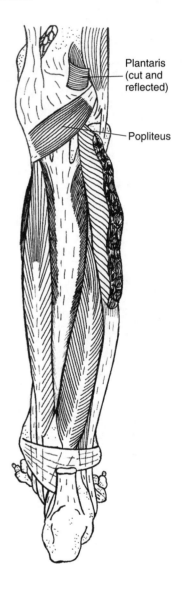

Plantaris
(cut and
reflected)

Popliteus

The proximal tendon of the popliteus travels within the capsule of the knee joint.

The popliteus is considered important for its rotation action at the knee joint, which is said to "unlock" the extended knee.

TIBIALIS POSTERIOR
(IN THE DEEP POSTERIOR COMPARTMENT)

tib-ee-**a**-lis pos-**tee**-ri-or

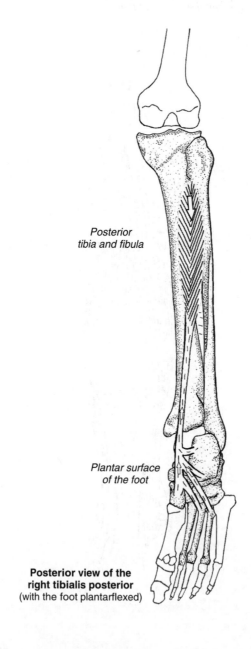

*Posterior
tibia and fibula*

*Plantar surface
of the foot*

**Posterior view of the
right tibialis posterior**
(with the foot plantarflexed)

Actions	**Innervation**	**Myofascial Meridians**
Plantarflexion of the foot at the ankle joint	The tibial nerve	Deep front line
Inversion of the foot at the subtalar joint	**Arterial Supply**	
	The posterior tibial artery	

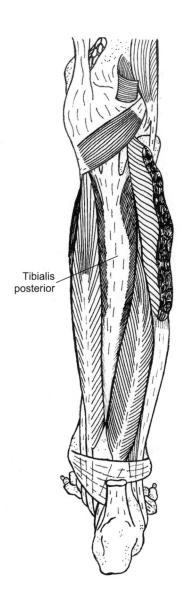

Tibialis posterior

DID YOU KNOW

The tibialis posterior is "Tom" of the "Tom, Dick, and Harry muscles." "Tom, Dick, and Harry muscles" are grouped together because their distal tendons all cross posterior to the medial malleolus of the tibia.

DID YOU KNOW

The tibialis posterior is the muscle most often involved in posterior shin splints.

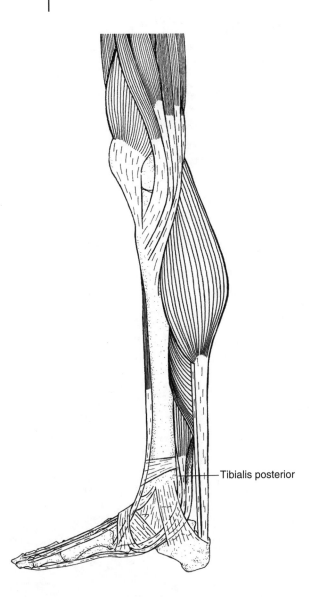

Tibialis posterior

FLEXOR DIGITORUM LONGUS
(IN THE DEEP POSTERIOR COMPARTMENT)
fleks-or dij-i-**toe**-rum **long**-us

Actions
Flexion of toes #2-5 at the metatarsophalan-
    geal joint and the proximal and distal
    interphalangeal joints
Plantarflexion of the foot at the ankle joint
Inversion of the foot at the subtalar joint

Innervation
The tibial nerve

Arterial Supply
The posterior tibial artery

Myofascial Meridians
Deep front line

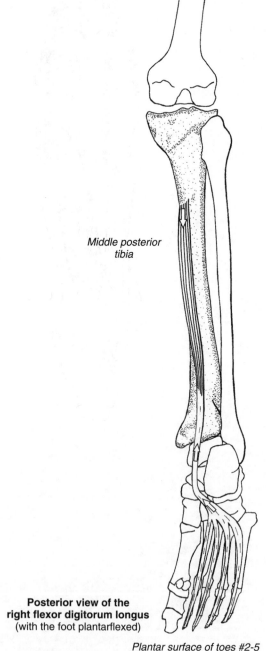

*Middle posterior
tibia*

**Posterior view of the
right flexor digitorum longus**
(with the foot plantarflexed)

Plantar surface of toes #2-5

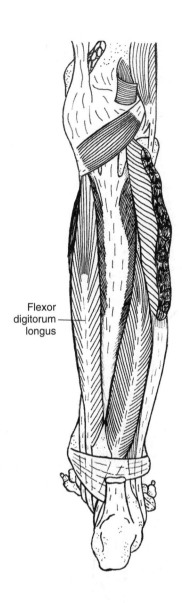

Flexor digitorum longus

DID YOU KNOW

The flexor digitorum longus is "Dick" of the "Tom, Dick, and Harry muscles." "Tom, Dick, and Harry muscles" are grouped together because their distal tendons all cross posterior to the medial malleolus of the tibia.

DID YOU KNOW

Because of the architecture of the distal tendon of the flexor digitorum longus, this muscle cannot independently control motion of toes 2-5.

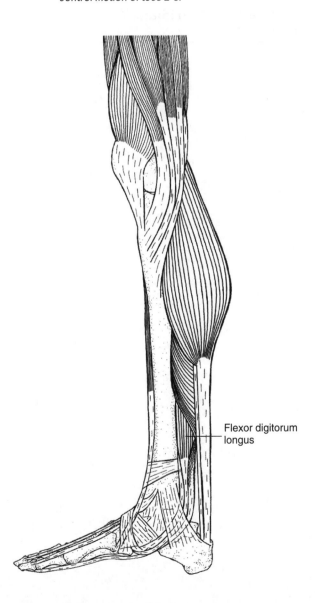

Flexor digitorum longus

FLEXOR HALLUCIS LONGUS
(IN THE DEEP POSTERIOR COMPARTMENT)

fleks-or hal-**oo**-sis **long**-us

Actions
Flexion of the big toe (toe #1) at the
    metatarsophalangeal joint and the
    interphalangeal joint
Plantarflexion of the foot at the ankle joint
Inversion of the foot at the subtalar joint

Innervation
The tibial nerve

Arterial Supply
The posterior tibial artery

Myofascial Meridians
Deep front line

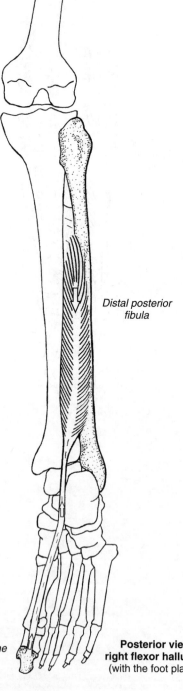

*Distal posterior
fibula*

*Plantar surface of the
big toe (toe #1)*

**Posterior view of the
right flexor hallucis longus**
(with the foot plantarflexed)

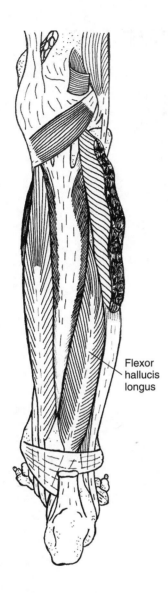

Flexor
hallucis
longus

DID YOU KNOW

*The flexor hallucis longus is "Harry"
of the "Tom, Dick, and Harry muscles."
"Tom, Dick, and Harry muscles" are
grouped together because their distal
tendons all cross posterior to the
medial malleolus of the tibia.*

DID YOU KNOW

*The role of flexion of the big toe by the
flexor hallucis longus is extremely important
during the toe-off phase of the gait cycle.*

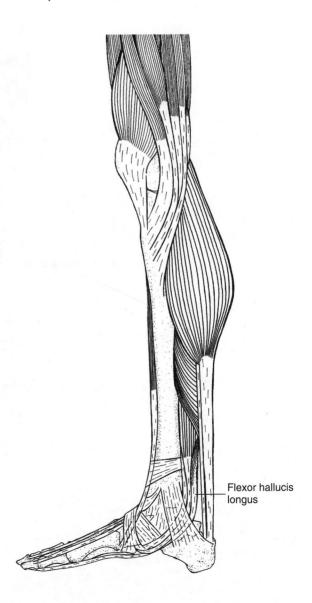

Flexor hallucis
longus

ANTERIOR VIEW OF THE RIGHT LEG

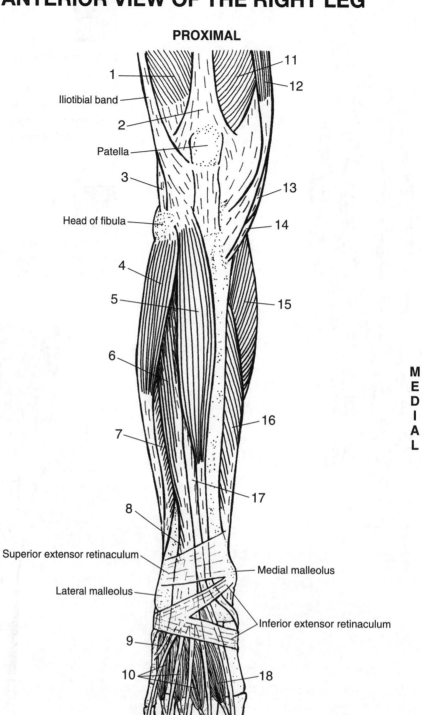

PROXIMAL

1

Iliotibial band

2

Patella

3

Head of fibula

4

5

6

7

8

Superior extensor retinaculum

Lateral malleolus

9

10

LATERAL

MEDIAL

11

12

13

14

15

16

17

Medial malleolus

Inferior extensor retinaculum

18

DISTAL

Answers to labeling exercises are on p. 487.

POSTERIOR VIEW OF THE RIGHT LEG (SUPERFICIAL)

PROXIMAL

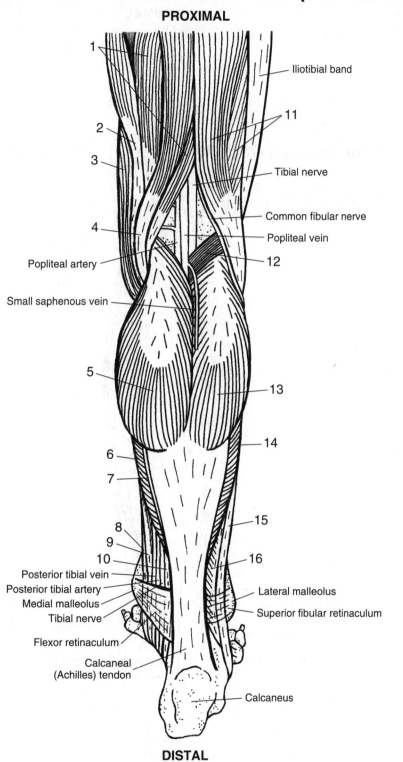

Iliotibial band

Tibial nerve

Common fibular nerve

Popliteal vein

Popliteal artery

Small saphenous vein

Posterior tibial vein

Posterior tibial artery

Medial malleolus

Tibial nerve

Flexor retinaculum

Calcaneal
(Achilles) tendon

Lateral malleolus

Superior fibular retinaculum

Calcaneus

MEDIAL

LATERAL

DISTAL

POSTERIOR VIEW OF THE RIGHT LEG (INTERMEDIATE)

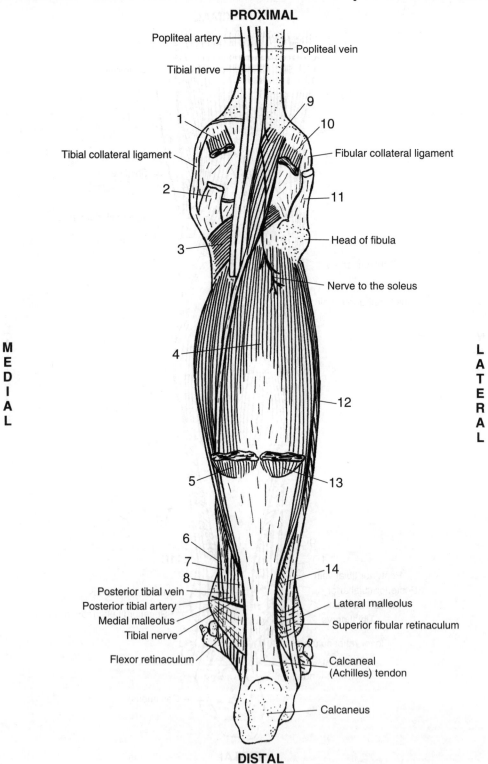

PROXIMAL

Popliteal artery

Popliteal vein

Tibial nerve

9

1

10

Tibial collateral ligament

Fibular collateral ligament

2

11

Head of fibula

3

Nerve to the soleus

MEDIAL

4

LATERAL

12

5

13

6

7

8

14

Posterior tibial vein

Posterior tibial artery

Lateral malleolus

Medial malleolus

Superior fibular retinaculum

Tibial nerve

Flexor retinaculum

Calcaneal (Achilles) tendon

Calcaneus

DISTAL

POSTERIOR VIEW OF THE RIGHT LEG (DEEP)

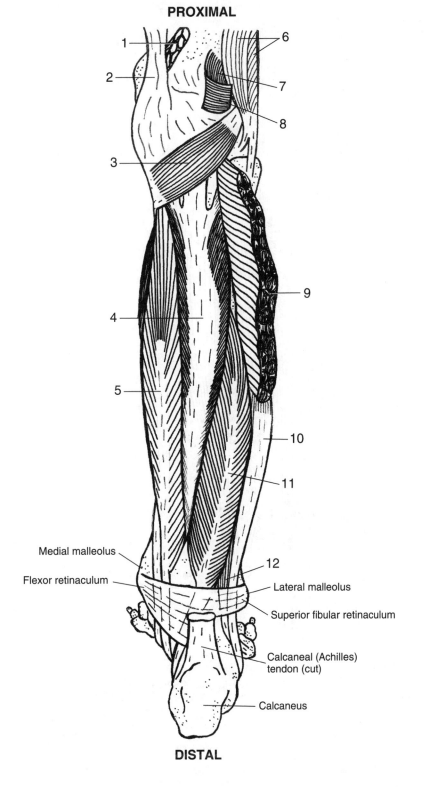

PROXIMAL

MEDIAL

LATERAL

1

2

3

4

5

6

7

8

9

10

11

12

Medial malleolus

Flexor retinaculum

Lateral malleolus

Superior fibular retinaculum

Calcaneal (Achilles) tendon (cut)

Calcaneus

DISTAL

LATERAL VIEW OF THE RIGHT LEG

PROXIMAL

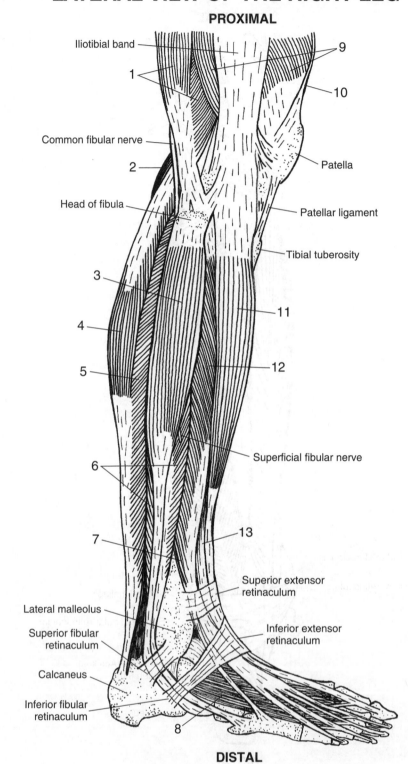

Iliotibial band

1

Common fibular nerve

2

Head of fibula

3

4

5

6

7

9

10

Patella

Patellar ligament

Tibial tuberosity

11

12

Superficial fibular nerve

13

Superior extensor retinaculum

Lateral malleolus

Superior fibular retinaculum

Calcaneus

Inferior fibular retinaculum

Inferior extensor retinaculum

8

POSTERIOR

ANTERIOR

DISTAL

MEDIAL VIEW OF THE RIGHT LEG

PROXIMAL

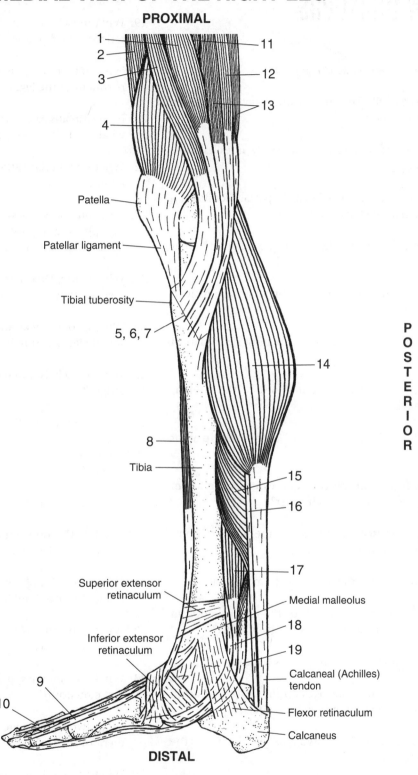

1
2
3
4

11
12
13

Patella

Patellar ligament

Tibial tuberosity

5, 6, 7

14

ANTERIOR

POSTERIOR

8

Tibia

15
16

17

Superior extensor
retinaculum

Medial malleolus

18
19

Inferior extensor
retinaculum

Calcaneal (Achilles)
tendon

9

Flexor retinaculum

10

Calcaneus

DISTAL

Review Questions

Muscles of the Leg
Answers to these questions are found on page 488.

1. How are the fibularis tertius and brevis synergistic with each other?

2. Where are the Tom, Dick, and Harry muscles most superficial?

3. What muscle is considered to be important for its rotation action at the knee joint?

4. All three fibularis muscles attach proximally to what bone?

5. How are the fibularis tertius and brevis antagonistic to each other?

6. The fibularis tertius is actually the most distal part of what muscle?

7. What action(s) would an antagonist to the fibularis longus have?

8. Which fibularis muscle travels in the deep plantar foot?

9. How are the tibialis anterior and extensor digitorum longus synergistic with each other?

10. What three muscles are located in the superficial posterior compartment of the leg?

11. What two muscles attach to the 5th metatarsal?

12. What happens to the length of the flexor digitorum longus when the knee joint is passively flexed?

13. What muscles make up the triceps surae group?

14. To which phalanx/phalanges do the flexor digitorum and flexor hallucis longus muscles attach?

15. The distal tendon of what two muscles is known as the Achilles tendon?

16. Who are the Tom, Dick, and Harry muscles?

17. Which muscle is deeper, the extensor digitorum longus or the extensor hallucis longus?

18. What muscle is immediately superficial to the plantaris?

19. What muscle is located superficially immediately posterior to the fibularis longus?

20. What four muscles are located in the anterior compartment of the leg?

21. If the tibialis anterior is concentrically contracting, what joint action(s) is/are occurring?

22. What two muscles attach to the lateral condyle of the femur?

23. If the big toe is flexed at the metatarsophalangeal and interphalangeal joints, what happens to the length of the extensor hallucis longus?

24. Which Tom, Dick, and Harry muscle lies closest to the medial malleolus of the tibia?

25. Which Tom, Dick, and Harry muscle has the most superficial exposure in the distal medial leg?

26. What muscle is immediately posterior to the fibularis longus?

27. What are the two stirrup muscles?

28. Is the tibialis anterior synergistic with or antagonistic to the gastrocnemius?

29. Which muscle is deeper, the fibularis longus or brevis?

30. What is the only muscle of the posterior compartments of the leg that does not cross the ankle joint?

31. How can the popliteus both medially and laterally rotate the knee joint?

32. What joint actions are shared by all three Tom, Dick, and Harry muscles?

33. What two muscles attach to the first metatarsal and first cuneiform?

34. What two muscles are located in the lateral compartment of the leg?

35. What muscle is immediately superficial to the Tom, Dick, and Harry muscles?

36. What muscle is antagonistic to both actions of the foot of the flexor hallucis longus?

37. What is the only tarsal bone to which the tibialis posterior does not attach?

38. What muscle lies immediately medial to the belly of the tibialis posterior?

39. If the fibularis longus and brevis are eccentrically contracting, what joint motion(s) is/are occurring?

40. From a posterior perspective, what muscle is immediately deep to the gastrocnemius?

41. What happens to the length of the tibialis posterior if the ankle joint is passively or actively plantarflexed?

42. What four muscles are located in the deep posterior compartment of the leg?

Intrinsic Muscles of the Foot 9

Note: Throughout this chapter, muscle attachments are indicated by italics.

☺ More review activities on Evolve at: http://evolve.elsevier.com/Muscolino/anatomycoloring/

DORSAL VIEW OF THE RIGHT FOOT

PROXIMAL

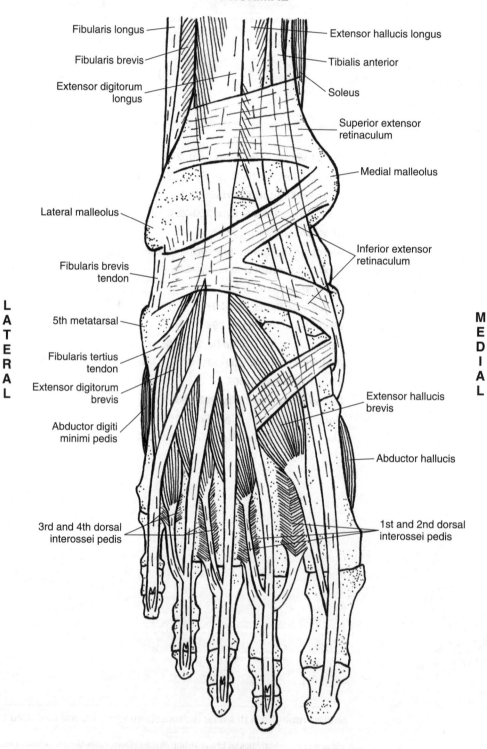

Fibularis longus

Fibularis brevis

Extensor digitorum longus

Lateral malleolus

Fibularis brevis tendon

5th metatarsal

Fibularis tertius tendon

Extensor digitorum brevis

Abductor digiti minimi pedis

3rd and 4th dorsal interossei pedis

Extensor hallucis longus

Tibialis anterior

Soleus

Superior extensor retinaculum

Medial malleolus

Inferior extensor retinaculum

Extensor hallucis brevis

Abductor hallucis

1st and 2nd dorsal interossei pedis

LATERAL

MEDIAL

DISTAL

PLANTAR VIEW OF THE RIGHT FOOT
(SUPERFICIAL MUSCULAR LAYER)

DISTAL

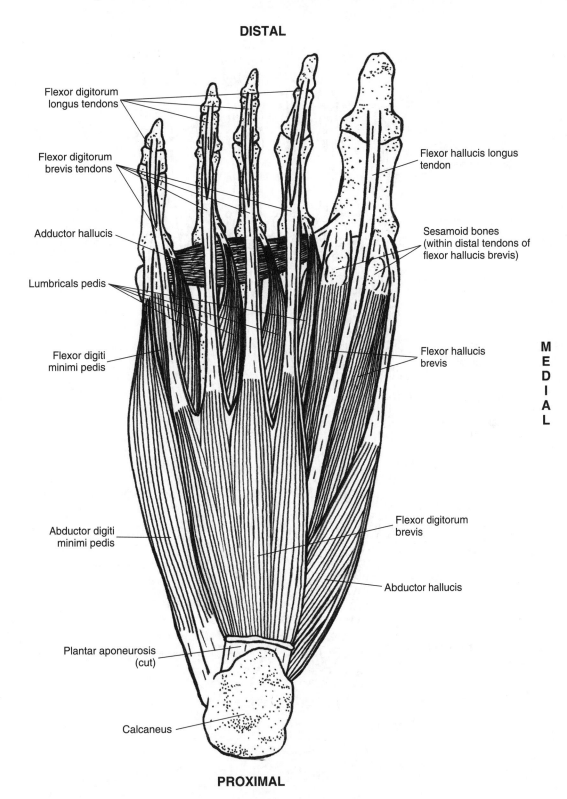

Flexor digitorum
longus tendons

Flexor digitorum
brevis tendons

Adductor hallucis

Lumbricals pedis

Flexor digiti
minimi pedis

Abductor digiti
minimi pedis

Plantar aponeurosis
(cut)

Calcaneus

Flexor hallucis longus
tendon

Sesamoid bones
(within distal tendons of
flexor hallucis brevis)

Flexor hallucis
brevis

Flexor digitorum
brevis

Abductor hallucis

**L
A
T
E
R
A
L**

**M
E
D
I
A
L**

PROXIMAL

PLANTAR VIEW OF THE RIGHT FOOT (INTERMEDIATE MUSCULAR LAYER)

DISTAL

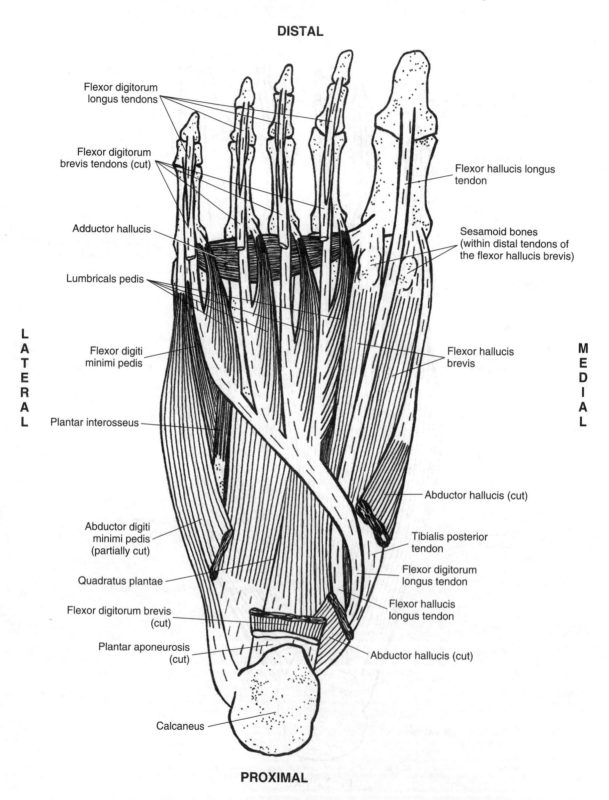

Flexor digitorum longus tendons

Flexor digitorum brevis tendons (cut)

Adductor hallucis

Lumbricals pedis

Flexor digiti minimi pedis

Plantar interosseus

Abductor digiti minimi pedis (partially cut)

Quadratus plantae

Flexor digitorum brevis (cut)

Plantar aponeurosis (cut)

Calcaneus

Flexor hallucis longus tendon

Sesamoid bones (within distal tendons of the flexor hallucis brevis)

Flexor hallucis brevis

Abductor hallucis (cut)

Tibialis posterior tendon

Flexor digitorum longus tendon

Flexor hallucis longus tendon

Abductor hallucis (cut)

LATERAL

MEDIAL

PROXIMAL

PLANTAR VIEW OF THE RIGHT FOOT
(DEEP MUSCULAR LAYER)

DISTAL

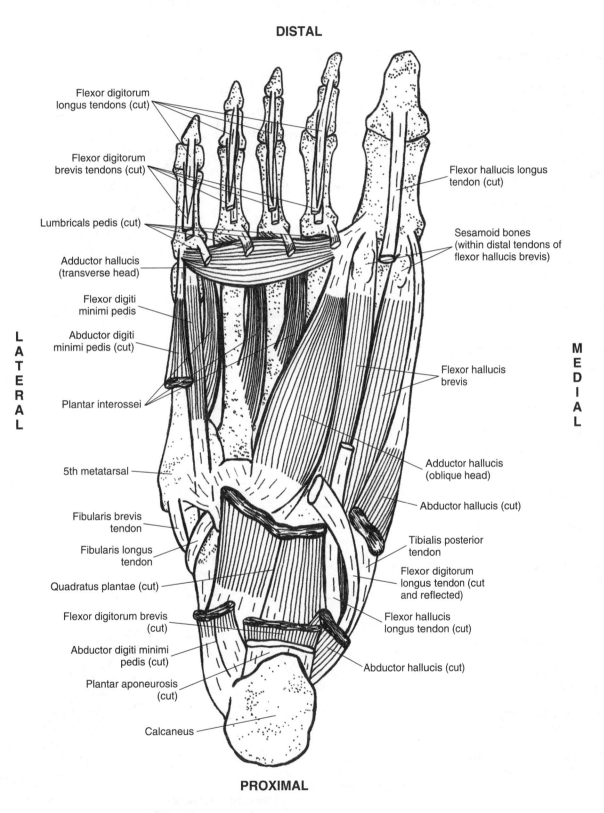

Flexor digitorum
longus tendons (cut)

Flexor digitorum
brevis tendons (cut)

Lumbricals pedis (cut)

Adductor hallucis
(transverse head)

Flexor digiti
minimi pedis

Abductor digiti
minimi pedis (cut)

Plantar interossei

5th metatarsal

Fibularis brevis
tendon

Fibularis longus
tendon

Quadratus plantae (cut)

Flexor digitorum brevis
(cut)

Abductor digiti minimi
pedis (cut)

Plantar aponeurosis
(cut)

Calcaneus

LATERAL

MEDIAL

Flexor hallucis longus
tendon (cut)

Sesamoid bones
(within distal tendons of
flexor hallucis brevis)

Flexor hallucis
brevis

Adductor hallucis
(oblique head)

Abductor hallucis (cut)

Tibialis posterior
tendon

Flexor digitorum
longus tendon (cut
and reflected)

Flexor hallucis
longus tendon (cut)

Abductor hallucis (cut)

PROXIMAL

EXTENSOR DIGITORUM BREVIS
(DORSAL SURFACE)

eks-**ten**-sor
dij-i-**toe**-rum **bre**-vis

Action
Extension of toes #2-4 at the metatarso-phalangeal and proximal and distal interphalangeal joints

Innervation
The deep fibular nerve

Arterial Supply
The dorsalis pedis artery

Myofascial Meridians
Superficial front line

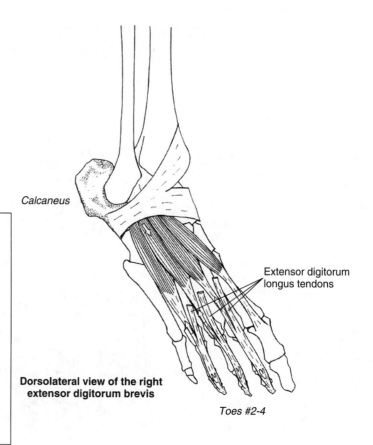

Calcaneus

Extensor digitorum longus tendons

Dorsolateral view of the right extensor digitorum brevis

Toes #2-4

EXTENSOR HALLUCIS BREVIS
(DORSAL SURFACE)

eks-**ten**-sor hal-**oo**-sis **bre**-vis

Action
Extension of the big toe (toe #1) at the metatarsophalangeal joint

Innervation
The deep fibular nerve

Arterial Supply
The dorsalis pedis artery

Myofascial Meridians
Superficial front line

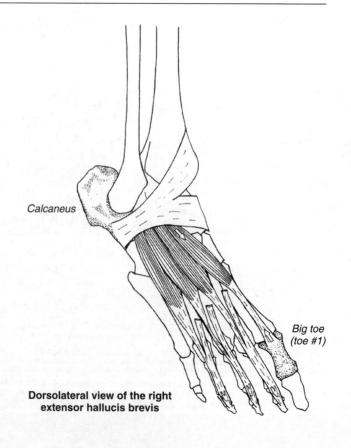

Calcaneus

Big toe (toe #1)

Dorsolateral view of the right extensor hallucis brevis

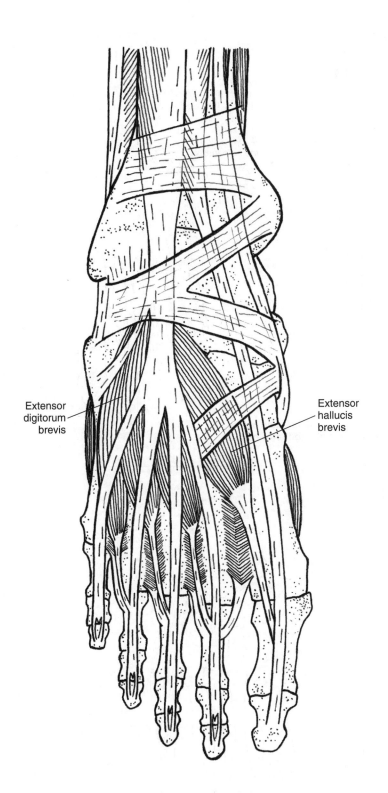

Extensor digitorum brevis

Extensor hallucis brevis

DID YOU KNOW

The extensor digitorum brevis and extensor hallucis brevis are actually parts of the same muscle. They are named as separate muscles because the distal attachment of the fibers of the extensor hallucis brevis are onto the big toe; and the distal attachments of the fibers of the extensor digitorum are onto the other toes. The extensor digitorum brevis is the only "digitorum" muscle that does not attach onto all digits 2-5; it does not attach onto the little toe (toe 5).

ABDUCTOR HALLUCIS

(PLANTAR SURFACE—LAYER I)

ab-**duk**-tor hal-**oo**-sis

Actions
Abduction of the big toe
(toe #1) at the meta-
tarsophalangeal joint
Flexion of the big toe
(toe #1) at the meta-
tarsophalangeal joint

Innervation
The medial plantar nerve

Arterial Supply
The medial plantar artery

Myofascial Meridians
Superficial back line

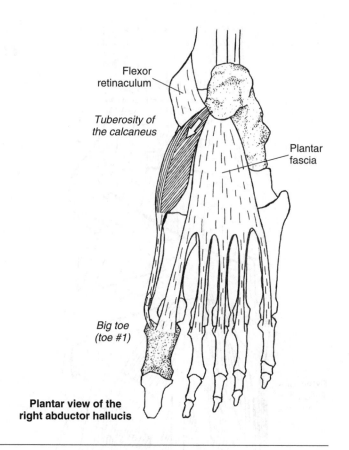

**Plantar view of the
right abductor hallucis**

ABDUCTOR DIGITI MINIMI PEDIS

(PLANTAR SURFACE—LAYER I)

ab-**duk**-tor **dij**-i-tee **min**-i-mee
peed-us

Actions
Abduction of the little
toe (toe #5) at the
metatarsophalangeal
joint
Flexion of the little toe
(toe #5) at the meta-
tarsophalangeal joint

Innervation
The lateral plantar nerve

Arterial Supply
The lateral plantar artery

Myofascial Meridians
Superficial back line

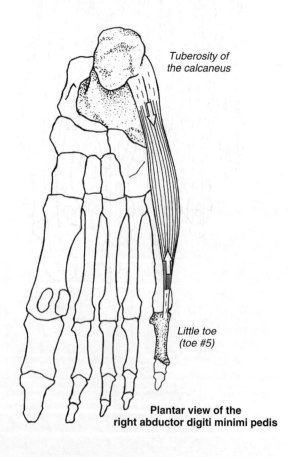

**Plantar view of the
right abductor digiti minimi pedis**

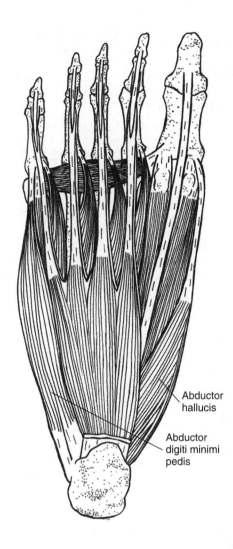

Abductor
hallucis

Abductor
digiti minimi
pedis

The abductor hallucis is easily palpable on the medial side of the plantar surface of the foot.

DID YOU KNOW

The abductor hallucis is an important muscle to strengthen in people who have hallux valgus (commonly known as bunion).

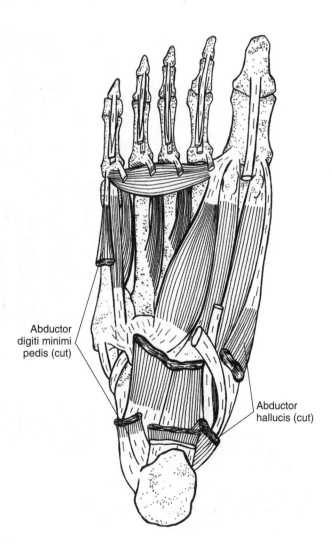

Abductor
digiti minimi
pedis (cut)

Abductor
hallucis (cut)

DID YOU KNOW

The abductor digiti minimi pedis is often known simply as the abductor digiti minimi. But there is an abductor digiti minimi (manus) of the hand as well, and confusion can result.

DID YOU KNOW

Abducting the little toe is important toward widening the foot to increase stability of stance.

FLEXOR DIGITORUM BREVIS
(PLANTAR SURFACE—LAYER I)

fleks-or dij-i-**toe**-rum **bre**-vis

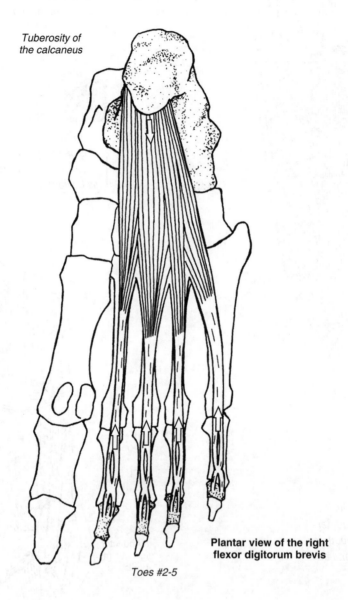

*Tuberosity of
the calcaneus*

**Plantar view of the right
flexor digitorum brevis**

Toes #2-5

Action
Flexion of toes #2-5 at the
metatarsophalangeal and the
proximal interphalangeal joints

Innervation
The medial plantar nerve

Arterial Supply
The medial and lateral plantar
arteries

Myofascial Meridians
Superficial back line

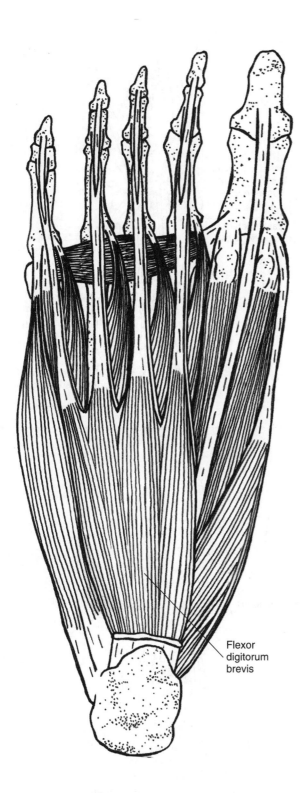

Flexor
digitorum
brevis

DID
YOU
KNOW

*The distal tendons of the flexor
digitorum brevis split to allow
passage of the distal tendons of the
flexor digitorum longus to the distal
phalanges of toes #2-5.*

DID
YOU
KNOW

*This arrangement is similar to the
relationship between the flexor
digitorum superficialis and flexor
digitorum profundus in the upper
extremity.*

QUADRATUS PLANTAE
(PLANTAR SURFACE—LAYER II)

kwod-**ray**-tus **plan**-tee

Action
Flexion of toes #2-5 at the metatarsophalangeal and the proximal and distal interphalangeal joints

Innervation
The lateral plantar nerve

Arterial Supply
The medial and lateral plantar arteries

Myofascial Meridians
Superficial back line

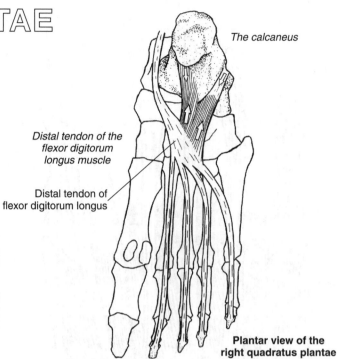

The calcaneus

Distal tendon of the flexor digitorum longus muscle

Distal tendon of flexor digitorum longus

Plantar view of the right quadratus plantae

LUMBRICALS PEDIS
(PLANTAR SURFACE—LAYER II)

(There are four lumbrical pedis muscles, named #1, #2, #3, and #4.)

lum-bri-kuls **peed**-us

Actions
Extension of toes #2-5 at the proximal and distal interphalangeal joints
Flexion of toes #2-5 at the metatarsophalangeal joint

Innervation
The medial and lateral plantar nerves

Arterial Supply
The medial and lateral plantar arteries

Myofascial Meridians
Involved: Superficial back line
Involved: Deep front line

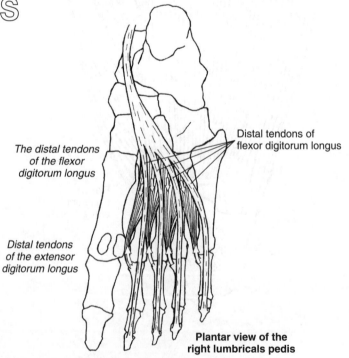

The distal tendons of the flexor digitorum longus

Distal tendons of flexor digitorum longus

Distal tendons of the extensor digitorum longus

Plantar view of the right lumbricals pedis

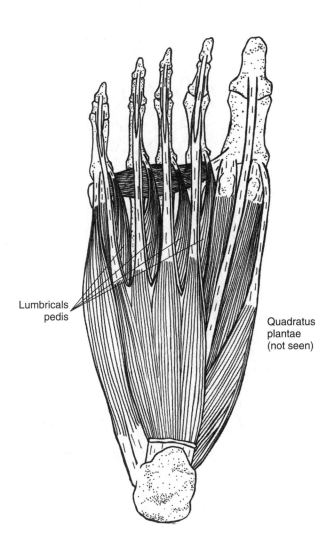

Lumbricals
pedis

Quadratus
plantae
(not seen)

DID YOU KNOW?

The quadratus plantae assists the flexor digitorum longus by straightening out the line of pull of this muscle upon the toes. For this reason, the quadratus plantae is also known as the flexor digitorum accessorius.

DID YOU KNOW?

Via its attachment into the distal tendon of the flexor digitorum longus, the quadratus plantae can flex toes 2-5 at all three of their joints.

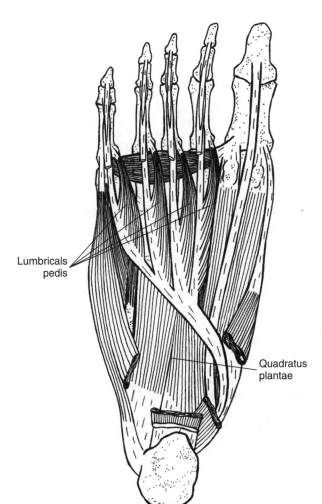

Lumbricals
pedis

Quadratus
plantae

DID YOU KNOW?

The lumbricals pedis are named for looking like earthworms; "lumbrical" is Latin for earthworm. There are four lumbricals pedis muscles in each foot.

DID YOU KNOW?

The lumbricals pedis muscles attach into their respective toes on the tibial/medial side.

FLEXOR HALLUCIS BREVIS

(PLANTAR SURFACE—LAYER III)

fleks-or hal-**oo**-sis **bre**-vis

Action
Flexion of the big toe (toe #1) at the metatarsophalangeal joint

Innervation
The medial plantar nerve

Arterial Supply
The medial plantar artery

Myofascial Meridians
Superficial back line

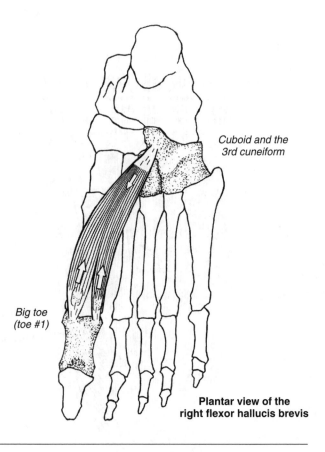

Cuboid and the 3rd cuneiform

Big toe (toe #1)

**Plantar view of the
right flexor hallucis brevis**

FLEXOR DIGITI MINIMI PEDIS

(PLANTAR SURFACE—LAYER III)

fleks-or **dij**-i-tee **min**-i-mee
peed-us

Action
Flexion of the little toe (toe #5) at the metatarsophalangeal joint

Innervation
The lateral plantar nerve

Arterial Supply
The lateral plantar artery

Myofascial Meridians
Superficial back line

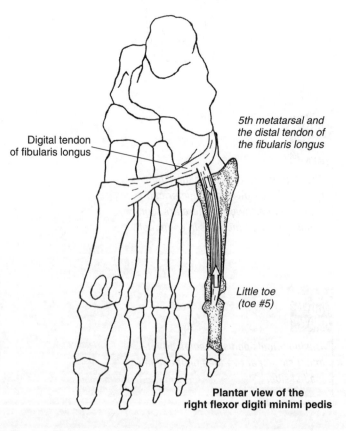

Digital tendon of fibularis longus

5th metatarsal and the distal tendon of the fibularis longus

Little toe (toe #5)

**Plantar view of the
right flexor digiti minimi pedis**

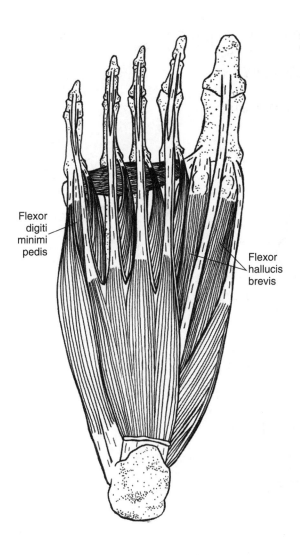

Flexor digiti minimi pedis

Flexor hallucis brevis

DID YOU KNOW

The flexor hallucis brevis has two heads: a medial head and a lateral head.

DID YOU KNOW

Distally, there is a sesamoid bone in the medial and lateral tendons of the flexor hallucis brevis.

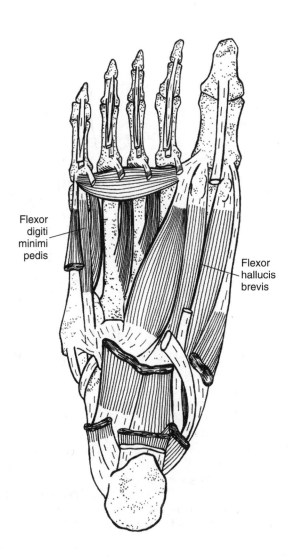

Flexor digiti minimi pedis

Flexor hallucis brevis

DID YOU KNOW

The flexor digiti minimi pedis is often known as simply the flexor digiti minimi or the flexor digiti minimi brevis. However, there is a flexor digiti minimi (manus) of the hand, and confusion can result.

DID YOU KNOW

Having a separate flexor muscle for the little toe allows for greater strength and independent motion of the little toe.

ADDUCTOR HALLUCIS

(PLANTAR SURFACE—LAYER III)

ad-**duk**-tor hal-**oo**-sis

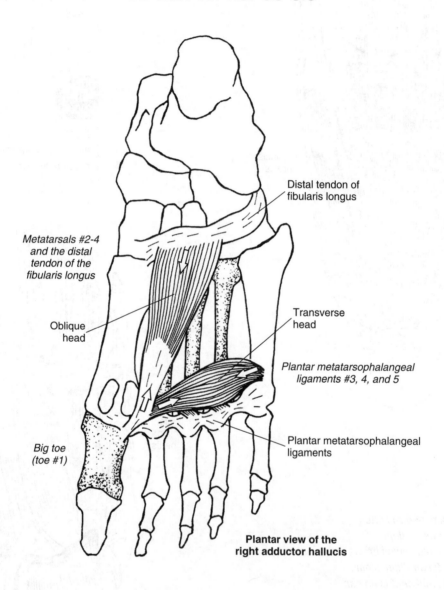

Distal tendon of
fibularis longus

*Metatarsals #2-4
and the distal
tendon of the
fibularis longus*

*Oblique
head*

Transverse
head

*Plantar metatarsophalangeal
ligaments #3, 4, and 5*

*Big toe
(toe #1)*

Plantar metatarsophalangeal
ligaments

**Plantar view of the
right adductor hallucis**

Actions	**Innervation**	**Myofascial Meridians**
Adduction of the big toe (toe #1) at the metatarsophalangeal joint	The lateral plantar nerve	Superficial back line
Flexion of the big toe (toe #1) at the metatarsophalangeal joint	**Arterial Supply** Branches of the plantar arch	

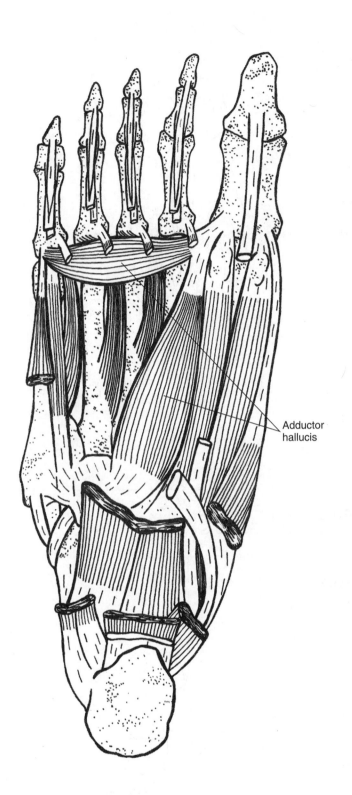

Adductor
hallucis

*The adductor hallucis occasionally
has attachments onto the 1st metatarsal that can create opposition of the
big toe toward the other toes. When
this occurs, this muscle is called the
opponens hallucis. This arrangement is
common in apes, whose feet are more
"handy" than ours ☺.*

*The adductor hallucis is often
excessively tight (overly facilitated)
in people who have hallux valgus
(commonly known as bunion).*

PLANTAR INTEROSSEI

(PLANTAR SURFACE—LAYER IV)

(There are three plantar interossei
muscles, named #1, #2, and #3.)

plan-tar in-ter-**oss**-ee-eye

Actions
Adduction of toes #3-5 at the
metatarsophalangeal joint
Flexion of toes #3-5 at the metatarsophalangeal
joint
Extension of toes #3-5 at the proximal and distal
interphalangeal joints

Innervation
The lateral plantar nerve

Arterial Supply
Branches of the plantar arch

Myofascial Meridians
Involved: Superficial back line
Involved: Deep front line

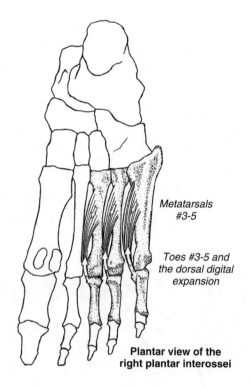

*Metatarsals
#3-5*

*Toes #3-5 and
the dorsal digital
expansion*

**Plantar view of the
right plantar interossei**

DORSAL INTEROSSEI PEDIS

(PLANTAR SURFACE—LAYER IV)

(There are four dorsal interossei pedis
muscles, named #1, #2, #3, and #4.)

plan-tar in-ter-**oss**-ee-eye **peed**-us

Actions
Abduction of toes #2-4 at the
metatarsophalangeal joint
Flexion of toes #2-4 at the metatarsophalangeal
joint at the metatarsophalangeal joint
Extension of toes #2-4 at the proximal and distal
interphalangeal joints

Innervation
The lateral plantar nerve

Arterial Supply
Branches of the plantar arch

Myofascial Meridians
Involved: Superficial back line
Involved: Deep front line

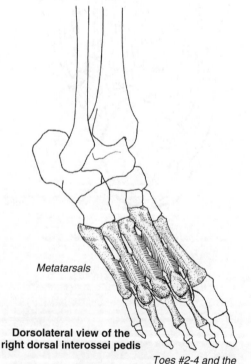

Metatarsals

**Dorsolateral view of the
right dorsal interossei pedis**

*Toes #2-4 and the
dorsal digital expansion*

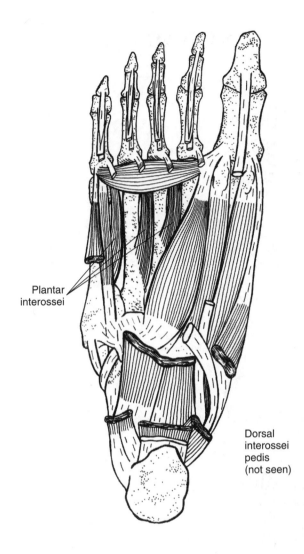

Plantar interossei

Dorsal interossei pedis (not seen)

The main action of the dorsal interossei pedis is abduction of the toes at the metatarsophalangeal joints. The main action of the plantar interossei is adduction of the toes at the metatarsophalangeal joints. The mnemonic to remember these actions is *DAB PAD*; *Dorsals **AB**duct, **P**lantars **AD**duct*.

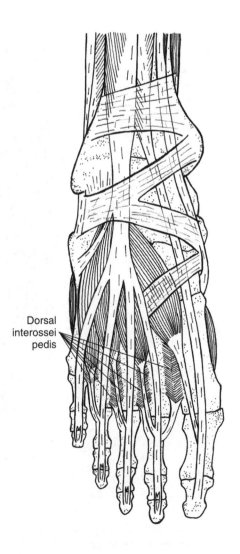

Dorsal interossei pedis

This arrangement is similar to the relationship between the palmar interossei and dorsal interossei manus of the hand.

DORSAL VIEW OF THE RIGHT FOOT

PROXIMAL

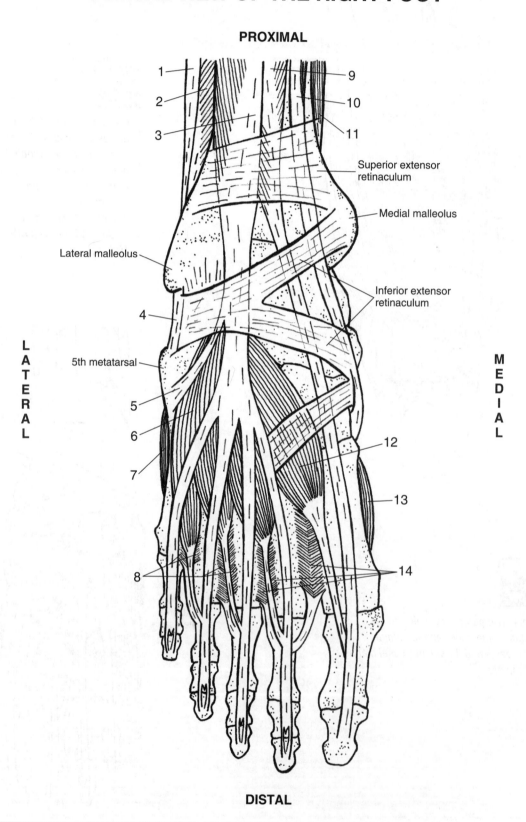

1

2

3

9

10

11

Superior extensor
retinaculum

Medial malleolus

Lateral malleolus

Inferior extensor
retinaculum

4

5th metatarsal

5

6

7

12

13

8

14

LATERAL

MEDIAL

DISTAL

PLANTAR VIEW OF THE RIGHT FOOT
(SUPERFICIAL MUSCULAR LAYER)

DISTAL

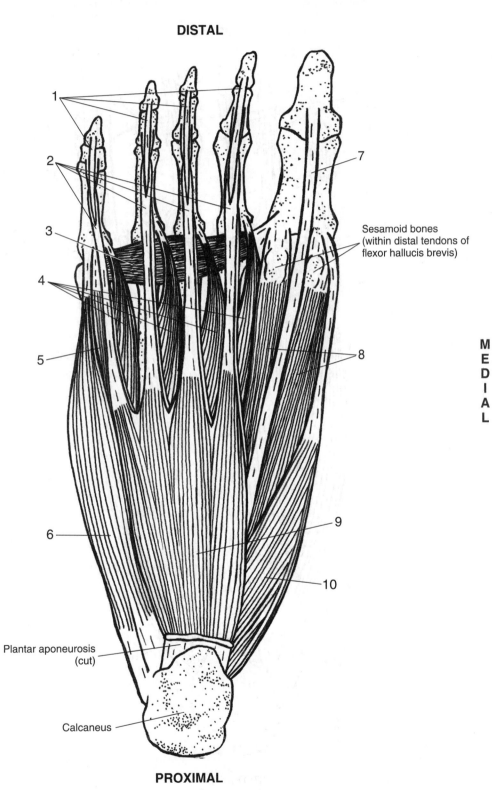

LATERAL

MEDIAL

Sesamoid bones
(within distal tendons of
flexor hallucis brevis)

Plantar aponeurosis
(cut)

Calcaneus

PROXIMAL

PLANTAR VIEW OF THE RIGHT FOOT (INTERMEDIATE MUSCULAR LAYER)

DISTAL

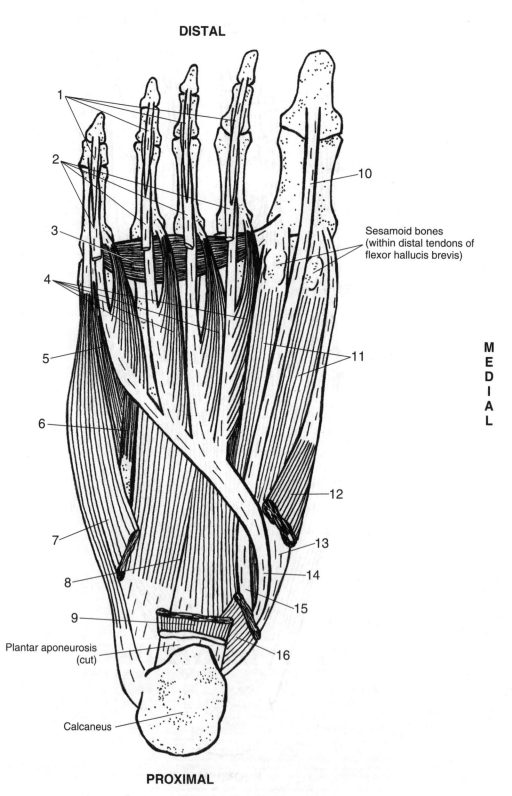

LATERAL

MEDIAL

Sesamoid bones
(within distal tendons of
flexor hallucis brevis)

Plantar aponeurosis
(cut)

Calcaneus

PROXIMAL

PLANTAR VIEW OF THE RIGHT FOOT
(DEEP MUSCULAR LAYER)

DISTAL

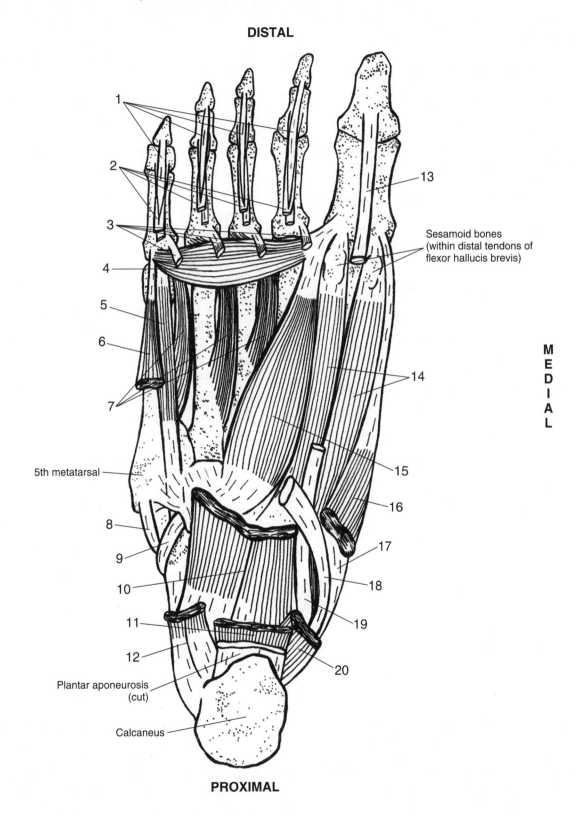

LATERAL

MEDIAL

Sesamoid bones
(within distal tendons of
flexor hallucis brevis)

5th metatarsal

Plantar aponeurosis
(cut)

Calcaneus

PROXIMAL

Review Questions

Intrinsic Muscles of the Foot
Answers to these questions are found on page 489.

1. What is another name for the quadratus plantae?

2. What muscle is synergistic with the extensor digitorum brevis?

3. What joint actions are occurring when the flexor digitorum brevis is concentrically contracting?

4. What two muscles are antagonistic to the flexor hallucis brevis?

5. What joint action occurs when the adductor hallucis concentrically contracts?

6. What muscle is antagonistic to the adductor hallucis?

7. If the big toe is passively extended at the metatarsophalangeal joint, what happens to the length of the extensor hallucis brevis?

8. Which interosseus muscle is lengthened if the 2nd toe tibially abducts?

9. What are the three muscles located in Layer III of the plantar foot?

10. What intrinsic muscle of the foot has sesamoid bones within its distal tendons?

11. What muscle is immediately medial to the oblique head of the adductor hallucis?

12. How many intrinsic muscles of the foot are located on the dorsal side?

13. What muscle is immediately deep to the transverse head of the adductor hallucis?

14. What three muscles are located in Layer I of the plantar foot?

15. What is the relationship of the lumbricals pedis to the transverse head of the adductor hallucis?

16. What is the mnemonic for the actions of the dorsal interossei pedis and plantar interossei?

17. In the proximal foot, what muscle is immediately deep to the flexor digitorum brevis?

18. What is the common proximal attachment of the extensors hallucis and digitorum brevis?

19. What muscle is antagonistic to the abductor digiti minimi pedis?

20. The tendons of what muscles are superficial to the extensor digitorum brevis?

21. What two muscles are located in Layer II of the plantar foot?

22. From the plantar perspective, which muscle group is deeper, the plantar interossei or the dorsal interossei pedis?

23. When the distal tendons of the flexor digitorum brevis split, what muscle's tendons pass through?

24. What is the common proximal attachment of the abductor hallucis and abductor digiti minimi pedis?

25. What are the names of the two heads of the adductor hallucis?

26. Which two dorsal interosseus pedis (DIP) muscles are antagonistic to each other?

27. What muscle is immediately medial to the abductor digiti minimi pedis?

28. In the proximal foot, what muscle is immediately lateral to the flexor digitorum brevis?

29. What three muscles attach to the tuberosity of the calcaneus?

30. What distal tendon of the foot serves as a proximal attachment of the flexor digiti minimi pedis?

31. What muscle is synergistic with the extensor hallucis brevis?

32. What muscle is superficial to the quadratus plantae?

33. What joint action(s) is/are occurring when the flexor digitorum brevis is lengthened?

34. What muscle is antagonistic to the adduction action of the plantar interosseus muscle of the little (5th) toe?

35. What muscle is antagonistic to the abductor hallucis?

36. What joint action occurs when the abductor hallucis eccentrically contracts?

37. What muscle is synergistic with the quadratus plantae's actions of flexion of toes #2-5 at the distal interphalangeal joint?

38. What is the proximal attachment of the lumbricals pedis?

39. What two muscles are located in Layer IV of the plantar foot?

40. What intrinsic muscle of the foot contains sesamoid bones?

41. What happens to the length of the flexor digiti minimi pedis when the little toe extends at the metatarsophalangeal joint?

42. Do the lumbricals flex and/or extend the toes (#2-5)?

Muscles of the Scapula/Arm 10

ANTERIOR VIEW OF THE RIGHT SHOULDER

SUPERIOR

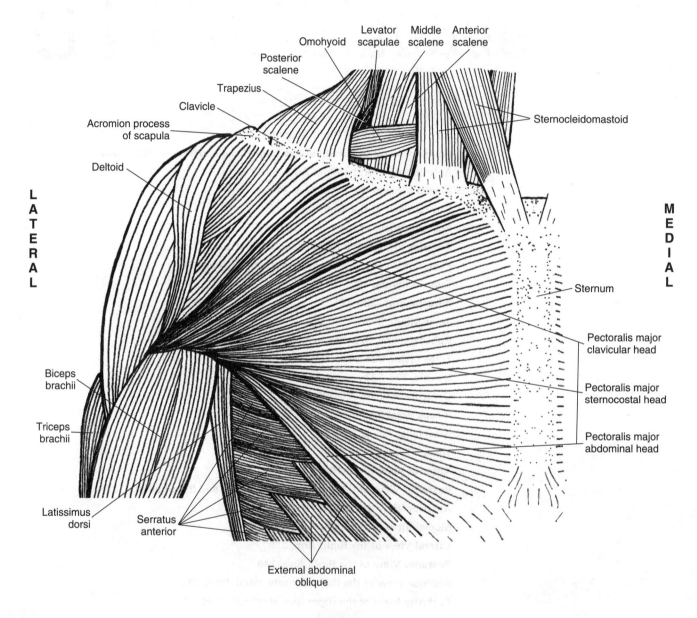

Omohyoid

Levator scapulae

Middle scalene

Anterior scalene

Posterior scalene

Trapezius

Clavicle

Acromion process of scapula

Deltoid

Sternocleidomastoid

Sternum

Pectoralis major clavicular head

Pectoralis major sternocostal head

Pectoralis major abdominal head

Biceps brachii

Triceps brachii

Latissimus dorsi

Serratus anterior

External abdominal oblique

LATERAL

MEDIAL

INFERIOR

POSTERIOR VIEW OF THE SHOULDERS (SUPERFICIAL AND INTERMEDIATE)

SUPERIOR

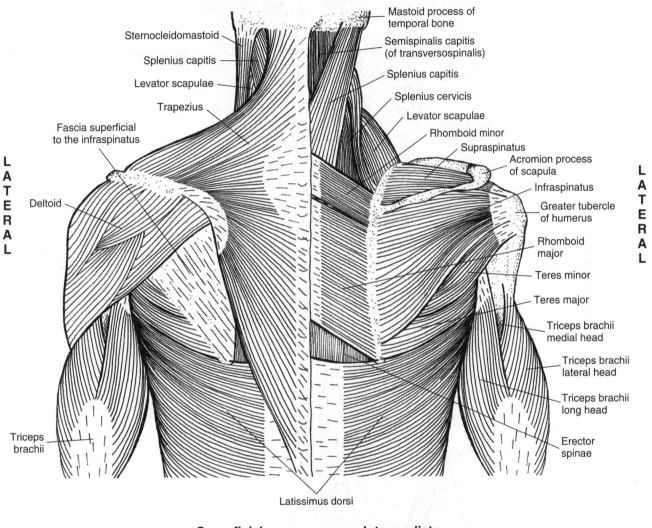

Sternocleidomastoid

Splenius capitis

Levator scapulae

Trapezius

Fascia superficial to the infraspinatus

Deltoid

Triceps brachii

Mastoid process of temporal bone

Semispinalis capitis (of transversospinalis)

Splenius capitis

Splenius cervicis

Levator scapulae

Rhomboid minor

Supraspinatus

Acromion process of scapula

Infraspinatus

Greater tubercle of humerus

Rhomboid major

Teres minor

Teres major

Triceps brachii medial head

Triceps brachii lateral head

Triceps brachii long head

Erector spinae

Latissimus dorsi

LATERAL

LATERAL

Superficial

Intermediate

INFERIOR

ANTERIOR VIEW OF THE RIGHT ARM (SUPERFICIAL)

PROXIMAL

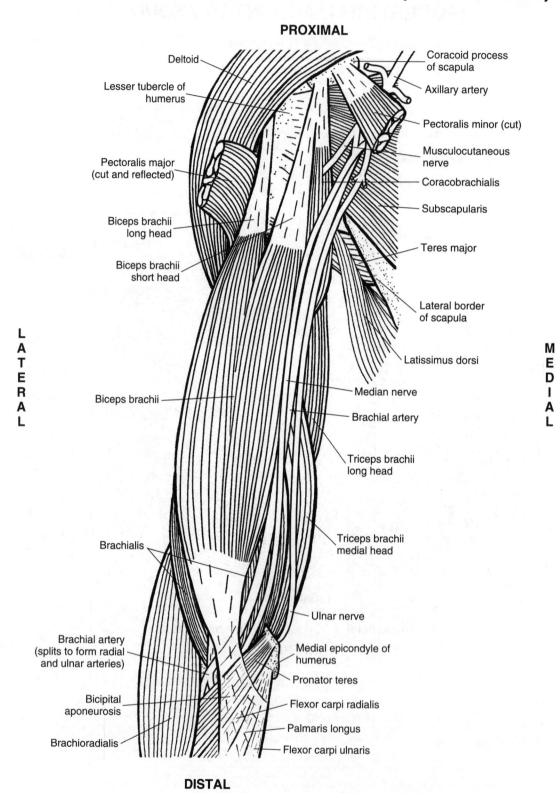

Deltoid

Lesser tubercle of
humerus

Pectoralis major
(cut and reflected)

Biceps brachii
long head

Biceps brachii
short head

Coracoid process
of scapula

Axillary artery

Pectoralis minor (cut)

Musculocutaneous
nerve

Coracobrachialis

Subscapularis

Teres major

Lateral border
of scapula

Latissimus dorsi

LATERAL

MEDIAL

Biceps brachii

Brachialis

Brachial artery
(splits to form radial
and ulnar arteries)

Bicipital
aponeurosis

Brachioradialis

Median nerve

Brachial artery

Triceps brachii
long head

Triceps brachii
medial head

Ulnar nerve

Medial epicondyle of
humerus

Pronator teres

Flexor carpi radialis

Palmaris longus

Flexor carpi ulnaris

DISTAL

ANTERIOR VIEW OF THE RIGHT ARM (DEEP)

PROXIMAL

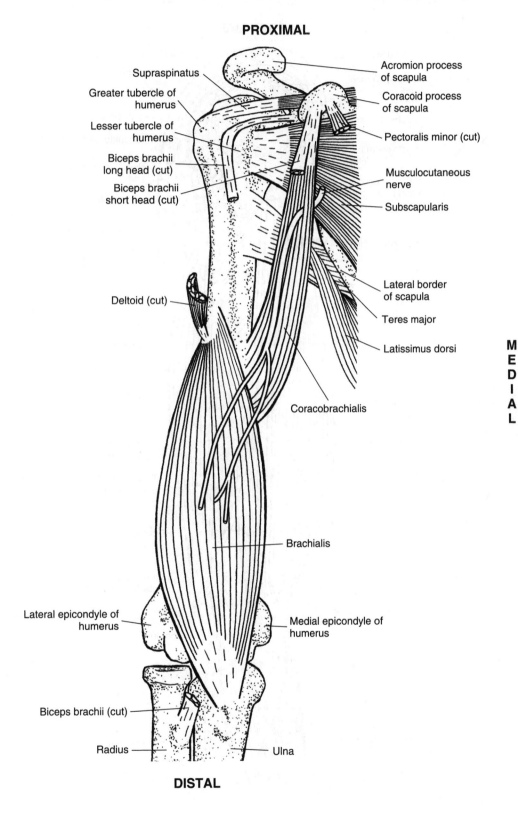

Supraspinatus

Greater tubercle of humerus

Lesser tubercle of humerus

Biceps brachii long head (cut)

Biceps brachii short head (cut)

Acromion process of scapula

Coracoid process of scapula

Pectoralis minor (cut)

Musculocutaneous nerve

Subscapularis

Deltoid (cut)

Lateral border of scapula

Teres major

Latissimus dorsi

L A T E R A L

M E D I A L

Coracobrachialis

Brachialis

Lateral epicondyle of humerus

Medial epicondyle of humerus

Biceps brachii (cut)

Radius

Ulna

DISTAL

MEDIAL VIEW OF THE RIGHT ARM

PROXIMAL

Subdeltoid bursa

Biceps brachii
long head (cut)

Subscapularis
(cut)

Pectoralis major
(cut)

Biceps brachii
short head (cut)

Coracobrachialis
(cut)

Median nerve

Biceps brachii

Bicipital aponeurosis
of biceps brachii

Brachioradialis

Flexor carpi radialis

Supraspinatus (cut)

Head of humerus

Bursa

Infraspinatus (cut)

Shoulder joint capsule

Teres minor (cut)

Deltoid (cut)

Teres major (cut)

Latissimus dorsi (cut)

Deep brachial artery

Brachial artery

Ulnar nerve

Humerus

Triceps brachii
long head

Triceps brachii
medial head

Brachialis

Superior ulnar
collateral artery

Pronator teres

Palmaris longus

Flexor carpi ulnaris

A N T E R I O R

P O S T E R I O R

DISTAL

LATERAL VIEW OF THE RIGHT ARM

PROXIMAL

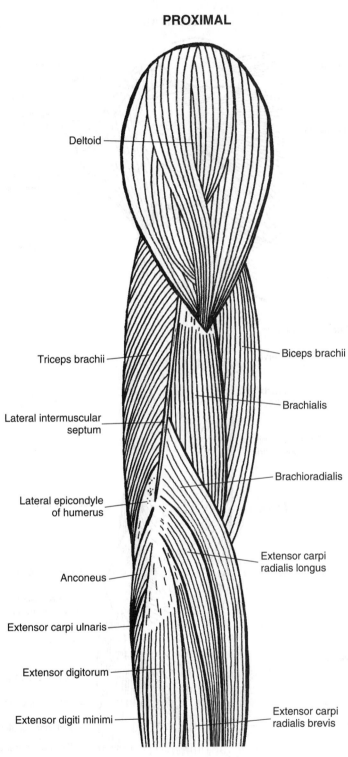

Deltoid

P O S T E R I O R

A N T E R I O R

Triceps brachii

Biceps brachii

Brachialis

Lateral intermuscular septum

Brachioradialis

Lateral epicondyle of humerus

Extensor carpi radialis longus

Anconeus

Extensor carpi ulnaris

Extensor digitorum

Extensor carpi radialis brevis

Extensor digiti minimi

DISTAL

POSTERIOR VIEW OF THE RIGHT ARM

PROXIMAL

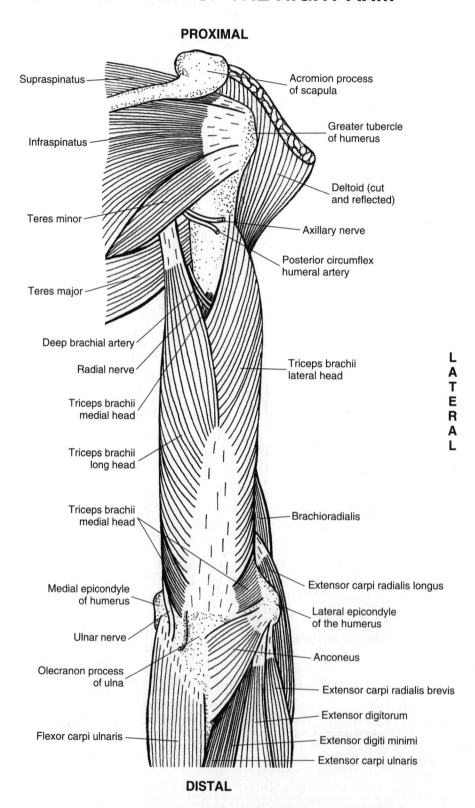

Supraspinatus

Infraspinatus

Teres minor

Teres major

Deep brachial artery

Radial nerve

Triceps brachii medial head

Triceps brachii long head

Triceps brachii medial head

Medial epicondyle of humerus

Ulnar nerve

Olecranon process of ulna

Flexor carpi ulnaris

Acromion process of scapula

Greater tubercle of humerus

Deltoid (cut and reflected)

Axillary nerve

Posterior circumflex humeral artery

Triceps brachii lateral head

Brachioradialis

Extensor carpi radialis longus

Lateral epicondyle of the humerus

Anconeus

Extensor carpi radialis brevis

Extensor digitorum

Extensor digiti minimi

Extensor carpi ulnaris

M E D I A L

L A T E R A L

DISTAL

ANTERIOR VIEW OF THE RIGHT GLENOHUMERAL JOINT

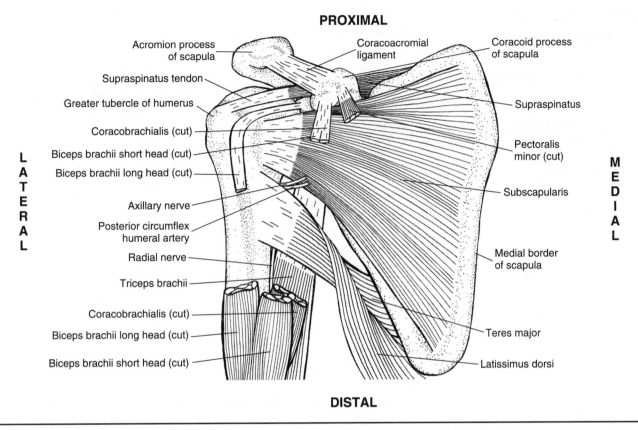

PROXIMAL

Acromion process of scapula

Supraspinatus tendon

Greater tubercle of humerus

Coracobrachialis (cut)

Biceps brachii short head (cut)

Biceps brachii long head (cut)

Axillary nerve

Posterior circumflex humeral artery

Radial nerve

Triceps brachii

Coracobrachialis (cut)

Biceps brachii long head (cut)

Biceps brachii short head (cut)

Coracoacromial ligament

Coracoid process of scapula

Supraspinatus

Pectoralis minor (cut)

Subscapularis

Medial border of scapula

Teres major

Latissimus dorsi

L A T E R A L

M E D I A L

DISTAL

POSTERIOR VIEW OF THE RIGHT GLENOHUMERAL JOINT

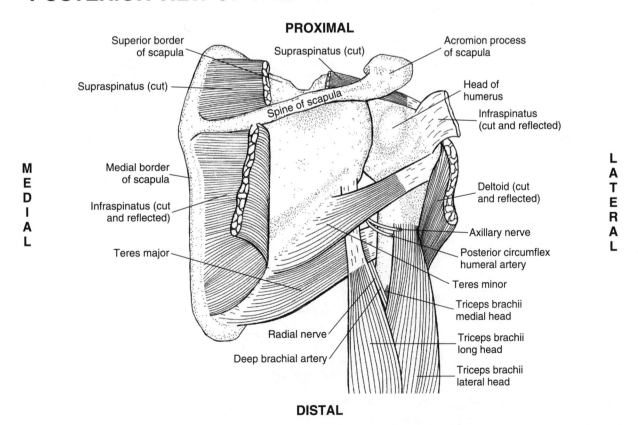

PROXIMAL

Superior border of scapula

Supraspinatus (cut)

Spine of scapula

Medial border of scapula

Infraspinatus (cut and reflected)

Teres major

Radial nerve

Deep brachial artery

Supraspinatus (cut)

Acromion process of scapula

Head of humerus

Infraspinatus (cut and reflected)

Deltoid (cut and reflected)

Axillary nerve

Posterior circumflex humeral artery

Teres minor

Triceps brachii medial head

Triceps brachii long head

Triceps brachii lateral head

M E D I A L

L A T E R A L

DISTAL

SUPRASPINATUS

(OF THE ROTATOR
CUFF GROUP)

soo-pra-spy-**nay**-tus

Action
Abduction of the arm at the shoulder joint
Innervation
The suprascapular nerve
Arterial Supply
The suprascapular artery
Myofascial Meridians
Deep back arm line

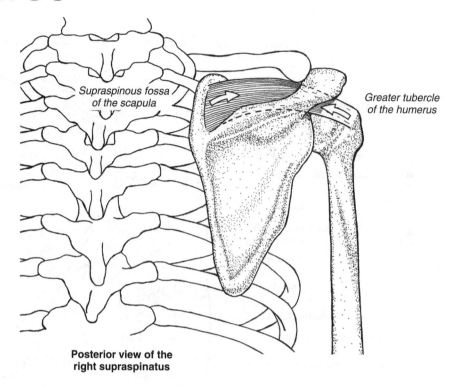

Posterior view of the right supraspinatus

INFRASPINATUS

(OF THE ROTATOR CUFF GROUP)

in-fra-spy-**nay**-tus

Action
Lateral rotation of the arm at the shoulder joint
Innervation
The suprascapular nerve
Arterial Supply
The suprascapular artery
Myofascial Meridians
Deep back arm line

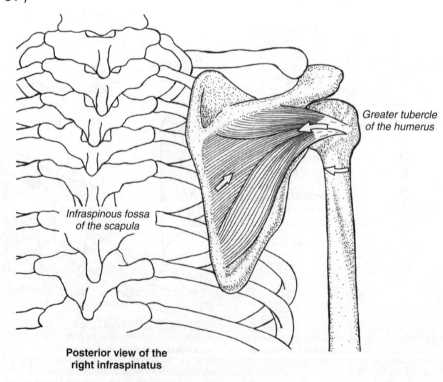

Posterior view of the right infraspinatus

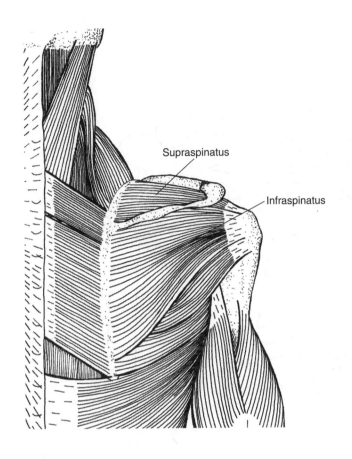

Supraspinatus

Infraspinatus

DID
YOU
KNOW

The distal tendon of the supraspinatus is the most commonly injured tendon of the rotator cuff group.

DID
YOU
KNOW

It is often impinged between the greater tubercle of the humerus and acromion process of the scapula.

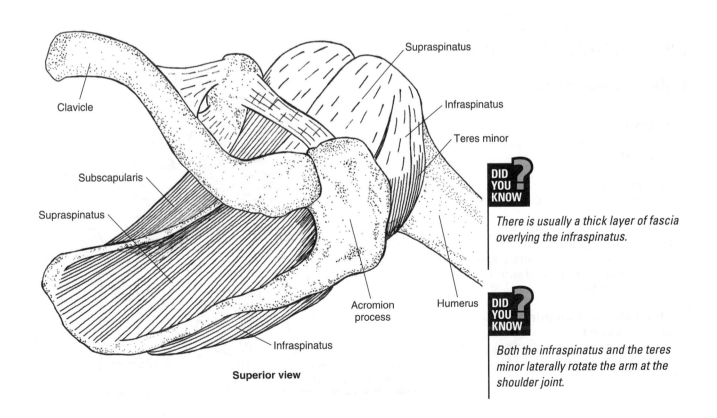

Clavicle

Subscapularis

Supraspinatus

Infraspinatus

Supraspinatus

Infraspinatus

Teres minor

Acromion
process

Humerus

Superior view

DID
YOU
KNOW

There is usually a thick layer of fascia overlying the infraspinatus.

DID
YOU
KNOW

Both the infraspinatus and the teres minor laterally rotate the arm at the shoulder joint.

TERES MINOR
(OF THE ROTATOR CUFF GROUP)

te-reez my-nor

Action
Lateral rotation of the arm at the shoulder joint
Adduction of the arm at the shoulder joint

Innervation
The axillary nerve

Arterial Supply
The circumflex scapular artery

Myofascial Meridians
Deep back arm line

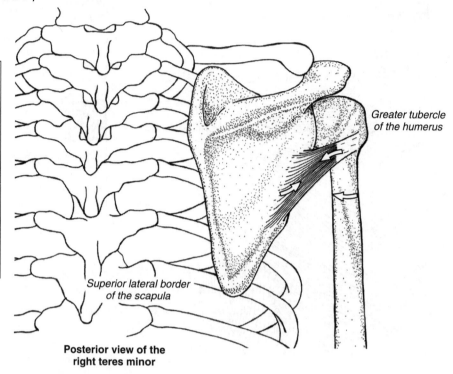

Greater tubercle of the humerus

Superior lateral border of the scapula

Posterior view of the right teres minor

SUBSCAPULARIS
(OF THE ROTATOR CUFF GROUP)

sub-skap-u-la-ris

Action
Medial rotation of the arm at the shoulder joint

Innervation
The upper and lower subscapular nerves

Arterial Supply
The circumflex scapular artery and the dorsal scapular and suprascapular arteries

Myofascial Meridians
Deep back arm line

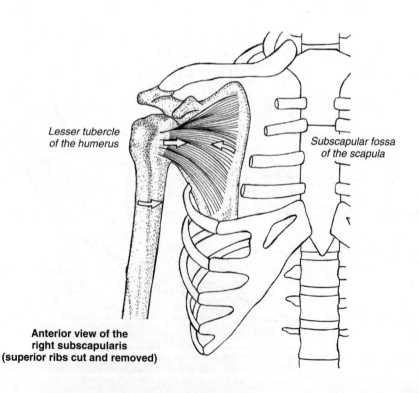

Lesser tubercle of the humerus

Subscapular fossa of the scapula

Anterior view of the right subscapularis (superior ribs cut and removed)

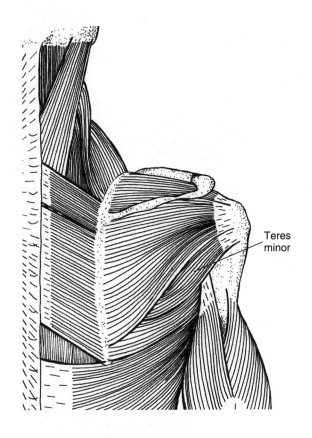

Teres minor

The teres minor often blends with the infraspinatus.

The teres minor and teres major are both round ("teres" means round) and next to each other; but are in antagonistic functional groups. The teres minor is a lateral rotator, and the teres major is a medial rotator.

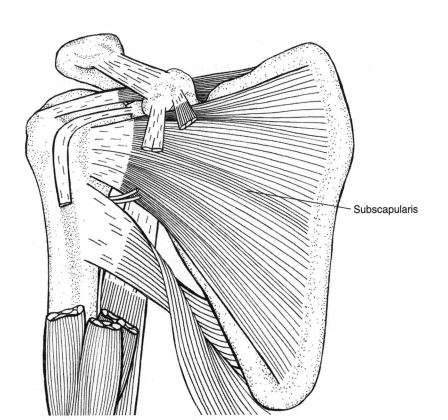

Subscapularis

The subscapularis is the only member of the rotator cuff group that attaches onto the anterior (subscapular) surface of the scapula and onto the lesser tubercle of the humerus.

TERES MAJOR

te-reez **may**-jor

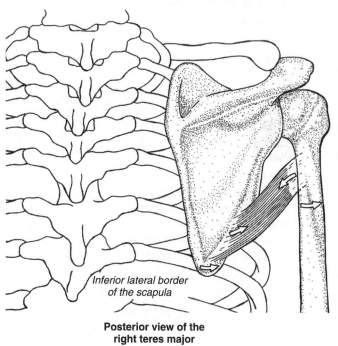

Inferior lateral border
of the scapula

**Posterior view of the
right teres major**

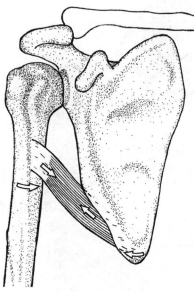

Medial lip of the
bicipital groove
of the humerus

**Anterior view of the
right teres major**

Actions
Medial rotation of the arm at the
    shoulder joint
Adduction of the arm at the
    shoulder joint
Extension of the arm at the
    shoulder joint
Upward rotation of the scapula at
    the scapulocostal joint

Innervation
The lower subscapular nerve

Arterial Supply
The circumflex scapular artery

Myofascial Meridians
Superficial front arm line
Involved: Deep back arm line

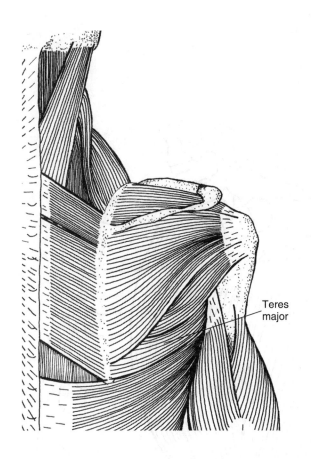

Teres
major

The teres major can do all three actions of the arm at the shoulder joint (extension, adduction, and medial rotation) that the latissimus dorsi can. Therefore, these muscles often work together.

The teres major and teres minor are antagonistic to each other. The teres major medially rotates the arm; the teres minor laterally rotates the arm.

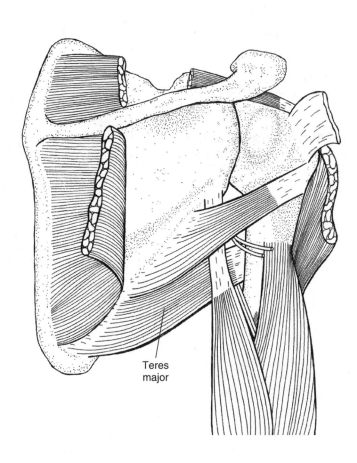

Teres
major

DELTOID

del-toid

Actions
Abduction of the arm at the shoulder joint (entire muscle)

Flexion of the arm at the shoulder joint (anterior deltoid)

Extension of the arm at the shoulder joint (posterior deltoid)

Medial rotation of the arm at the shoulder joint (anterior deltoid)

Lateral rotation of the arm at the shoulder joint (posterior deltoid)

Downward rotation of the scapula at the scapulocostal joint (entire muscle)

Ipsilateral rotation of the trunk at the shoulder joint (anterior deltoid)

Contralateral rotation of the trunk at the shoulder joint (posterior deltoid)

Innervation
The axillary nerve

Arterial Supply
The anterior and posterior circumflex humeral arteries

Myofascial Meridians
Superficial back arm line

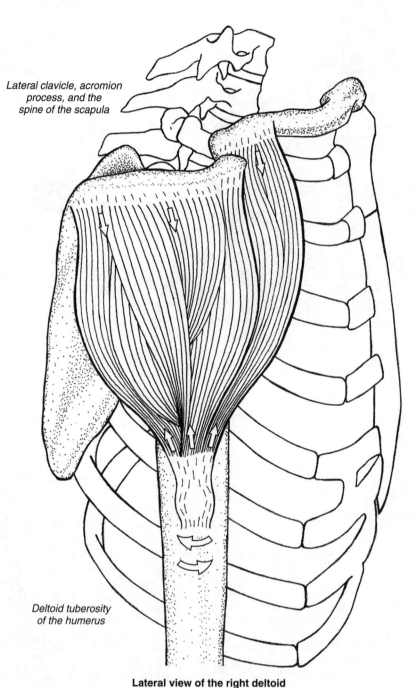

Lateral clavicle, acromion process, and the spine of the scapula

Deltoid tuberosity of the humerus

Lateral view of the right deltoid

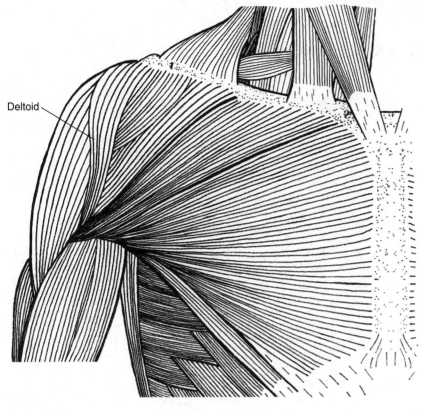

Deltoid

DID YOU KNOW ?

The name "deltoid" tells us that it has a triangular shape like the Greek letter delta (Δ).

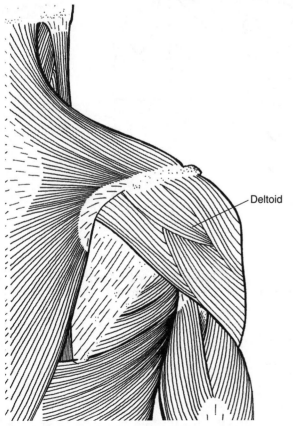

Deltoid

DID YOU KNOW ?

The deltoid has three heads: anterior, posterior, and middle.

CORACOBRACHIALIS

kor-a-ko-**bray**-key-**al**-is

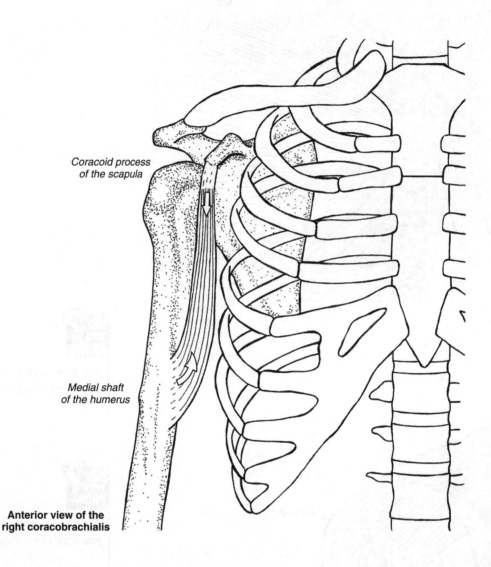

Coracoid process
of the scapula

Medial shaft
of the humerus

**Anterior view of the
right coracobrachialis**

Actions	**Innervation**	**Myofascial Meridians**
Flexion of the arm at the shoulder joint	The musculocutaneous nerve	Deep front arm line
Adduction of the arm at the shoulder joint	**Arterial Supply**	
	The muscular branches of the brachial artery	

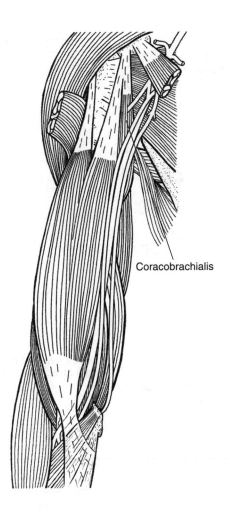

Coracobrachialis

DID YOU KNOW

The name coracobrachialis tells us that this muscle attaches from the coracoid process of the scapula to the brachium (arm). That, in turn, tells us that it crosses the shoulder joint, so its actions must be at the shoulder joint.

DID YOU KNOW

The coracobrachialis blends with the short head of the biceps brachii.

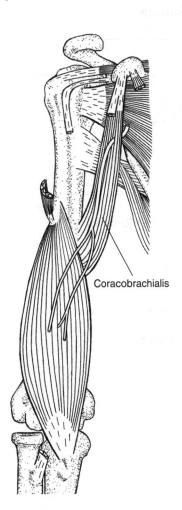

Coracobrachialis

BICEPS BRACHII

by-seps **bray**-key-eye

Actions
Flexion of the forearm at the elbow joint (entire muscle)
Supination of the forearm at the radioulnar joints (entire muscle)
Flexion of the arm at the shoulder joint (entire muscle)
Abduction of the arm at the shoulder joint (long head)
Adduction of the arm at the shoulder joint (short head)

Innervation
The musculocutaneous nerve

Arterial Supply
The muscular branches of the brachial artery

Myofascial Meridians
Deep front arm line

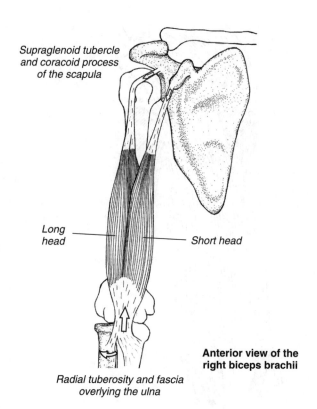

Supraglenoid tubercle and coracoid process of the scapula

Long head   *Short head*

Anterior view of the right biceps brachii

Radial tuberosity and fascia overlying the ulna

BRACHIALIS

bray-key-**al**-is

Action
Flexion of the forearm at the elbow joint

Innervation
The musculocutaneous nerve

Arterial Supply
Muscular branches of the brachial artery

Myofascial Meridians
Deep front arm line

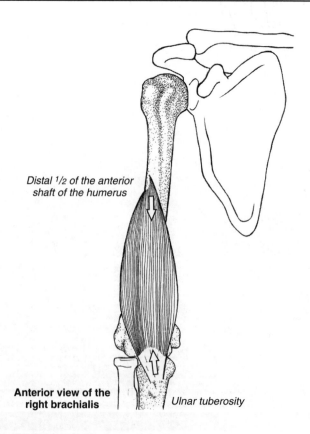

Distal 1/2 of the anterior shaft of the humerus

Anterior view of the right brachialis

Ulnar tuberosity

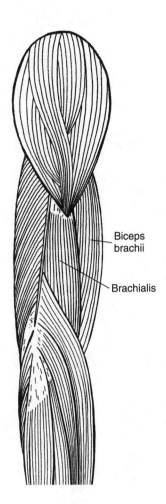

Biceps brachii

Brachialis

DID
YOU
KNOW

The bicipital groove of the humerus is so named because the long head of the biceps brachii courses through it.

DID
YOU
KNOW

The short head of the biceps brachii is one of three muscles that attach onto the coracoid process of the scapula (along with the coracobrachialis and pectoralis minor).

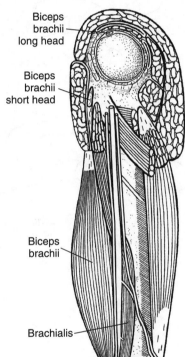

Biceps brachii long head

Biceps brachii short head

Biceps brachii

Brachialis

Biceps brachii bicipital aponeurosis

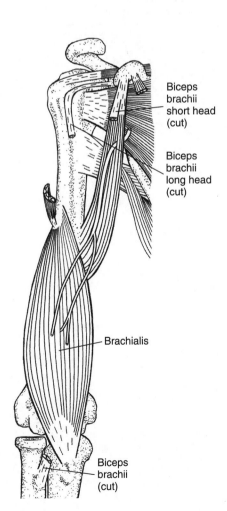

Biceps brachii short head (cut)

Biceps brachii long head (cut)

Brachialis

Biceps brachii (cut)

DID
YOU
KNOW

The brachialis is a strong and fairly large muscle, which accounts for much of the contour of the biceps brachii being so visible. Behind every great biceps brachii is a great brachialis ☺.

DID
YOU
KNOW

The brachialis is one of the "3Bs of elbow joint flexion," along with the biceps brachii and brachioradialis.

TRICEPS BRACHII

try-seps **bray**-key-eye

Actions
Extension of the forearm
  at the elbow joint
  (entire muscle)
Adduction of the arm
  at the shoulder joint
  (long head)
Extension of the arm
  at the shoulder joint
  (long head)

Innervation
The radial nerve

Arterial Supply
The deep brachial artery

**Myofascial
Meridians**
Deep back arm line

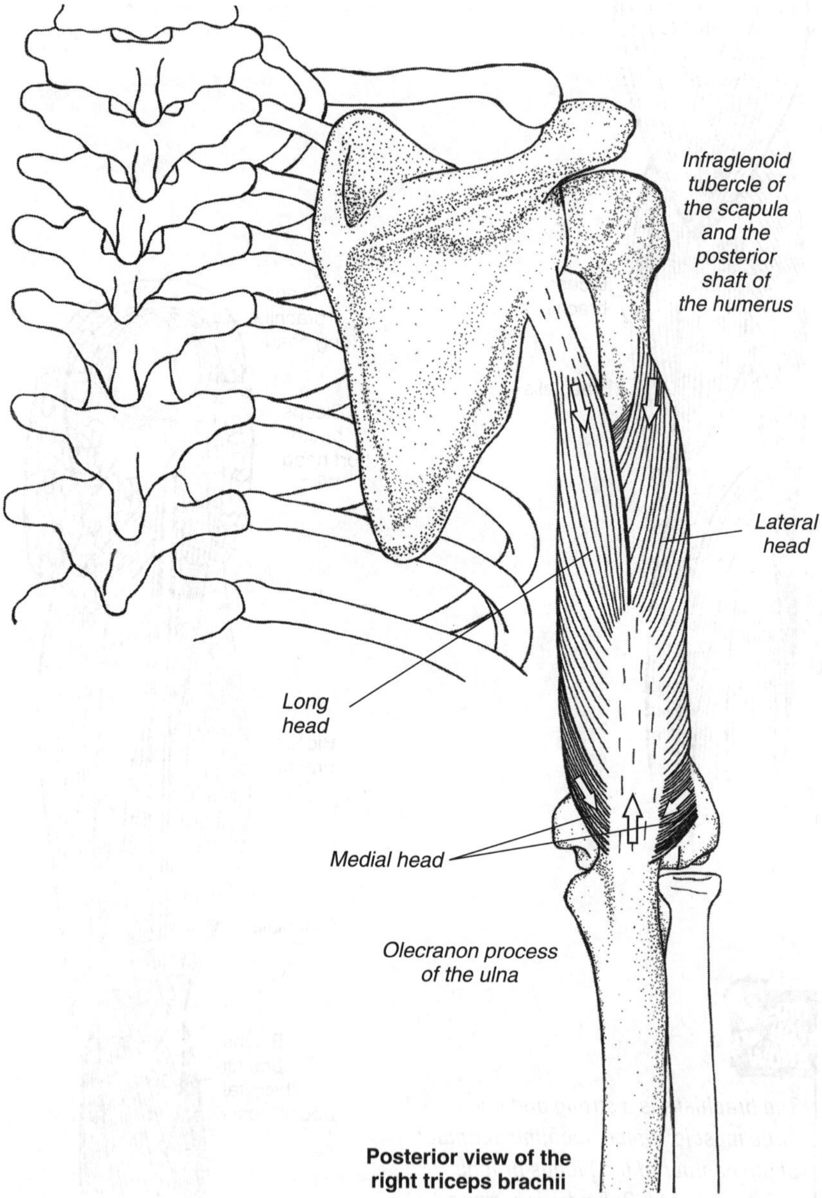

Infraglenoid
tubercle of
the scapula
and the
posterior
shaft of
the humerus

Lateral
head

Long
head

Medial head

Olecranon process
of the ulna

**Posterior view of the
right triceps brachii**

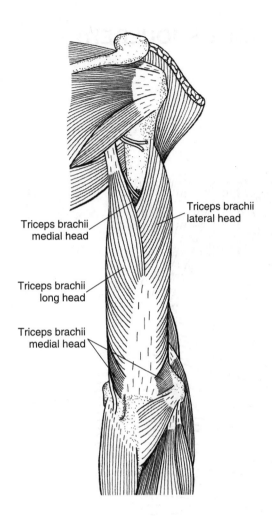

Triceps brachii
medial head

Triceps brachii
lateral head

Triceps brachii
long head

Triceps brachii
medial head

*The triceps brachii has three heads,
the lateral, medial, and long heads;
only the long head crosses, and
therefore can move, the shoulder joint.*

*Sometimes the medial head is named
the deep head because the majority of
it lies deep to the other two heads.*

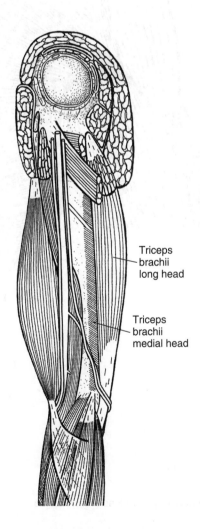

Triceps
brachii
long head

Triceps
brachii
medial head

ANTERIOR VIEW OF THE RIGHT SHOULDER

SUPERIOR

LATERAL

MEDIAL

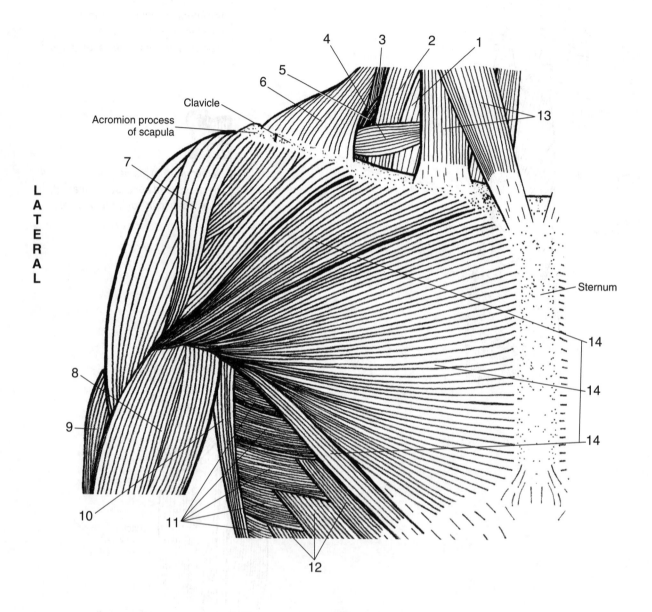

Clavicle

Acromion process
of scapula

Sternum

INFERIOR

POSTERIOR VIEW OF THE SHOULDERS
(SUPERFICIAL AND INTERMEDIATE)

SUPERIOR

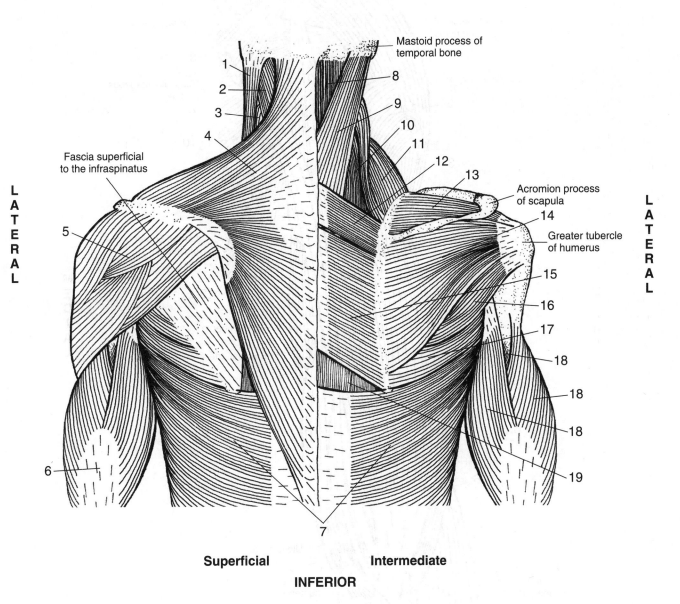

LATERAL

LATERAL

Mastoid process of
temporal bone

Fascia superficial
to the infraspinatus

Acromion process
of scapula

Greater tubercle
of humerus

Superficial   Intermediate

INFERIOR

ANTERIOR VIEW OF THE RIGHT ARM (SUPERFICIAL)

PROXIMAL

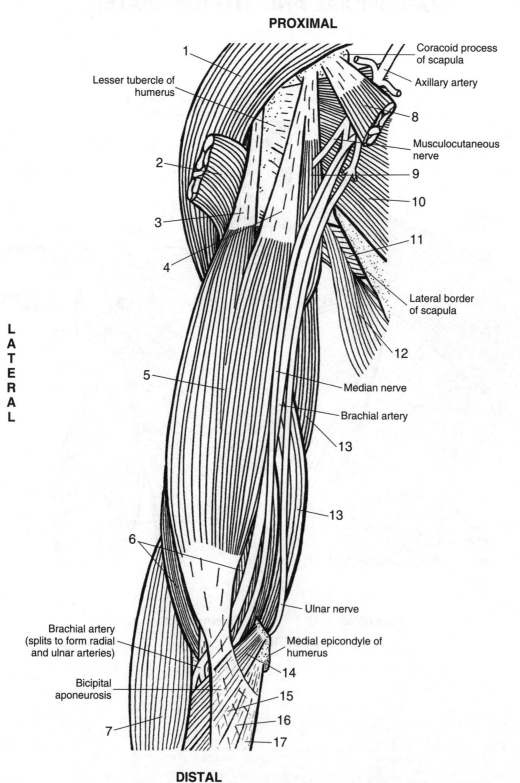

Lesser tubercle of humerus

Coracoid process of scapula

Axillary artery

Musculocutaneous nerve

Lateral border of scapula

LATERAL

MEDIAL

Median nerve

Brachial artery

Ulnar nerve

Brachial artery (splits to form radial and ulnar arteries)

Bicipital aponeurosis

Medial epicondyle of humerus

1
2
3
4
5
6
7
8
9
10
11
12
13
13
14
15
16
17

DISTAL

ANTERIOR VIEW OF THE RIGHT ARM (DEEP)

PROXIMAL

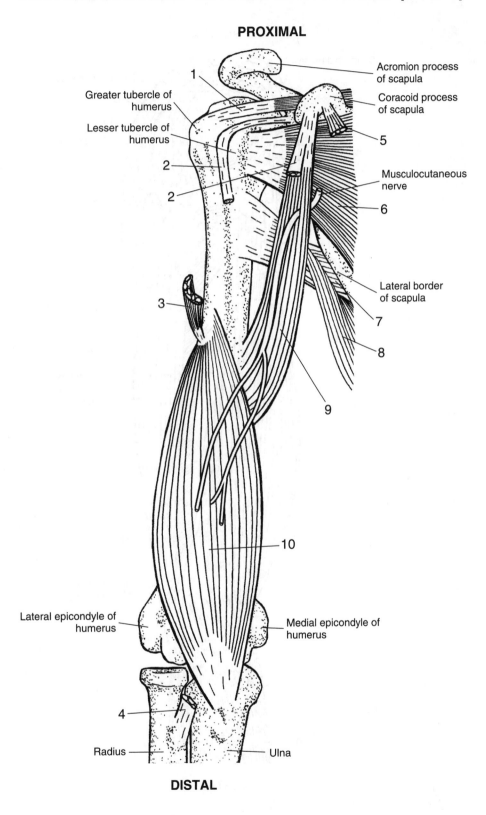

1

Greater tubercle of
humerus

Lesser tubercle of
humerus

2

2

3

LATERAL

Acromion process
of scapula

Coracoid process
of scapula

5

Musculocutaneous
nerve

6

Lateral border
of scapula

7

8

9

MEDIAL

10

Lateral epicondyle of
humerus

Medial epicondyle of
humerus

4

Radius

Ulna

DISTAL

MEDIAL VIEW OF THE RIGHT ARM

PROXIMAL

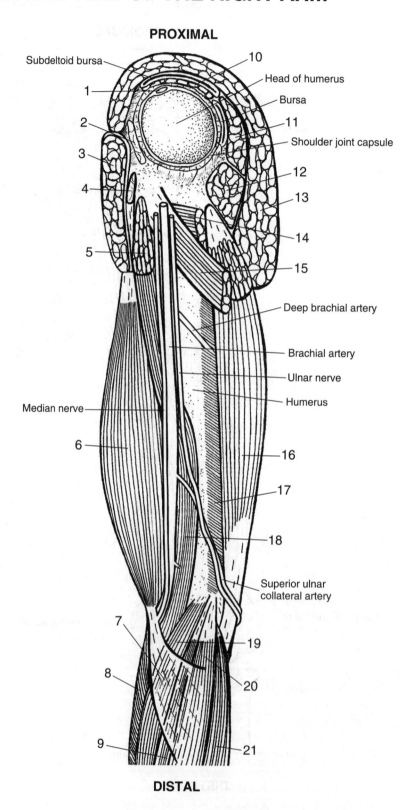

Subdeltoid bursa

10

Head of humerus

1

Bursa

2

11

Shoulder joint capsule

3

12

4

13

5

14

15

Deep brachial artery

A N T E R I O R

Brachial artery

Ulnar nerve

Median nerve

Humerus

6

16

17

18

Superior ulnar collateral artery

7

19

8

20

9

21

P O S T E R I O R

DISTAL

LATERAL VIEW OF THE RIGHT ARM

PROXIMAL

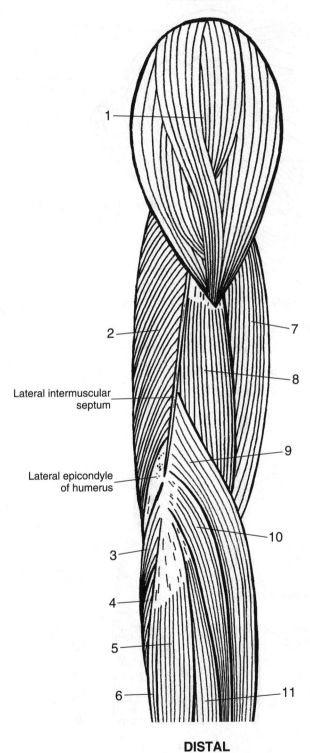

Lateral intermuscular
septum

Lateral epicondyle
of humerus

**P
O
S
T
E
R
I
O
R**

**A
N
T
E
R
I
O
R**

DISTAL

POSTERIOR VIEW OF THE RIGHT ARM

PROXIMAL

M E D I A L

L A T E R A L

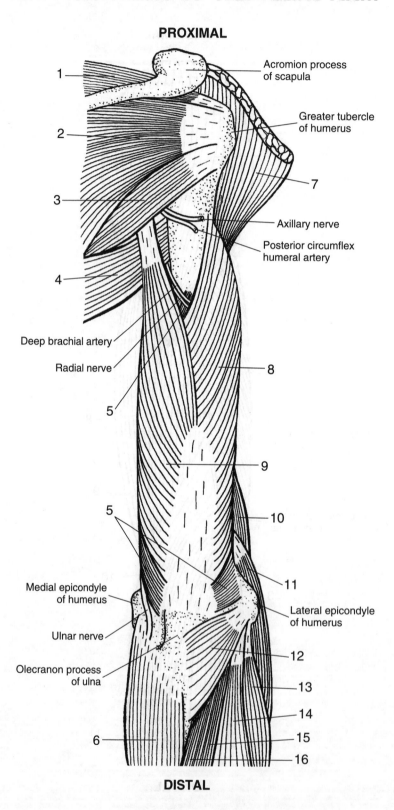

1

Acromion process
of scapula

2

Greater tubercle
of humerus

3

7

Axillary nerve

Posterior circumflex
humeral artery

4

Deep brachial artery

Radial nerve

5

8

9

5

10

11

Medial epicondyle
of humerus

Lateral epicondyle
of humerus

Ulnar nerve

12

Olecranon process
of ulna

13

14

6

15

16

DISTAL

ANTERIOR VIEW OF THE RIGHT GLENOHUMERAL JOINT

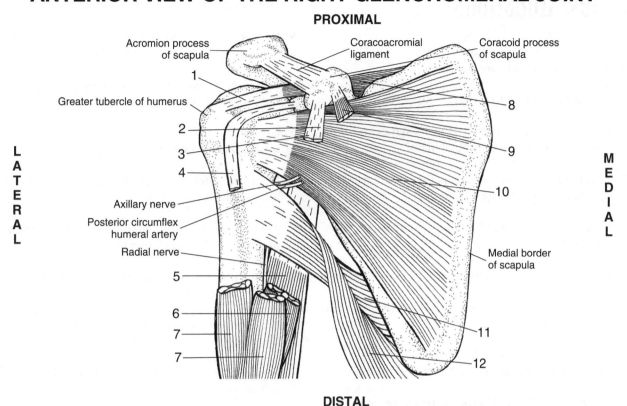

PROXIMAL

Acromion process of scapula

Coracoacromial ligament

Coracoid process of scapula

1

Greater tubercle of humerus

2

3

4

Axillary nerve

Posterior circumflex humeral artery

Radial nerve

5

6

7

7

8

9

10

Medial border of scapula

11

12

L A T E R A L

M E D I A L

DISTAL

POSTERIOR VIEW OF THE RIGHT GLENOHUMERAL JOINT

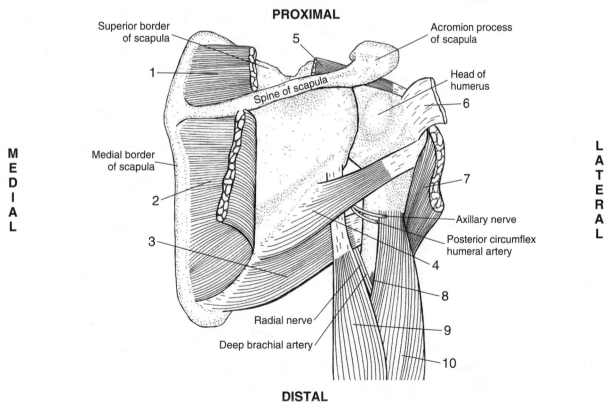

PROXIMAL

Superior border of scapula

5

Acromion process of scapula

1

Spine of scapula

Head of humerus

6

Medial border of scapula

2

7

3

Axillary nerve

Posterior circumflex humeral artery

4

Radial nerve

8

Deep brachial artery

9

10

M E D I A L

L A T E R A L

DISTAL

Review Questions

Muscles of the Scapula/Arm
Answers to these questions are found on page 490.

1. Name an antagonist to the brachialis.

2. Is the short head of the biceps brachii synergistic with or antagonistic to the coracobrachialis?

3. From the anterior perspective, is the coracobrachialis superficial or deep to the subscapularis?

4. What joint action would lengthen and stretch the infraspinatus?

5. How is the deltoid synergistic with the supraspinatus?

6. The long head of the triceps brachii passes between which two muscles?

7. From a posterior perspective, where is the teres major compared to the long head of the triceps brachii?

8. Which is the deepest head of the triceps brachii?

9. How are the anterior and posterior fibers of the deltoid antagonistic to each other?

10. Which portion of the deltoid attaches to the lateral clavicle?

11. The distal attachments of the supraspinatus and infraspinatus are deep to what muscle?

12. Name three muscles that attach to the coracoid process of the scapula.

13. Name a rotator cuff muscle that is synergistic to the teres major.

14. Which head of the triceps brachii will be stretched if the shoulder joint is flexed?

15. Where is the scapular attachment of the teres major relative to the teres minor?

16. Is the pronator teres synergistic with or antagonistic to the triceps brachii?

17. What muscle is immediately anterior to the triceps brachii on the lateral side?

18. Will passive lateral rotation of the arm at the shoulder joint shorten or lengthen the teres minor?

19. If the forearm is pronated at the radioulnar joints, will the brachialis be shortened or lengthened?

20. If the arm is passively flexed at the shoulder joint, will the coracobrachialis be shortened or lengthened?

21. From the anterior perspective, is the coracobrachialis superficial or deep to the deltoid?

22. From the anterior perspective, which is deeper, the biceps brachii or the brachialis?

23. Are the biceps brachii and brachialis synergistic with or antagonistic to each other?

24. What humeral joint actions would lengthen and stretch the teres major?

25. Besides the teres major, what other muscle attaches to the medial lip of the bicipital groove of the humerus?

26. Which rotator cuff muscle runs deep to the acromion process of the scapula?

27. From which perspective is the greatest amount of the brachialis superficial?

28. How many joints does the biceps brachii cross?

29. What two other muscles share the same distal attachment with the infraspinatus?

30. If the elbow joint is passively extended, will the triceps brachii be shortened or lengthened?

31. What four muscles comprise the rotator cuff group?

32. Are the teres minor and teres major synergistic or antagonistic to each other?

33. What rotator cuff muscle is synergistic with the teres minor?

34. How are the anterior fibers and posterior fibers of the deltoid synergistic with each other?

35. Name three muscles that attach to the greater tubercle of the humerus.

36. Which portion of the pectoralis major is adjacent to the deltoid?

37. What joint actions at the shoulder joint would stretch the coracobrachialis?

38. Is the infraspinatus superior or inferior to the supraspinatus?

39. Where is the teres minor relative to the teres major?

40. What muscle from the pelvis and back shares the same humeral joint actions with the teres major?

41. What two muscles attach to the lateral clavicle, acromion process, and spine of the scapula?

42. What muscle is named for being triangular in shape?

Muscles of the Forearm 11

Note: Throughout this chapter, muscle attachments are indicated by italics.

☺ More review activities on Evolve at: http://evolve.elsevier.com/Muscolino/anatomycoloring/

ANTERIOR VIEW OF THE RIGHT FOREARM (SUPERFICIAL)

PROXIMAL

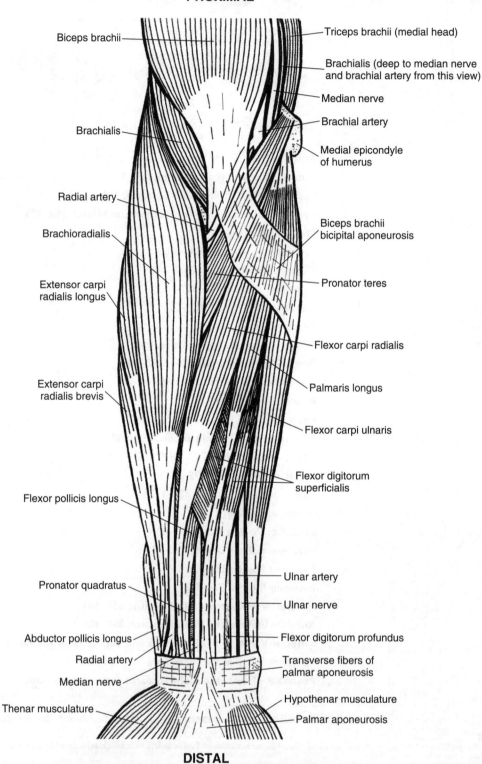

Biceps brachii

Brachialis

Radial artery

Brachioradialis

Extensor carpi
radialis longus

Extensor carpi
radialis brevis

Flexor pollicis longus

Pronator quadratus

Abductor pollicis longus

Radial artery

Median nerve

Thenar musculature

Triceps brachii (medial head)

Brachialis (deep to median nerve
and brachial artery from this view)

Median nerve

Brachial artery

Medial epicondyle
of humerus

Biceps brachii
bicipital aponeurosis

Pronator teres

Flexor carpi radialis

Palmaris longus

Flexor carpi ulnaris

Flexor digitorum
superficialis

Ulnar artery

Ulnar nerve

Flexor digitorum profundus

Transverse fibers of
palmar aponeurosis

Hypothenar musculature

Palmar aponeurosis

LATERAL   RADIAL

ULNAR   MEDIAL

DISTAL

ANTERIOR VIEW OF THE RIGHT FOREARM (INTERMEDIATE)

PROXIMAL

Biceps brachii

Brachial artery (splits to form radial and ulnar arteries)

Brachialis

Radial nerve

Head of the radius

Brachialis tendon

Biceps brachii tendon

Supinator

Brachioradialis

Pronator teres (cut)

Flexor pollicis longus

Abductor pollicis longus

Pronator quadratus

Radial artery

Flexor carpi radialis (cut)

Palmaris longus cut and in reflected fibers of transverse fibers of palmar aponeurosis

Thenar musculature

Median nerve

Triceps brachii medial head

Pronator teres humeral head (cut and reflected)

Medial epicondyle of humerus

Brachialis

Flexor carpi radialis (cut)

Palmaris longus (cut)

Pronator teres ulnar head (cut)

Flexor digitorum profundus

Flexor carpi ulnaris

Flexor digitorum superficialis

Median nerve

Ulnar artery

Ulnar nerve

Flexor digitorum profundus

Flexor retinaculum (transverse carpal ligament)

Hypothenar musculature

L A T E R A L

R A D I A L

U L N A R

M E D I A L

DISTAL

ANTERIOR VIEW OF THE RIGHT FOREARM (DEEP)

PROXIMAL

Brachial artery

Brachialis

Lateral epicondyle
of humerus

Radial nerve

Biceps brachii

Supinator

Flexor digitorum
superficialis (cut)

Pronator teres
(cut and reflected)

Flexor pollicis
longus (cut)

Radius

Pronator quadratus

Radial artery

Brachioradialis (cut)

Flexor carpi radialis (cut)

Flexor pollicis longus (cut)

Median nerve

Ulnar nerve

Triceps brachii

Pronator teres
humeral head
(cut and reflected)

Medial epicondyle
of humerus

Flexor carpi radialis
(cut and reflected)

Palmaris longus (cut)

Flexor carpi ulnaris (cut)

Flexor digitorum superficialis
humeroulnar head (cut)

Pronator teres
ulnar head (cut)

Ulnar artery

Ulnar nerve

Flexor digitorum
profundus (cut)

Flexor carpi ulnaris
(cut)

L A T E R A L

R A D I A L

U L N A R

M E D I A L

DISTAL

ANTERIOR VIEW OF THE PRONATORS AND SUPINATOR OF THE RIGHT RADIUS

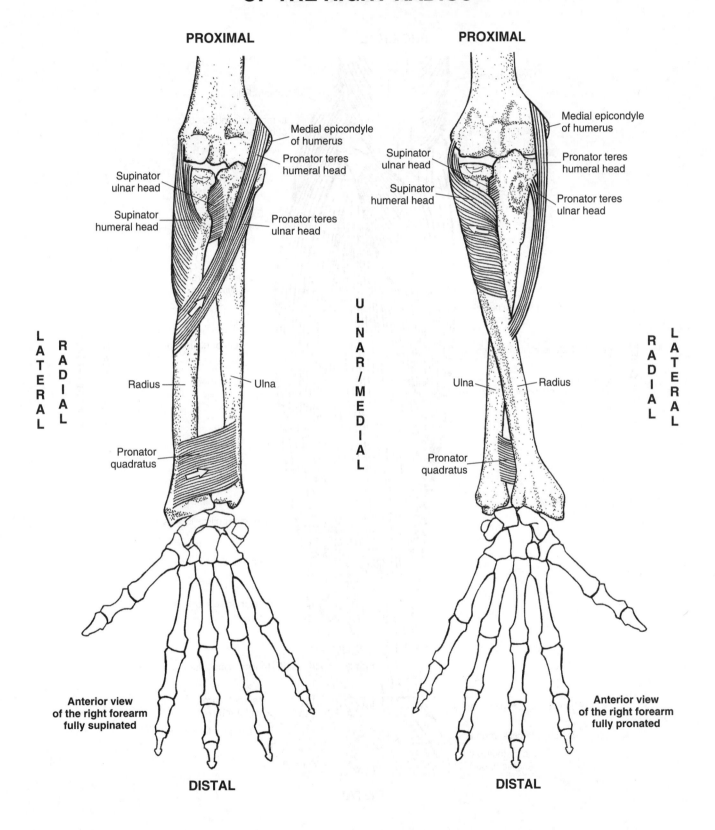

PROXIMAL

Medial epicondyle of humerus

Pronator teres humeral head

Supinator ulnar head

Supinator humeral head

Pronator teres ulnar head

LATERAL

RADIAL

Radius — Ulna

Pronator quadratus

Anterior view of the right forearm fully supinated

DISTAL

ULNAR/MEDIAL

PROXIMAL

Medial epicondyle of humerus

Supinator ulnar head

Pronator teres humeral head

Supinator humeral head

Pronator teres ulnar head

RADIAL

LATERAL

Ulna — Radius

Pronator quadratus

Anterior view of the right forearm fully pronated

DISTAL

POSTERIOR VIEW OF THE RIGHT FOREARM (SUPERFICIAL)

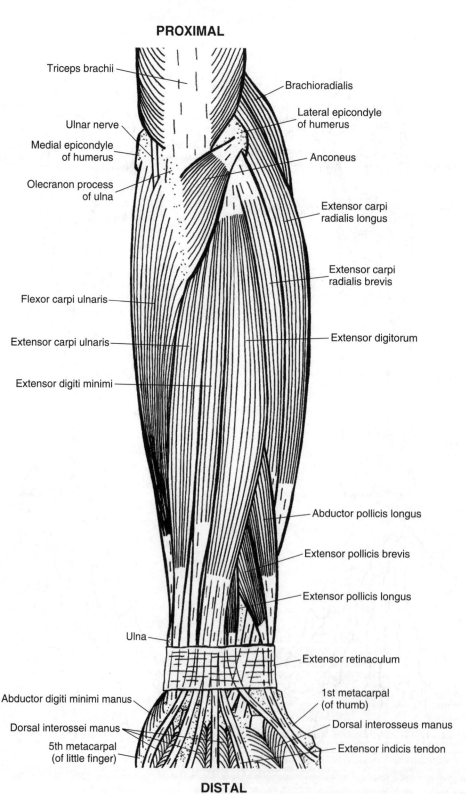

PROXIMAL

Triceps brachii

Ulnar nerve

Medial epicondyle of humerus

Olecranon process of ulna

Flexor carpi ulnaris

Extensor carpi ulnaris

Extensor digiti minimi

Brachioradialis

Lateral epicondyle of humerus

Anconeus

Extensor carpi radialis longus

Extensor carpi radialis brevis

Extensor digitorum

M E D I A L

U L N A R

R A D I A L

L A T E R A L

Abductor pollicis longus

Extensor pollicis brevis

Extensor pollicis longus

Ulna

Extensor retinaculum

Abductor digiti minimi manus

1st metacarpal (of thumb)

Dorsal interossei manus

Dorsal interosseus manus

5th metacarpal (of little finger)

Extensor indicis tendon

DISTAL

POSTERIOR VIEW OF THE RIGHT FOREARM (DEEP)

PROXIMAL

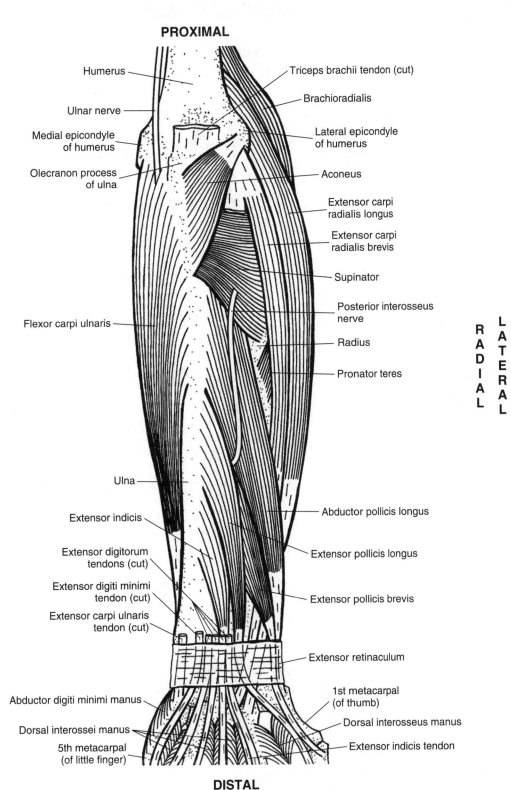

Humerus

Triceps brachii tendon (cut)

Ulnar nerve

Brachioradialis

Medial epicondyle
of humerus

Lateral epicondyle
of humerus

Olecranon process
of ulna

Aconeus

Extensor carpi
radialis longus

Extensor carpi
radialis brevis

Supinator

Flexor carpi ulnaris

Posterior interosseus
nerve

Radius

Pronator teres

M E D I A L **U L N A R**

R A D I A L **L A T E R A L**

Ulna

Extensor indicis

Abductor pollicis longus

Extensor digitorum
tendons (cut)

Extensor pollicis longus

Extensor digiti minimi
tendon (cut)

Extensor carpi ulnaris
tendon (cut)

Extensor pollicis brevis

Extensor retinaculum

Abductor digiti minimi manus

1st metacarpal
(of thumb)

Dorsal interossei manus

Dorsal interosseus manus

5th metacarpal
(of little finger)

Extensor indicis tendon

DISTAL

POSTERIOR VIEW OF THE RIGHT FOREARM AND HAND (SUPERFICIAL)

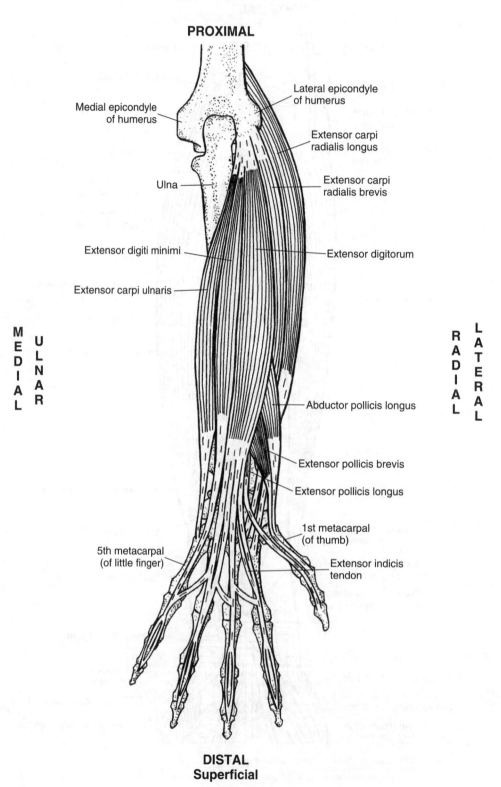

PROXIMAL

Medial epicondyle of humerus

Lateral epicondyle of humerus

Extensor carpi radialis longus

Ulna

Extensor carpi radialis brevis

Extensor digiti minimi

Extensor digitorum

Extensor carpi ulnaris

M E D I A L

U L N A R

R A D I A L

L A T E R A L

Abductor pollicis longus

Extensor pollicis brevis

Extensor pollicis longus

1st metacarpal (of thumb)

5th metacarpal (of little finger)

Extensor indicis tendon

DISTAL
Superficial

POSTERIOR VIEW OF THE RIGHT FOREARM AND HAND (DEEP)

PROXIMAL

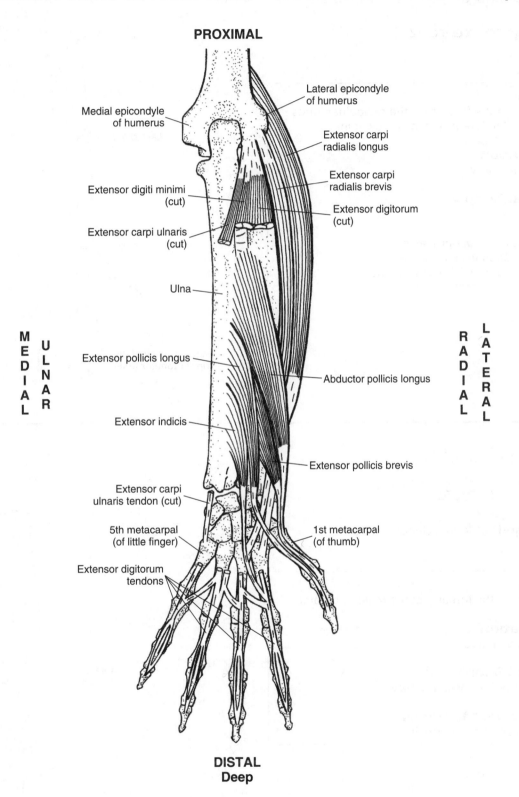

Lateral epicondyle
of humerus

Medial epicondyle
of humerus

Extensor carpi
radialis longus

Extensor carpi
radialis brevis

Extensor digiti minimi
(cut)

Extensor digitorum
(cut)

Extensor carpi ulnaris
(cut)

Ulna

M E D I A L   **U L N A R**

R A D I A L   **L A T E R A L**

Extensor pollicis longus

Abductor pollicis longus

Extensor indicis

Extensor pollicis brevis

Extensor carpi
ulnaris tendon (cut)

5th metacarpal
(of little finger)

1st metacarpal
(of thumb)

Extensor digitorum
tendons

DISTAL
Deep

PRONATOR TERES

pro-**nay**-tor **te**-reez

Actions
Pronation of the forearm at the radioulnar joints
Flexion of the forearm at the elbow joint

Innervation
The median nerve

Arterial Supply
The ulnar artery

Myofascial Meridians
Involved: Deep front arm line
Involved: Superficial back arm line

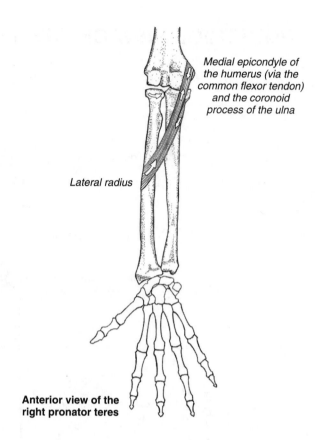

Medial epicondyle of the humerus (via the common flexor tendon) and the coronoid process of the ulna

Lateral radius

Anterior view of the right pronator teres

PRONATOR QUADRATUS

pro-**nay**-tor kwod-**ray**-tus

Action
Pronation of the forearm at the radioulnar joints

Innervation
The median nerve

Arterial Supply
The anterior interosseus artery

Myofascial Meridians
Involved: Deep front arm line

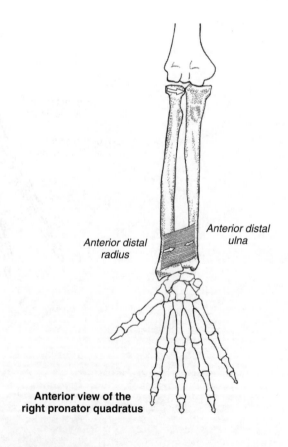

Anterior distal ulna

Anterior distal radius

Anterior view of the right pronator quadratus

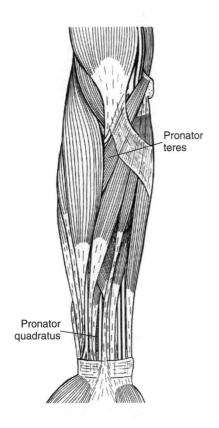

Pronator
teres

Pronator
quadratus

*The median nerve runs between the
two heads of the pronator teres and
can be compressed there, resulting in
pronator teres syndrome.*

*The pronator teres is one of five
muscles of the common flexor belly/
tendon.*

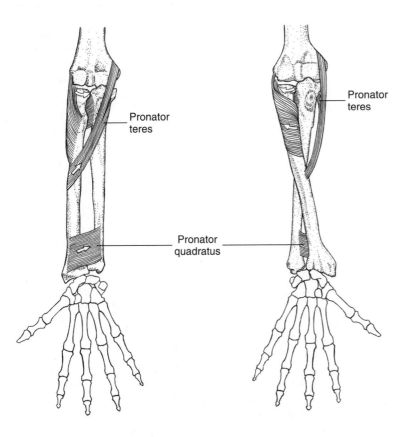

Pronator
teres

Pronator
teres

Pronator
quadratus

*Although it is not very large, the
pronator quadratus is considered by
most sources to be the prime mover
of pronation of the forearm at the
radioulnar joints.*

*The pronator quadratus lies in the deep
anterior compartment of the forearm.*

FLEXOR CARPI RADIALIS

(OF THE WRIST FLEXOR GROUP)

fleks-or **kar**-pie **ray**-dee-a-lis

Actions
Flexion of the hand at the wrist joint
Radial deviation (abduction) of the hand at the
    wrist joint
Flexion of the forearm at the elbow joint
Pronation of the forearm at the radioulnar joints

Innervation
The median nerve

Arterial Supply
The ulnar and radial arteries

Myofascial Meridians
Superficial front arm line

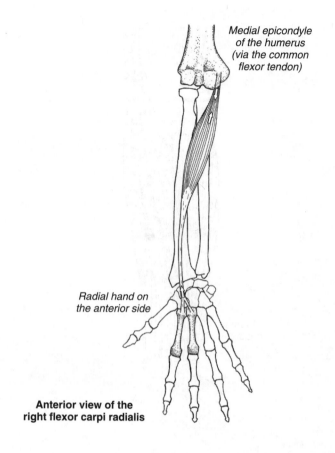

Medial epicondyle of the humerus (via the common flexor tendon)

Radial hand on the anterior side

**Anterior view of the
right flexor carpi radialis**

PALMARIS LONGUS

(OF THE WRIST FLEXOR GROUP)

pall-**ma**-ris **long**-us

Actions
Flexion of the hand at the wrist joint
Flexion of the forearm at the elbow joint
Pronation of the forearm at the radioulnar joints
Wrinkles the skin of the palm

Innervation
The median nerve

Arterial Supply
The ulnar artery

Myofascial Meridians
Superficial front arm line

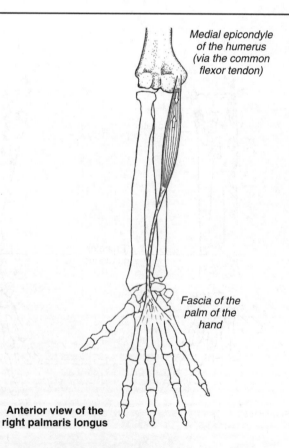

Medial epicondyle of the humerus (via the common flexor tendon)

Fascia of the palm of the hand

**Anterior view of the
right palmaris longus**

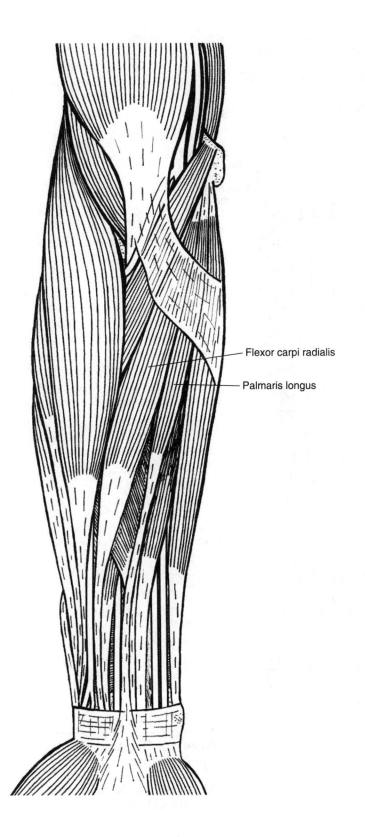

Flexor carpi radialis

Palmaris longus

Irritation and inflammation of the medial condyle of the humerus and/or the common flexor belly/tendon is known as medial elbow tendinopathy, medial epicondylosis, or medial epicondylitis; and is often called golfer's elbow.

The palmaris longus is often missing, sometimes unilaterally, sometimes bilaterally.

If there is a palmaris longus, there will be a palmaris brevis.

FLEXOR CARPI ULNARIS
(OF THE WRIST FLEXOR GROUP)

fleks-or **kar**-pie ul-**na**-ris

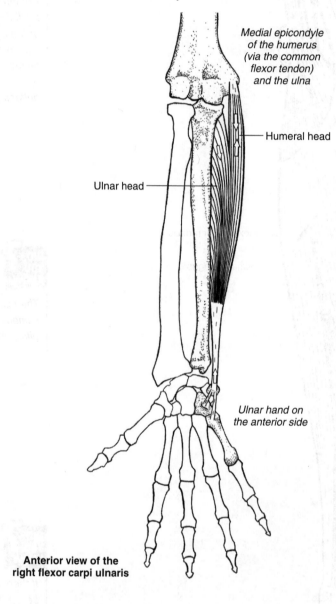

Medial epicondyle of the humerus (via the common flexor tendon) and the ulna

Humeral head

Ulnar head

Ulnar hand on the anterior side

Anterior view of the right flexor carpi ulnaris

Actions	**Innervation**	**Arterial Supply**
Flexion of the hand at the wrist joint	The ulnar nerve	The ulnar artery
Ulnar deviation (adduction) of the hand at the wrist joint		**Myofascial Meridians**
Flexion of the forearm at the elbow joint		Superficial front arm line

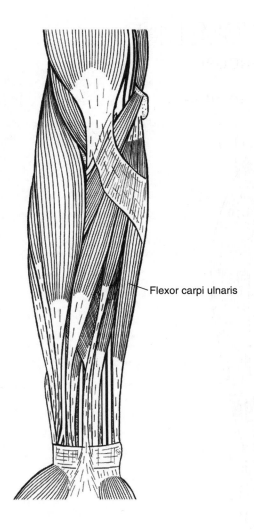

Flexor carpi ulnaris

DID YOU KNOW?

All three wrist flexor group muscles (flexor carpi radialis, palmaris longus, and flexor carpi ulnaris) attach onto the medial epicondyle of the humerus via the common flexor belly/tendon. Only the flexor carpi ulnaris has an additional proximal attachment (onto the ulna). Similarly, the extensor carpi ulnaris is the only wrist extensor that has an additional proximal attachment (onto the ulna).

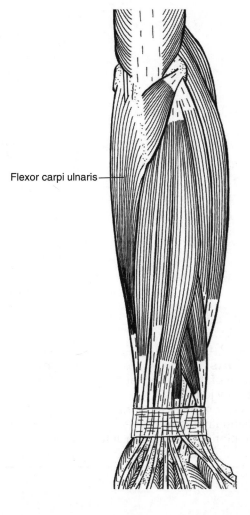

Flexor carpi ulnaris

BRACHIORADIALIS
(OF THE RADIAL GROUP)

bray-key-o-**ray**-dee-**al**-is

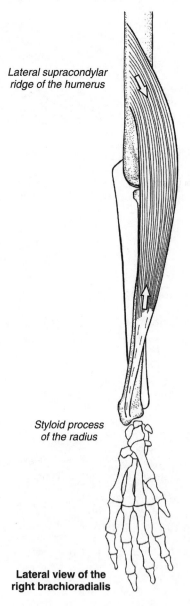

Lateral supracondylar
ridge of the humerus

Styloid process
of the radius

**Lateral view of the
right brachioradialis**

Actions	**Innervation**	**Arterial Supply**
Flexion of the forearm at the elbow joint	The radial nerve	Branches of the brachial artery and the radial artery
Supination of the forearm at the radioulnar joints		
Pronation of the forearm at the radioulnar joints		**Myofascial Meridians**
		Superficial back arm line
		Deep back arm line

Brachioradialis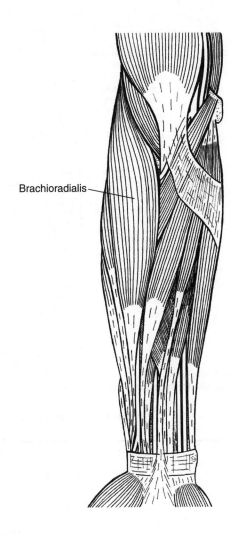

The brachioradialis can either pronate or supinate the forearm at the radioulnar joints. But it can only create these actions to a halfway position. The brachioradialis is one of the "3Bs of elbow joint flexion," along with the biceps brachii and brachialis.

Brachioradialis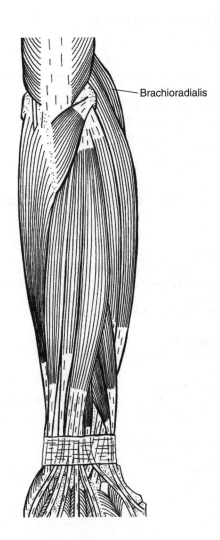

FLEXOR DIGITORUM SUPERFICIALIS

fleks-or dij-i-**toe**-rum
soo-per-fish-ee-**a**-lis

Actions
Flexion of fingers #2-5 at the
   metacarpophalangeal and proximal
   interphalangeal joints
Flexion of the hand at the wrist joint
Flexion of the forearm at the elbow joint

Innervation
The median nerve

Arterial Supply
The ulnar and radial arteries

Myofascial Meridians
Superficial front arm line

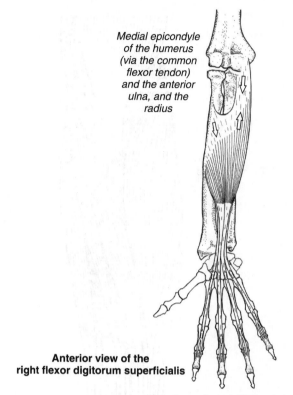

*Medial epicondyle
of the humerus
(via the common
flexor tendon)
and the anterior
ulna, and the
radius*

**Anterior view of the
right flexor digitorum superficialis**

Anterior surfaces of fingers #2-5

FLEXOR DIGITORUM PROFUNDUS

fleks-or dij-i-**toe**-rum pro-**fun**-dus

Actions
Flexion of fingers #2-5 at the
   metacarpophalangeal and proximal and distal
   interphalangeal joints
Flexion of the hand at the wrist joint

Innervation
The median and the ulnar nerves

Arterial Supply
The ulnar and radial arteries and the anterior
   interosseus artery

Myofascial Meridians
Superficial front arm line

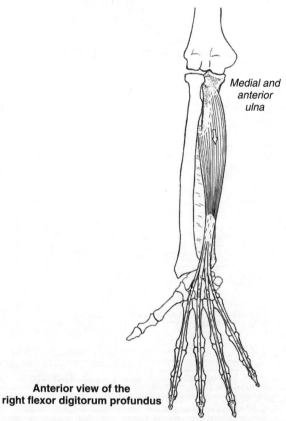

*Medial and
anterior
ulna*

**Anterior view of the
right flexor digitorum profundus**

Anterior surfaces of fingers #2-5

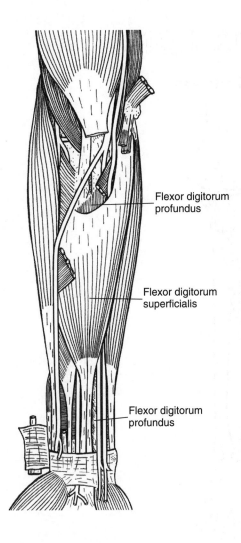

Flexor digitorum profundus

Flexor digitorum superficialis

Flexor digitorum profundus

The distal tendons of the flexor digitorum superficialis split to allow passage of the distal tendons of the flexor digitorum profundus to the distal phalanges of fingers #2-5.

The flexor digitorum superficialis is the only muscle of the common flexor belly/tendon that is in the intermediate compartment of the anterior forearm.

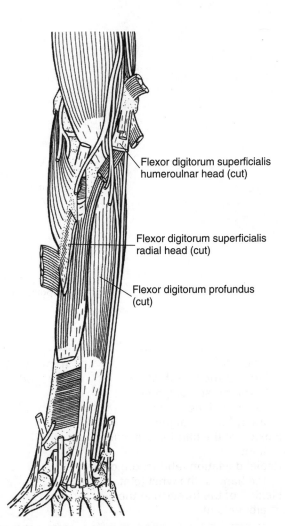

Flexor digitorum superficialis humeroulnar head (cut)

Flexor digitorum superficialis radial head (cut)

Flexor digitorum profundus (cut)

The flexor digitorum profundus is the only muscle that can flex the distal phalanges of fingers #2-5 at the distal interphalangeal joints.

The distal tendons of the flexor digitorum profundus pass between the split distal tendons of the flexor digitorum superficialis.

FLEXOR POLLICIS LONGUS

fleks-or **pol**-i-sis **long**-us

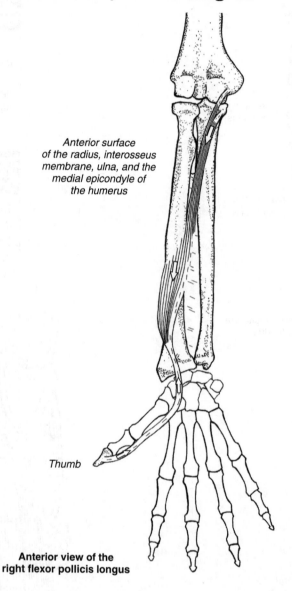

Anterior surface
of the radius, interosseus
membrane, ulna, and the
medial epicondyle of
the humerus

Thumb

**Anterior view of the
right flexor pollicis longus**

Actions
Flexion of the thumb at the
carpometacarpal, meta-
carpophalangeal, and
interphalangeal joints
Flexion of the hand at the wrist
joint
Radial deviation (abduction) of
the hand at the wrist joint
Flexion of the forearm at the
elbow joint

Innervation
The median nerve

Arterial Supply
The radial artery and the anterior
interosseus artery

Myofascial Meridians
Superficial front arm line

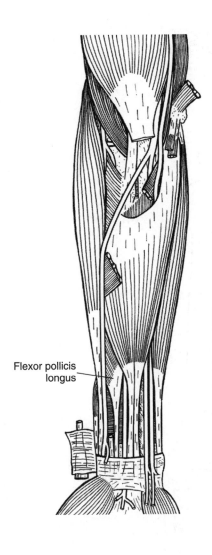

Flexor pollicis
longus

*The flexor pollicis longus has a
common variation wherein it is missing
its humeroulnar head.*

*The flexor pollicis longus is the only
muscle that can flex the thumb at the
interphalangeal joint.*

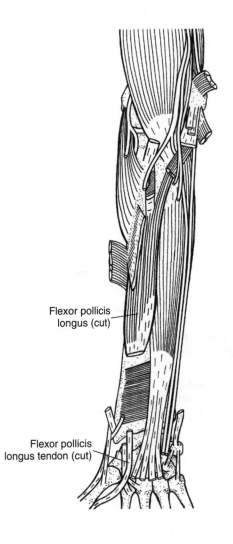

Flexor pollicis
longus (cut)

Flexor pollicis
longus tendon (cut)

ANCONEUS

an-**ko**-nee-us

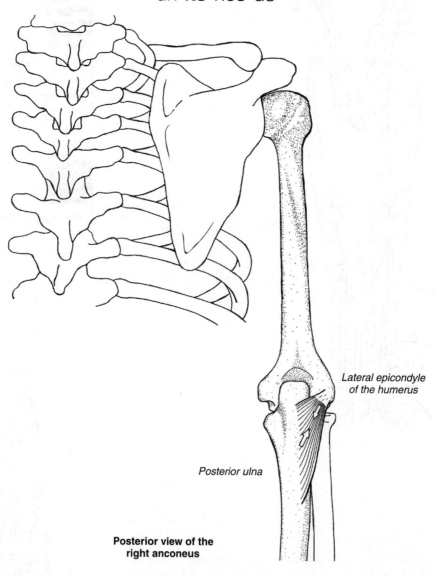

Lateral epicondyle
of the humerus

Posterior ulna

**Posterior view of the
right anconeus**

Action	**Arterial Supply**	**Myofascial Meridians**
Extension of the forearm at the elbow joint	The deep brachial artery	Deep back arm line
Innervation		
The radial nerve		

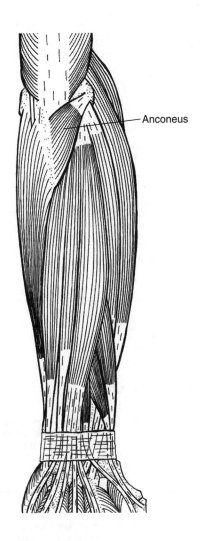

Anconeus

DID YOU KNOW

The anconeus is easily palpable in the posterior proximal forearm just distal to a point that is halfway between the olecranon process of the ulna and the lateral epicondyle of the humerus.

DID YOU KNOW

Because it extends the elbow joint, the anconeus is often described as an assistant to the triceps brachii.

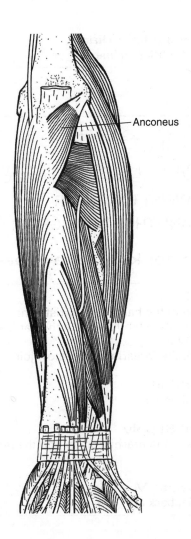

Anconeus

EXTENSOR CARPI RADIALIS LONGUS

(OF THE WRIST EXTENSOR GROUP AND THE RADIAL GROUP)

eks-**ten**-sor **kar**-pie **ray**-dee-**a**-lis **long**-us

Actions
Extension of the hand at the wrist joint
Radial deviation (abduction) of the hand at the wrist joint
Flexion of the forearm at the elbow joint
Pronation of the forearm at the radioulnar joints

Innervation
The radial nerve

Arterial Supply
Branches of the brachial artery and the radial artery

Myofascial Meridians
Superficial back arm line

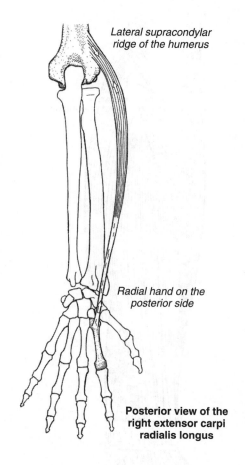

Lateral supracondylar ridge of the humerus

Radial hand on the posterior side

Posterior view of the right extensor carpi radialis longus

EXTENSOR CARPI RADIALIS BREVIS

(OF THE WRIST EXTENSOR GROUP AND THE RADIAL GROUP)

eks-**ten**-sor **kar**-pie **ray**-dee-**a**-lis **bre**-vis

Actions
Extension of the hand at the wrist joint
Radial deviation (abduction) of the hand at the wrist joint
Flexion of the forearm at the elbow joint

Innervation
The radial nerve

Arterial Supply
Branches of the brachial artery and the radial artery

Myofascial Meridians
Superficial back arm line

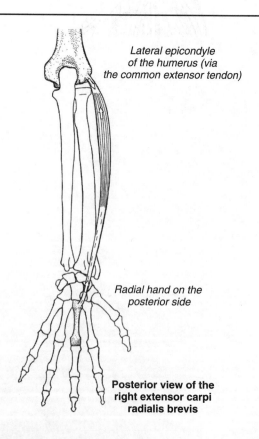

Lateral epicondyle of the humerus (via the common extensor tendon)

Radial hand on the posterior side

Posterior view of the right extensor carpi radialis brevis

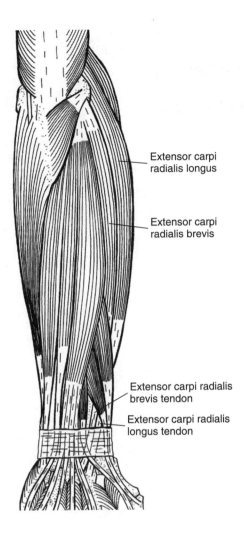

Extensor carpi
radialis longus

Extensor carpi
radialis brevis

Extensor carpi radialis
brevis tendon

Extensor carpi radialis
longus tendon

The extensor carpi radialis longus is the only one of the wrist extensor group muscles (extensor carpi radialis longus, extensor carpi radialis brevis, and extensor carpi ulnaris) that attaches onto the lateral supracondylar ridge of the humerus.

The brachioradialis also attaches onto the lateral supracondylar ridge.

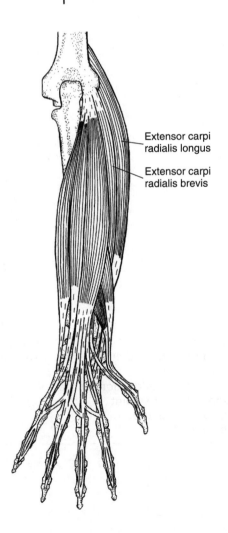

Extensor carpi
radialis longus

Extensor carpi
radialis brevis

Irritation and inflammation of the lateral condyle of the humerus and/or the common extensor belly/tendon are known as lateral elbow tendinopathy, lateral epicondylosis, or lateral epicondylitis; often called tennis elbow.

EXTENSOR CARPI ULNARIS
(OF THE WRIST EXTENSOR GROUP)

eks-**ten**-sor **kar**-pie ul-**na**-ris

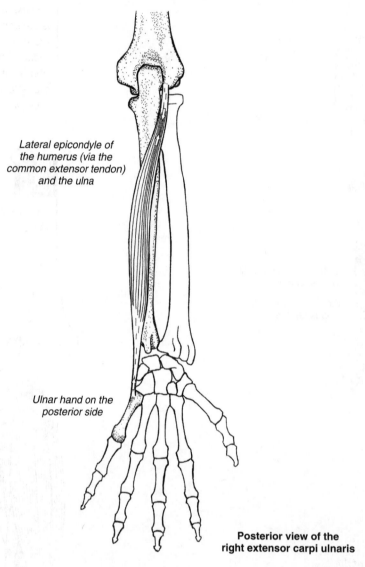

Lateral epicondyle of the humerus (via the common extensor tendon) and the ulna

Ulnar hand on the posterior side

Posterior view of the right extensor carpi ulnaris

Actions
Extension of the hand at the wrist joint
Ulnar deviation (adduction) of the hand at the wrist joint
Extension of the forearm at the elbow joint

Innervation
The radial nerve

Arterial Supply
The posterior interosseus artery

Myofascial Meridians
Superficial back arm line

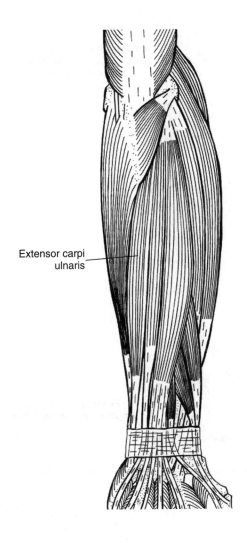

Extensor carpi
ulnaris

DID
YOU
KNOW

*The extensor carpi ulnaris is the
only one of the wrist extensor group
muscles (extensor carpi radialis
longus, extensor carpi radialis brevis,
and extensor carpi ulnaris) that has an
additional proximal attachment (onto
the ulna). Similarly, the flexor carpi
ulnaris is the only member of the wrist
flexor group that has an additional
proximal attachment (onto the ulna).*

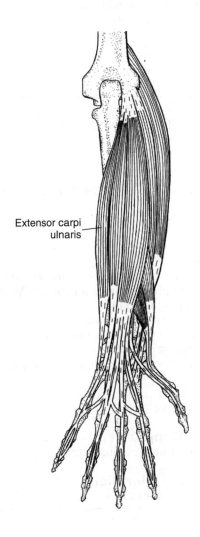

Extensor carpi
ulnaris

EXTENSOR DIGITORUM

eks-**ten**-sor dij-i-**toe**-rum

Actions
Extension of fingers #2-5 at the
    metacarpophalangeal and proximal and distal
    interphalangeal joints
Extension of the hand at the wrist joint
Medial rotation of the little finger (finger #5) at the
    carpometacarpal joint
Extension of the forearm at the elbow joint

Innervation
The radial nerve

Arterial Supply
The posterior interosseus artery

Myofascial Meridians
Superficial back arm line

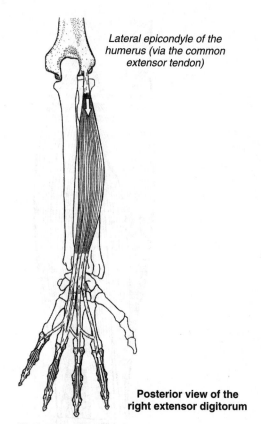

Lateral epicondyle of the humerus (via the common extensor tendon)

Posterior view of the right extensor digitorum

Phalanges of fingers #2-5

EXTENSOR DIGITI MINIMI

eks-**ten**-sor **dij**-i-tee **min**-i-mee

Actions
Extension of the little finger (finger #5) at the
    metacarpophalangeal and proximal and distal
    interphalangeal joints
Extension of the hand at the wrist joint
Medial rotation of the little finger (finger #5) at the
    carpometacarpal joint
Extension of the forearm at the elbow joint

Innervation
The radial nerve

Arterial Supply
The posterior interosseus artery

Myofascial Meridians
Superficial back arm line

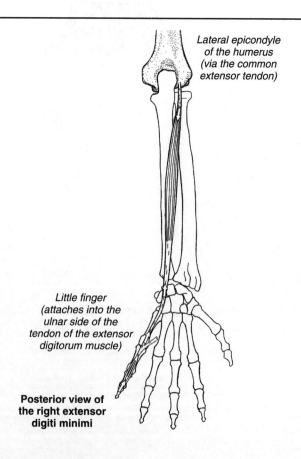

Lateral epicondyle of the humerus (via the common extensor tendon)

Little finger (attaches into the ulnar side of the tendon of the extensor digitorum muscle)

Posterior view of the right extensor digiti minimi

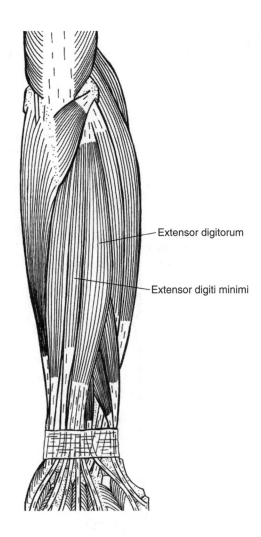

Extensor digitorum

Extensor digiti minimi

DID YOU KNOW?

The distal attachment of the extensor digitorum creates a structure called the dorsal digital expansion, which is an attachment site for many intrinsic muscles of the hand.

DID YOU KNOW?

The distal tendon of the extensor digiti minimi joints into the ulnar side of the distal tendon of the extensor digitorum that goes to the little finger. Only the index and little fingers have an additional extensor muscle.

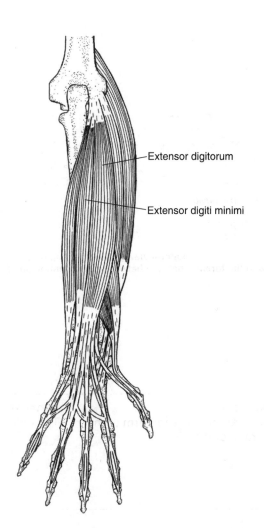

Extensor digitorum

Extensor digiti minimi

SUPINATOR

sue-pin-**a**-tor

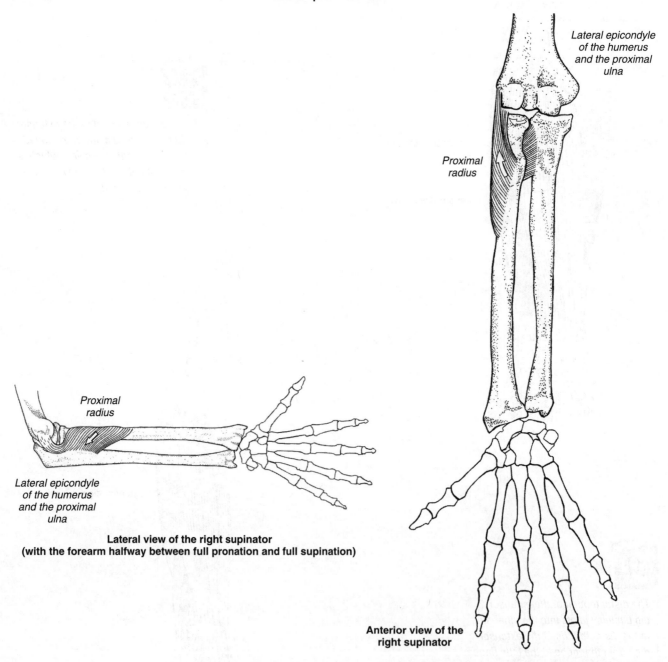

Lateral epicondyle
of the humerus
and the proximal
ulna

Proximal
radius

Proximal
radius

Lateral epicondyle
of the humerus
and the proximal
ulna

Lateral view of the right supinator
(with the forearm halfway between full pronation and full supination)

**Anterior view of the
right supinator**

Action Supination of the forearm at the radioulnar joints	**Innervation** The radial nerve	**Arterial Supply** Branches of the radial artery and the interosseus recurrent and posterior interosseus arteries
		Myofascial Meridians Deep front arm line

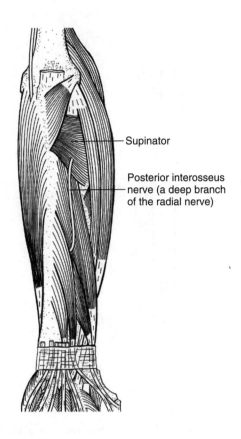

Supinator

Posterior interosseus nerve (a deep branch of the radial nerve)

A deep branch of the radial nerve runs between the two layers of the supinator and may be compressed there.

The supinator lies in the deep compartment of the posterior forearm.

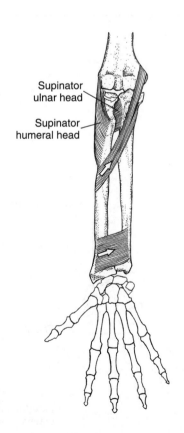

Supinator ulnar head

Supinator humeral head

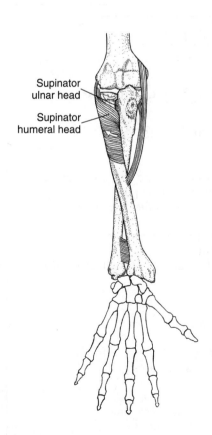

Supinator ulnar head

Supinator humeral head

ABDUCTOR POLLICIS LONGUS
(OF THE DEEP DISTAL FOUR GROUP)

ab-**duk**-tor **pol**-i-sis **long**-us

Actions
Abduction of the thumb at the carpometacarpal
joint
Extension of the thumb at the carpometacarpal
joint
Lateral rotation of the thumb at the
carpometacarpal joint
Radial deviation (abduction) of the hand at the
wrist joint
Flexion of the hand at the wrist joint
Supination of the forearm at the radioulnar joints

Innervation
The radial nerve

Arterial Supply
The posterior interosseus artery

Myofascial Meridians
Involved: Superficial back arm line
Involved: Deep front arm line

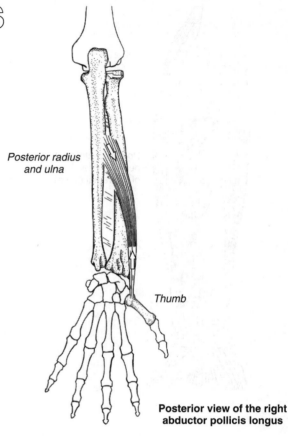

*Posterior radius
and ulna*

Thumb

**Posterior view of the right
abductor pollicis longus**

EXTENSOR POLLICIS BREVIS
(OF THE DEEP DISTAL FOUR GROUP)

eks-**ten**-sor **pol**-i-sis **bre**-vis

Actions
Extension of the thumb at the carpometacarpal
and metacarpophalangeal joints
Abduction of the thumb at the carpometacarpal
joint
Lateral rotation of the thumb at the carpometacarpal joint
Radial deviation (abduction) of the hand at the
wrist joint

Innervation
The radial nerve

Arterial Supply
The posterior interosseus artery

Myofascial Meridians
Involved: Superficial back arm line
Involved: Deep front arm line

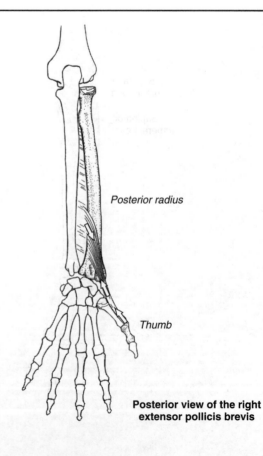

Posterior radius

Thumb

**Posterior view of the right
extensor pollicis brevis**

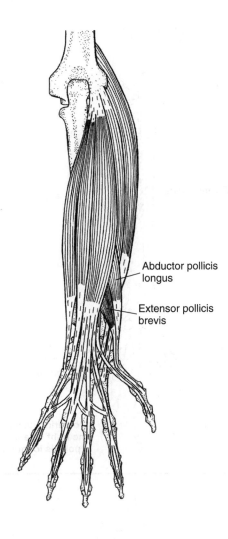

Abductor pollicis
longus

Extensor pollicis
brevis

*The distal tendons of these two
muscles form the lateral (radial) border
of the anatomic snuffbox.*

*These two muscles share a common
synovial sheath that can be involved
in a condition known as de Quervain's
condition.*

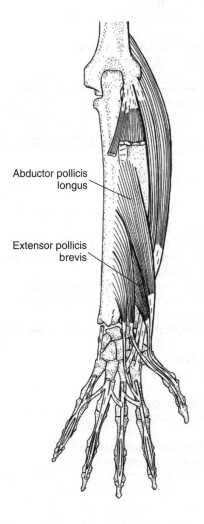

Abductor pollicis
longus

Extensor pollicis
brevis

EXTENSOR POLLICIS LONGUS
(OF THE DEEP DISTAL FOUR GROUP)

eks-**ten**-sor **pol**-i-sis **long**-us

Actions
Extension of the thumb at the carpometacarpal, metacarpophalangeal, and interphalangeal joints

Lateral rotation of the thumb at the carpo-metacarpal joint

Extension of the hand at the wrist joint

Radial deviation (abduction) of the hand at the wrist joint

Supination of the forearm at the radioulnar joints

Innervation
The radial nerve

Arterial Supply
The posterior interosseus artery

Myofascial Meridians
Superficial back arm line

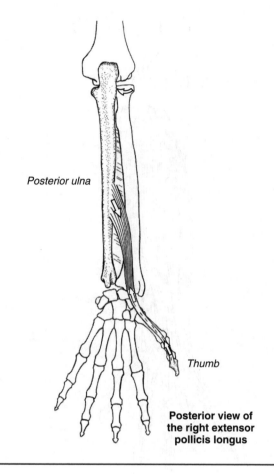

Posterior ulna

Thumb

Posterior view of the right extensor pollicis longus

EXTENSOR INDICIS
(OF THE DEEP DISTAL FOUR GROUP)

eks-**ten**-sor **in**-di-sis

Actions
Extension of the index finger (finger #2) at the metacarpophalangeal and proximal and distal interphalangeal joints

Extension of the hand at the wrist joint

Adduction of the index finger (finger #2) at the metacarpophalangeal joint

Supination of the forearm at the radioulnar joints

Innervation
The radial nerve

Arterial Supply
The posterior interosseus artery

Myofascial Meridians
Superficial back arm line

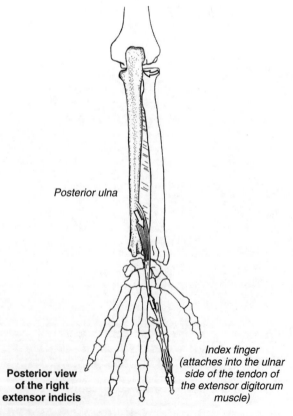

Posterior ulna

Posterior view of the right extensor indicis

Index finger (attaches into the ulnar side of the tendon of the extensor digitorum muscle)

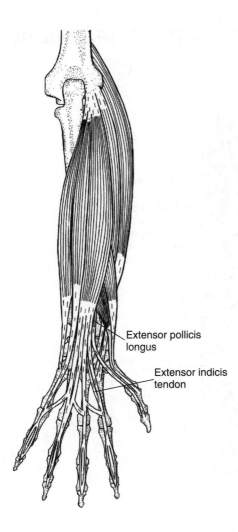

Extensor pollicis
longus

Extensor indicis
tendon

The distal tendon of the extensor pollicis longus forms the medial (ulnar) border of the anatomic snuffbox.

The scaphoid bone can be palpated in the anatomic snuffbox.

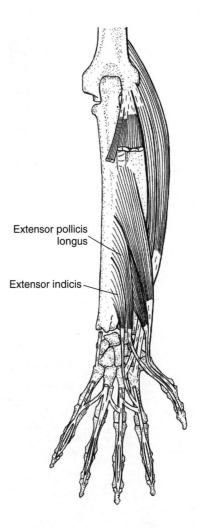

Extensor pollicis
longus

Extensor indicis

The extensor indicis aids the extensor digitorum in extending the index finger, which allows us to point out, i.e., indicate things.

The extensor indicis is the only member of the deep distal four group that does not attach onto the thumb; it attaches onto the index finger.

ANTERIOR VIEW OF THE RIGHT FOREARM (SUPERFICIAL)

PROXIMAL

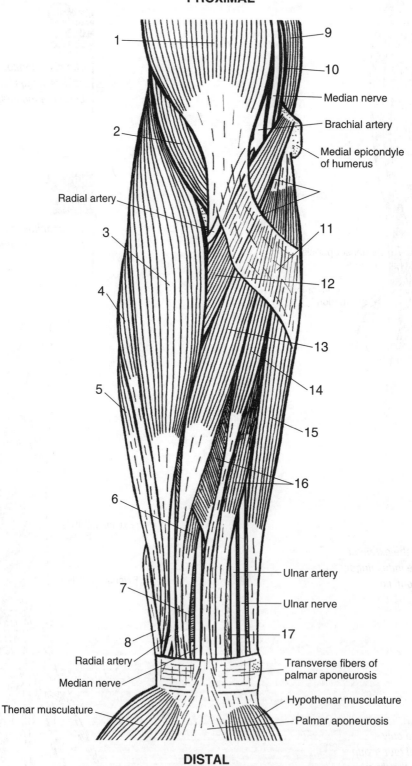

1

9

10

Median nerve

2

Brachial artery

Medial epicondyle
of humerus

Radial artery

3

11

12

4

**L
A
T
E
R
A
L**

**R
A
D
I
A
L**

**M
E
D
I
A
L**

**U
L
N
A
R**

13

14

5

15

16

6

7

Ulnar artery

Ulnar nerve

17

8

Radial artery

Transverse fibers of
palmar aponeurosis

Median nerve

Hypothenar musculature

Thenar musculature

Palmar aponeurosis

DISTAL

ANTERIOR VIEW OF THE RIGHT FOREARM (INTERMEDIATE)

PROXIMAL

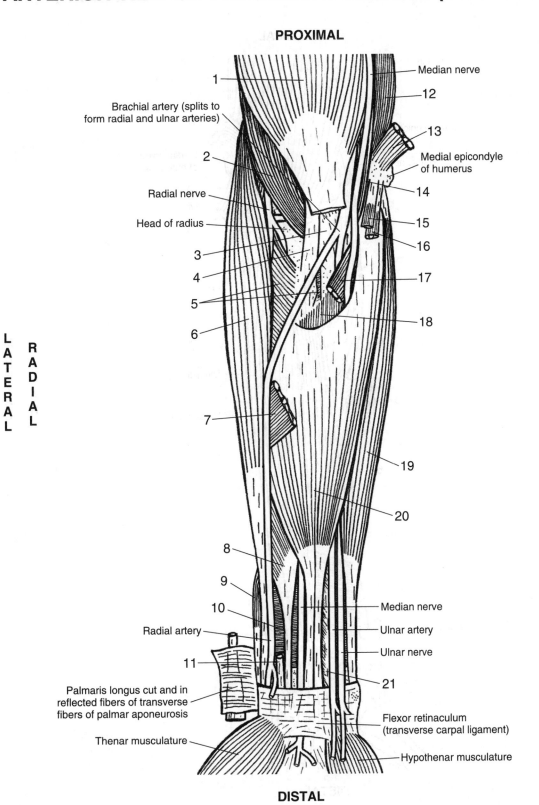

1

Brachial artery (splits to
form radial and ulnar arteries)

2

Radial nerve

Head of radius

3

4

5

6

7

8

9

10

Radial artery

11

Palmaris longus cut and in
reflected fibers of transverse
fibers of palmar aponeurosis

Thenar musculature

Median nerve

12

13

Medial epicondyle
of humerus

14

15

16

17

18

L
A
T
E
R
A
L

R
A
D
I
A
L

19

20

M
E
D
I
A
L

U
L
N
A
R

Median nerve

Ulnar artery

Ulnar nerve

21

Flexor retinaculum
(transverse carpal ligament)

Hypothenar musculature

DISTAL

ANTERIOR VIEW OF THE RIGHT FOREARM (DEEP)

PROXIMAL

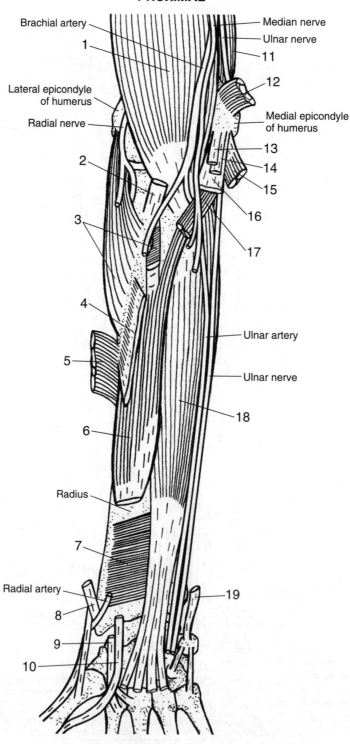

Brachial artery

1

Lateral epicondyle
of humerus

Radial nerve

2

3

4

5

6

Radius

7

Radial artery

8

9

10

Median nerve

Ulnar nerve

11

12

Medial epicondyle
of humerus

13

14

15

16

17

Ulnar artery

Ulnar nerve

18

19

LATERAL

RADIAL

ULNAR

MEDIAL

DISTAL

ANTERIOR VIEWS OF THE PRONATORS AND SUPINATOR OF THE RIGHT RADIUS

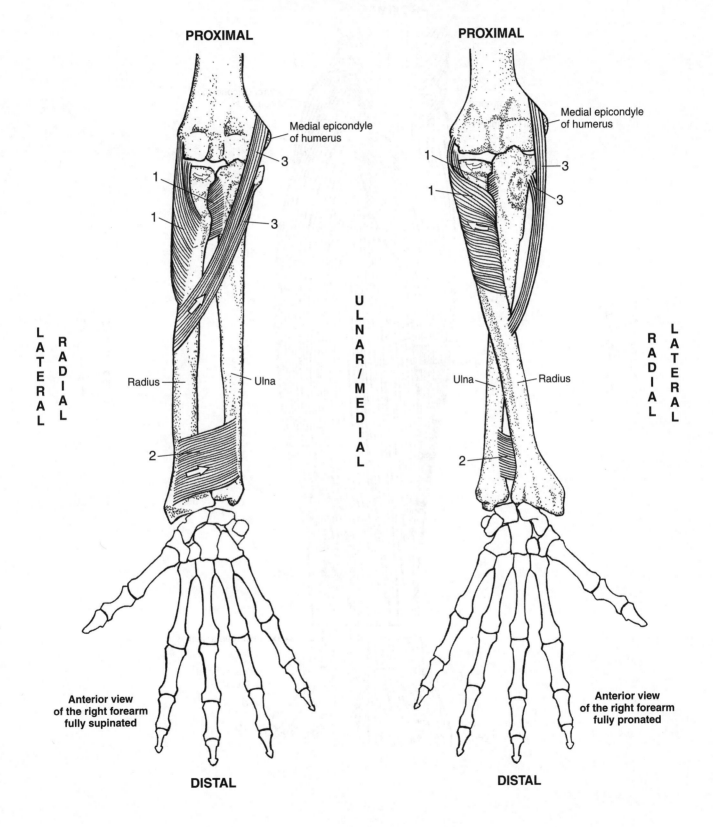

PROXIMAL

PROXIMAL

Medial epicondyle of humerus

1

1

3

3

L A T E R A L

R A D I A L

Radius

Ulna

2

Anterior view of the right forearm fully supinated

DISTAL

U L N A R / M E D I A L

Medial epicondyle of humerus

1

1

3

3

Ulna

Radius

R A D I A L

L A T E R A L

2

Anterior view of the right forearm fully pronated

DISTAL

POSTERIOR VIEW OF THE RIGHT FOREARM (SUPERFICIAL)

PROXIMAL

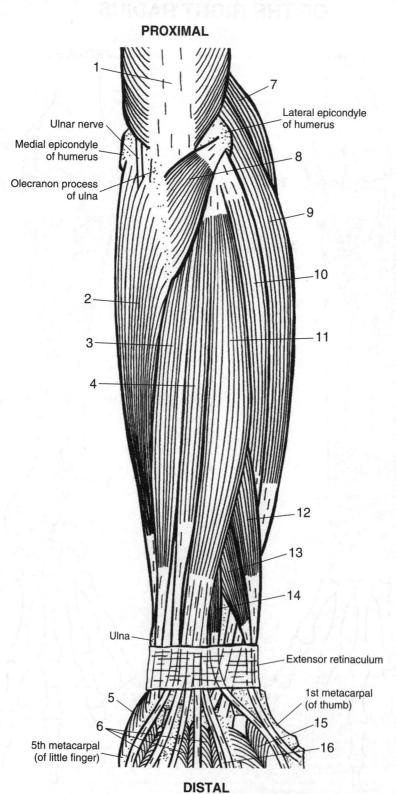

1

7

Ulnar nerve

Lateral epicondyle
of humerus

Medial epicondyle
of humerus

8

Olecranon process
of ulna

9

10

2

3

11

4

L A T E R A L

R A D I A L

U L N A R

M E D I A L

12

13

14

Ulna

Extensor retinaculum

1st metacarpal
(of thumb)

5

6

15

5th metacarpal
(of little finger)

16

DISTAL

POSTERIOR VIEW OF THE RIGHT FOREARM (DEEP)

PROXIMAL

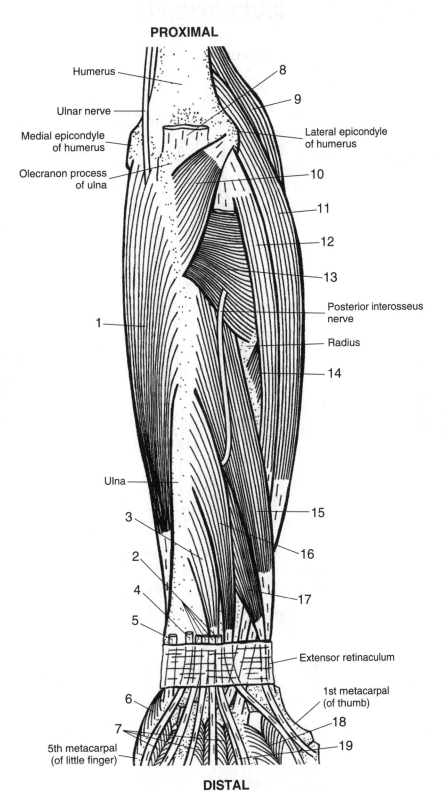

Humerus

Ulnar nerve

Medial epicondyle
of humerus

Olecranon process
of ulna

8

9

Lateral epicondyle
of humerus

10

11

12

13

Posterior interosseus
nerve

Radius

14

1

MEDIAL ULNAR

RADIAL LATERAL

Ulna

3

2

4

5

15

16

17

Extensor retinaculum

6

1st metacarpal
(of thumb)

18

7

19

5th metacarpal
(of little finger)

DISTAL

POSTERIOR VIEW OF THE RIGHT FOREARM AND HAND (SUPERFICIAL)

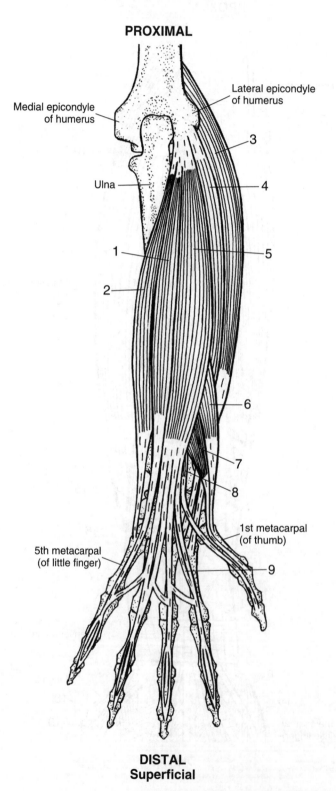

PROXIMAL

Medial epicondyle of humerus

Lateral epicondyle of humerus

Ulna

3

4

1

5

2

6

7

8

MEDIAL ULNAR

RADIAL LATERAL

5th metacarpal (of little finger)

1st metacarpal (of thumb)

9

DISTAL
Superficial

POSTERIOR VIEW OF THE RIGHT FOREARM AND HAND (DEEP)

PROXIMAL

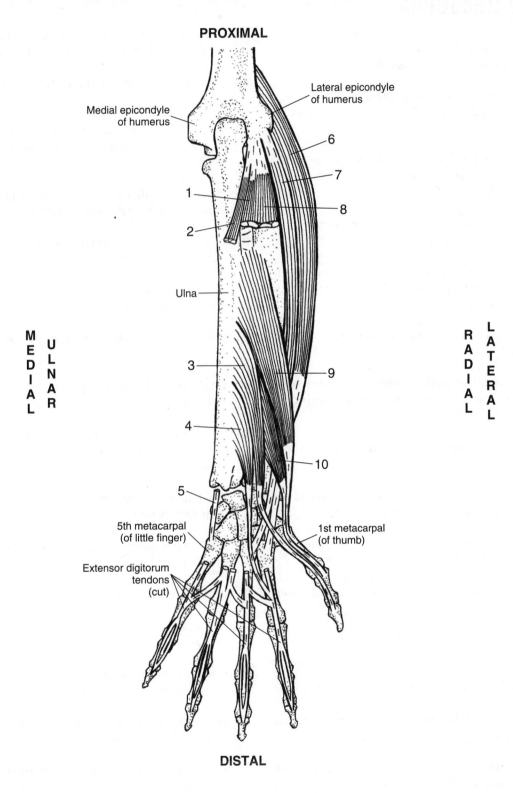

Lateral epicondyle
of humerus

Medial epicondyle
of humerus

6

7

1

8

2

Ulna

3

9

4

10

5

5th metacarpal
(of little finger)

1st metacarpal
(of thumb)

Extensor digitorum
tendons
(cut)

MEDIAL

ULNAR

RADIAL

LATERAL

DISTAL

Review Questions

Muscles of the Forearm
Answers to these questions are found on page 491.

1. The distal tendons of what muscle split, allowing passage of the tendons of the flexor digitorum profundus to the distal phalanges?

2. From an anterior perspective, where is the radial attachment of the pronator teres relative to the brachioradialis?

3. Where they overlap, which muscle is deeper, the anconeus or the extensor carpi ulnaris?

4. At the wrist, the distal tendon of the flexor pollicis longus can be found between the distal tendons of which two wrist flexor muscles?

5. The distal attachment of the pronator teres is deep to what muscle?

6. What joint action(s) is/are occurring at the wrist joint when the extensor carpi ulnaris is concentrically contracting?

7. What six muscles attach to the lateral epicondyle of the humerus?

8. The extensors carpi radialis longus and brevis and the extensor carpi ulnaris attach onto which metacarpals?

9. What joint actions would lengthen and stretch the flexor carpi radialis?

10. What is the major antagonist to the flexor digitorum profundus?

11. Why is the flexor carpi radialis antagonistic to the anconeus?

12. How is the brachioradialis synergistic to the supinator?

13. What muscle is immediately medial to the extensor digiti minimi?

14. Where they overlap, which muscle is deeper, the flexor digitorum superficialis or the flexor pollicis longus?

15. What two muscles attach to the lateral supracondylar ridge of the humerus?

16. What joint action would stretch the pronator teres but not the pronator quadratus?

17. From an anterior perspective, which muscle is deeper, the flexor digitorum superficialis or profundus?

18. What nerve runs between the two heads of the pronator teres?

19. Golfer's elbow (also known as medial epicondylitis or medial epicondylosis) involves what tendon of the forearm?

20. What is the only muscle in the body that can flex the thumb at the interphalangeal joint?

21. What muscle is immediately lateral to the extensor carpi radialis brevis?

22. How are the flexor carpi radialis and palmaris longus synergistic with each other?

23. What three muscles comprise the wrist extensor group?

24. What muscle is immediately medial to the extensor carpi ulnaris?

25. What two muscles attach to the lateral epicondyle of the humerus but not via the common extensor tendon?

26. What muscle of the deep distal four group attaches the most proximally?

27. What two muscles attach distally into a tendon of the extensor digitorum?

28. What three muscles border the anatomic snuffbox?

29. The abductor pollicis longus becomes superficial by emerging between what two muscles?

30. How are the extensor pollicis brevis and extensor carpi ulnaris antagonistic to each other?

31. The distal attachment of the supinator is immediately deep to what three muscles?

32. What motion of the hand at the wrist joint might occur when the extensor pollicis brevis concentrically contracts?

33. The proximal attachment of the supinator is deep to what muscle?

34. What is the only muscle of the deep distal four group that does not cross the radioulnar joints?

35. Which four muscles comprise the deep distal four group of the forearm?

36. What muscle is antagonistic to the extensor indicis at the distal interphalangeal joint of the index finger?

37. The distal tendons of what two muscles pass deep to the extensor pollicis longus?

38. What happens to the length of the abductor pollicis longus when the thumb flexes at the carpometacarpal joint?

39. Which muscle of the deep distal four group is the deepest?

40. What muscle is immediately deep to the ulnar head of the flexor carpi ulnaris?

41. What three muscles comprise the radial group?

42. What is the major synergist to the anconeus?

43. What muscle is immediately anterior to the extensor carpi ulnaris?

44. How are the flexor carpi radialis (FCR) and flexor carpi ulnaris (FCU) antagonistic to each other?

45. Which "pronator" muscle shares its proximal attachment with the wrist flexor group?

46. What are the two major antagonists to the supinator?

47. What is the common distal attachment of both the pronator teres and quadratus?

48. What happens to the length of the extensors carpi radialis longus and brevis when the hand radially deviates at the wrist joint?

49. What happens to the length of the extensor digitorum as the hand extends at the wrist joint?

50. What four muscles can flex the thumb at the carpometacarpal joint?

51. What is the common proximal attachment of the flexors carpi radialis and ulnaris, and the palmaris longus?

52. What muscle is immediately proximal to the anconeus?

53. What three muscles comprise the wrist flexor group?

54. Which "pronator" muscle crosses the elbow joint as well as the radioulnar joints?

55. How are the flexor carpi radialis and flexor carpi ulnaris synergistic with each other?

56. What five muscles are deep to the extensors digitorum and digiti minimi?

57. What muscle is immediately posterior to the flexor carpi ulnaris?

58. Name a synergist to the finger actions of the flexor digitorum superficialis.

59. What muscle is immediately medial to the extensor carpi radialis brevis in the proximal forearm?

60. Name a muscle that is synergistic to the supinator.

61. Name three powerful synergists to the brachioradialis' action at the elbow joint.

62. What muscle is antagonistic to all three joint actions of the extensor carpi ulnaris?

63. Which muscle is deeper, the flexor pollicis longus or the pronator quadratus?

64. What are the two major antagonists to the extensor digitorum?

65. What joint action occurs when the supinator eccentrically contracts?

66. What muscles attach to the lateral epicondyle via the common extensor tendon?

67. The belly of what muscle is immediately deep to the bellies of the flexor carpi radialis and palmaris longus?

68. What happens to the length of the brachioradialis if the elbow joint is passively flexed?

69. What muscle is immediately posterior to the brachioradialis?

70. What action(s) at the wrist joint are occurring if the flexor carpi ulnaris is eccentrically contracting?

71. What happens to the length of the extensor digitorum as the fingers flex at the metacarpophalangeal and interphalangeal joints?

72. The distal attachment of what muscle creates the dorsal digital expansion?

73. What happens to the length of the extensors carpi radialis longus and brevis when the hand ulnar deviates at the wrist joint?

74. What happens to the length of the flexor carpi ulnaris when the wrist joint is actively extended?

75. What joint action is occurring when the anconeus is shortening?

76. What happens to the length of the flexor pollicis longus if the hand is flexed at the wrist joint?

77. What joint actions may be occurring if the flexor digitorum superficialis is eccentrically contracting?

78. Which finger flexor muscle of the forearm crosses the distal interphalangeal joints?

Muscles of the Hand 12

Note: Throughout this chapter, muscle attachments are indicated by italics.

⊖ More review activities on Evolve at: http://evolve.elsevier.com/Muscolino/anatomycoloring/

PALMAR VIEW OF THE RIGHT HAND (SUPERFICIAL)

PROXIMAL

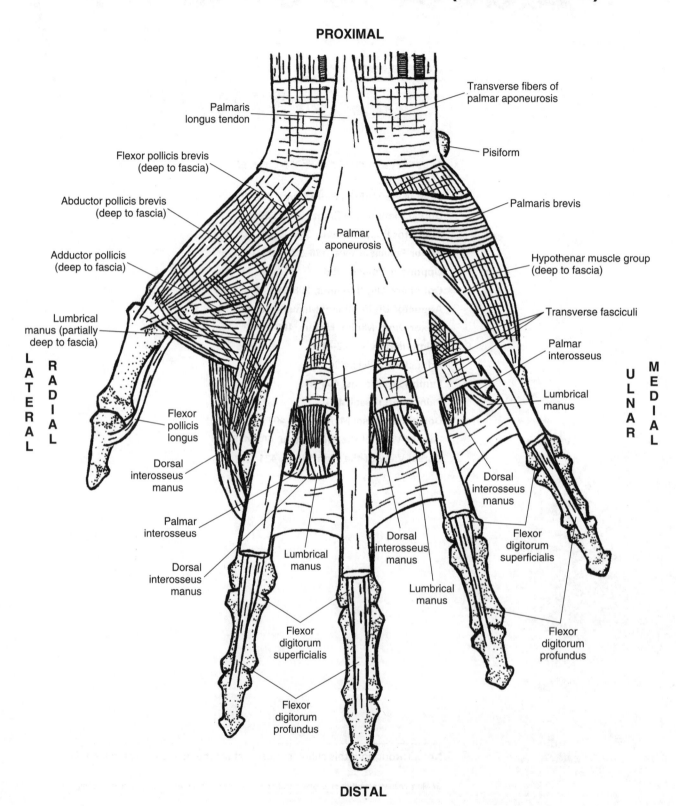

Palmaris
longus tendon

Transverse fibers of
palmar aponeurosis

Flexor pollicis brevis
(deep to fascia)

Pisiform

Abductor pollicis brevis
(deep to fascia)

Palmaris brevis

Adductor pollicis
(deep to fascia)

Palmar
aponeurosis

Hypothenar muscle group
(deep to fascia)

Lumbrical
manus (partially
deep to fascia)

Transverse fasciculi

Palmar
interosseus

L A T E R A L

R A D I A L

U L N A R

M E D I A L

Lumbrical
manus

Flexor
pollicis
longus

Dorsal
interosseus
manus

Palmar
interosseus

Dorsal
interosseus
manus

Dorsal
interosseus
manus

Flexor
digitorum
superficialis

Lumbrical
manus

Dorsal
interosseus
manus

Lumbrical
manus

Dorsal
interosseus
manus

Flexor
digitorum
profundus

Flexor
digitorum
superficialis

Flexor
digitorum
profundus

Flexor
digitorum
profundus

DISTAL

PALMAR VIEW OF THE RIGHT HAND
(SUPERFICIAL MUSCULAR LAYER)

PROXIMAL

Transverse fibers of
palmar aponeurosis

Scaphoid

Pisiform

Flexor
pollicis
brevis

Flexor retaniculum

Abductor pollicis
brevis

Opponens
digiti minimi

Abductor digiti
minimi manus

Sesamoid bone

Flexor digiti
minimi manus

Adductor pollicis
(deep to fascia)

Lumbrical
manus

Palmar
interosseus

L A T E R A L
R A D I A L

U L N A R
M E D I A L

Dorsal
interosseus
manus

Lumbrical
manus

Dorsal
interosseus
manus

Palmar interosseus

Dorsal
interosseus
manus

Flexor
digitorum
superficialis

Dorsal
interosseus
manus

Flexor
digitorum
superficialis

Flexor
digitorum
profundus

Flexor
digitorum
profundus

DISTAL

PALMAR VIEW OF THE RIGHT HAND
(DEEP MUSCULAR LAYER)

PROXIMAL

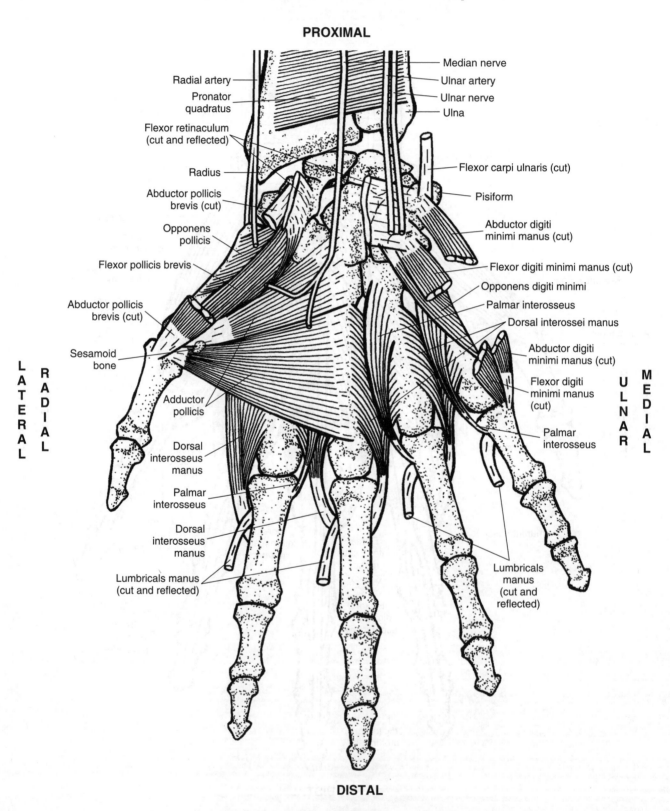

Radial artery

Pronator quadratus

Flexor retinaculum (cut and reflected)

Radius

Abductor pollicis brevis (cut)

Opponens pollicis

Flexor pollicis brevis

Abductor pollicis brevis (cut)

Sesamoid bone

Adductor pollicis

Dorsal interosseus manus

Palmar interosseus

Dorsal interosseus manus

Lumbricals manus (cut and reflected)

Median nerve

Ulnar artery

Ulnar nerve

Ulna

Flexor carpi ulnaris (cut)

Pisiform

Abductor digiti minimi manus (cut)

Flexor digiti minimi manus (cut)

Opponens digiti minimi

Palmar interosseus

Dorsal interossei manus

Abductor digiti minimi manus (cut)

Flexor digiti minimi manus (cut)

Palmar interosseus

Lumbricals manus (cut and reflected)

L A T E R A L

R A D I A L

U L N A R

M E D I A L

DISTAL

DORSAL VIEW OF THE RIGHT HAND

PROXIMAL

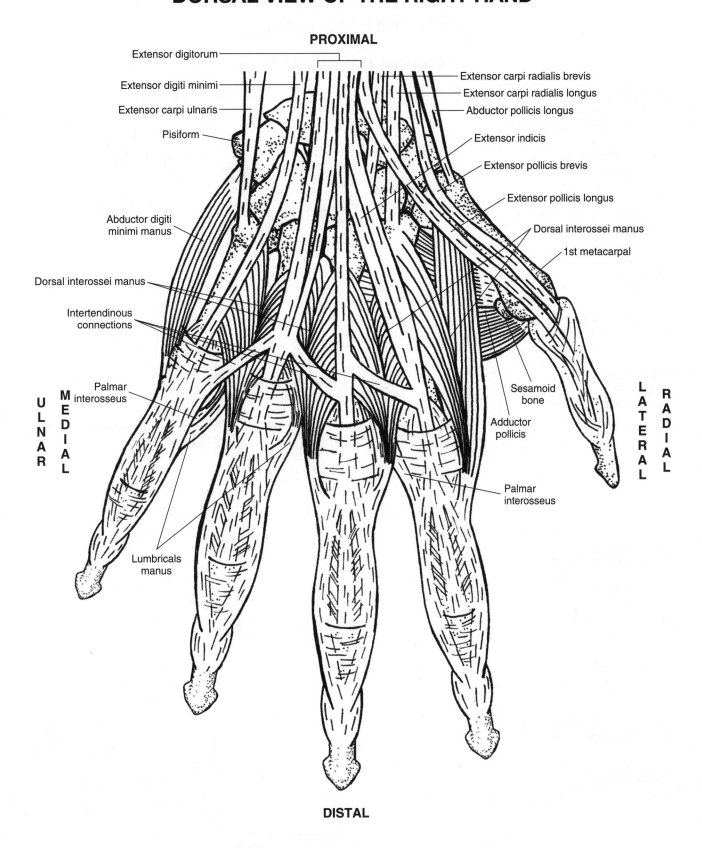

Extensor digitorum

Extensor digiti minimi

Extensor carpi ulnaris

Pisiform

Abductor digiti
minimi manus

Dorsal interossei manus

Intertendinous
connections

Palmar
interosseus

Lumbricals
manus

Extensor carpi radialis brevis

Extensor carpi radialis longus

Abductor pollicis longus

Extensor indicis

Extensor pollicis brevis

Extensor pollicis longus

Dorsal interossei manus

1st metacarpal

Sesamoid
bone

Adductor
pollicis

Palmar
interosseus

U L N A R

M E D I A L

L A T E R A L

R A D I A L

DISTAL

ABDUCTOR POLLICIS BREVIS
(OF THE THENAR EMINENCE)

ab-**duk**-tor **pol**-i-sis **bre**-vis

Actions
Abduction of the thumb
    at the carpometacarpal
    joint
Flexion of the thumb at
    the metacarpophalan-
    geal joint
Extension of the thumb
    at the carpometacarpal
    and interphalangeal
    joints

Innervation
The median nerve

Arterial Supply
Branches of the radial
    artery

**Myofascial
Meridians**
Deep front arm line

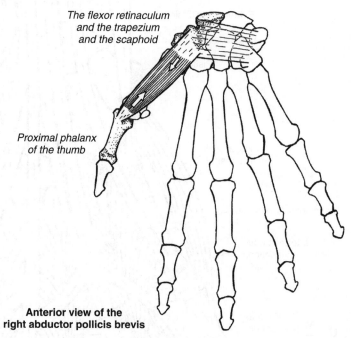

*The flexor retinaculum
and the trapezium
and the scaphoid*

*Proximal phalanx
of the thumb*

**Anterior view of the
right abductor pollicis brevis**

FLEXOR POLLICIS BREVIS
(OF THE THENAR EMINENCE)

fleks-or **pol**-i-sis **bre**-vis

Actions
Flexion of the thumb at the
    carpometacarpal and the
    metacarpophalangeal
    joints
Abduction of the thumb at
    the carpometacarpal joint

Innervation
The median and ulnar
    nerves

Arterial Supply
Branches of the radial artery

**Myofascial
Meridians**
Deep front arm line

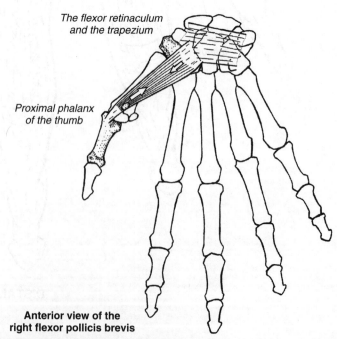

*The flexor retinaculum
and the trapezium*

*Proximal phalanx
of the thumb*

**Anterior view of the
right flexor pollicis brevis**

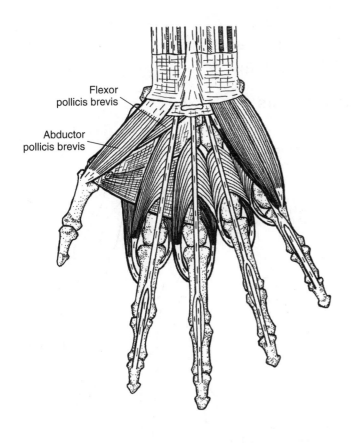

Flexor pollicis brevis

Abductor pollicis brevis

The abductor pollicis brevis is the most superficial of the three muscles of the thenar eminence group.

The abductor pollicis brevis abducts the thumb in the sagittal plane. Because the thumb rotated evolutionarily 90 degrees to be opposable, it flexes and extends in the frontal plane and abducts and adducts in the sagittal plane

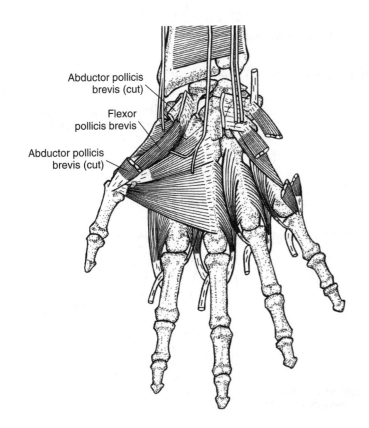

Abductor pollicis brevis (cut)

Flexor pollicis brevis

Abductor pollicis brevis (cut)

The flexor pollicis brevis of the thenar eminence group has a sesamoid bone in its distal tendon.

The flexor pollicis brevis flexes the thumb in the frontal plane.

OPPONENS POLLICIS
(OF THE THENAR EMINENCE)

op-**po**-nens **pol**-i-sis

Actions
Opposition of the thumb at the
    carpometacarpal joint
Flexion of the thumb at the
    carpometacarpal joint
Medial rotation of the thumb at the
    carpometacarpal joint
Abduction of the thumb at the
    carpometacarpal joint

Innervation
The median and ulnar nerves

Arterial Supply
Branches of the radial artery

Myofascial Meridians
Deep front arm line

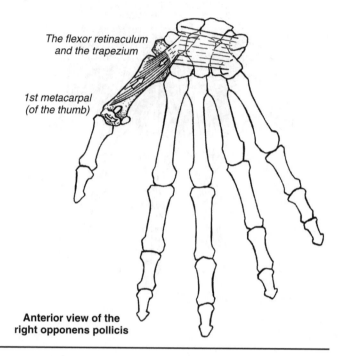

The flexor retinaculum
and the trapezium

1st metacarpal
(of the thumb)

**Anterior view of the
right opponens pollicis**

OPPONENS DIGITI MINIMI
(OF THE HYPOTHENAR EMINENCE)

op-**po**-nens **dij**-i-tee **min**-i-mee

Actions
Opposition of the little finger
    (finger #5) at the
    carpometacarpal joint
Flexion of the little finger (finger #5)
    at the carpometacarpal joint
Adduction of the little finger (finger
    #5) at the carpometacarpal joint
Lateral rotation of the little
    finger (finger #5) at the
    carpometacarpal joint

Innervation
The ulnar nerve

Arterial Supply
Branches of the ulnar artery

Myofascial Meridians
Deep back arm line

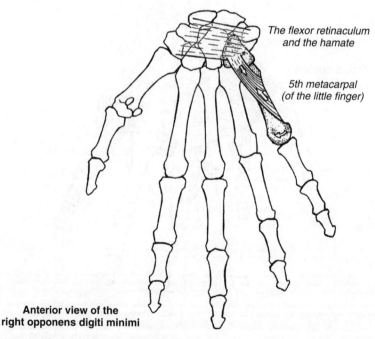

The flexor retinaculum
and the hamate

5th metacarpal
(of the little finger)

**Anterior view of the
right opponens digiti minimi**

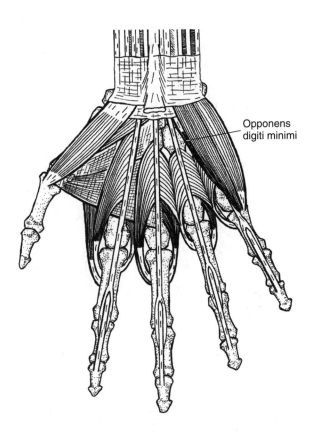

Opponens
digiti minimi

The opponens pollicis is the only muscle of the thenar eminence group that attaches onto the metacarpal of the thumb instead of the proximal phalanx of the thumb.

The opponens pollicis can oppose the thumb against the pad of the other fingers.

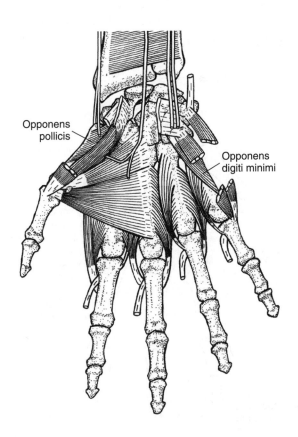

Opponens
pollicis

Opponens
digiti minimi

The thumb is not the only opposable finger; the opponens digiti minimi of the hypothenar group opposes the little finger.

Some people have an opponens digiti minimi of the little toe of the foot.

ABDUCTOR DIGITI MINIMI MANUS
(OF THE HYPOTHENAR EMINENCE)

ab-**duk**-tor **dij**-i-tee **min**-i-mee **man**-us

Actions
Abduction of the little
   finger (finger #5) at the
   carpometacarpal and
   metacarpophalangeal
   joints
Extension of the little
   finger (finger #5) at the
   proximal and distal
   interphalangeal joints

Innervation
The ulnar nerve

Arterial Supply
Branches of the ulnar
   artery

**Myofascial
Meridians**
Deep back arm line

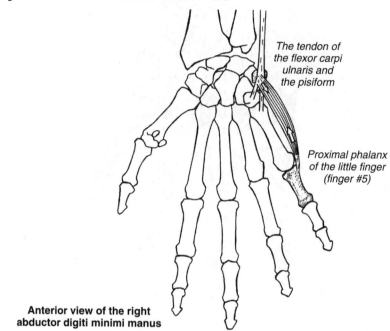

*The tendon of
the flexor carpi
ulnaris and
the pisiform*

*Proximal phalanx
of the little finger
(finger #5)*

**Anterior view of the right
abductor digiti minimi manus**

FLEXOR DIGITI MINIMI MANUS
(OF THE HYPOTHENAR EMINENCE)

fleks-or **dij**-i-tee **min**-i-mee **man**-us

Action
Flexion of the little finger
   (finger #5) at the
   metacarpophalangeal joint

Innervation
The ulnar nerve

Arterial Supply
Branches of the ulnar artery

Myofascial Meridians
Superficial front arm line

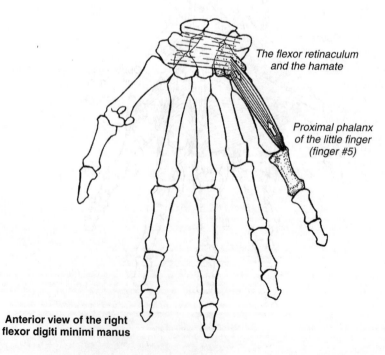

*The flexor retinaculum
and the hamate*

*Proximal phalanx
of the little finger
(finger #5)*

**Anterior view of the right
flexor digiti minimi manus**

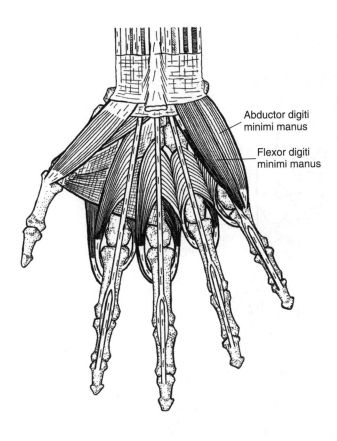

Abductor digiti
minimi manus

Flexor digiti
minimi manus

The abductor digiti minimi manus is the
most superficial of the three muscles of
the hypothenar eminence group.

Engaging the abductor digiti minimi
manus to abduct the little finger
requires the flexor carpi ulnaris to
isometrically contract to stabilize the
pisiform bone.

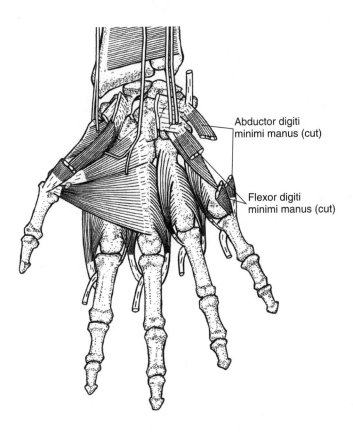

Abductor digiti
minimi manus (cut)

Flexor digiti
minimi manus (cut)

The flexor digiti minimi manus of the
hypothenar eminence group is often
known simply as the flexor digiti minimi
or the flexor digiti minimi brevis.

If there is a flexor digiti minimi manus,
there will be a flexor digiti minimi pedis
(of the foot).

PALMARIS BREVIS

pall-**ma**-ris **bre**-vis

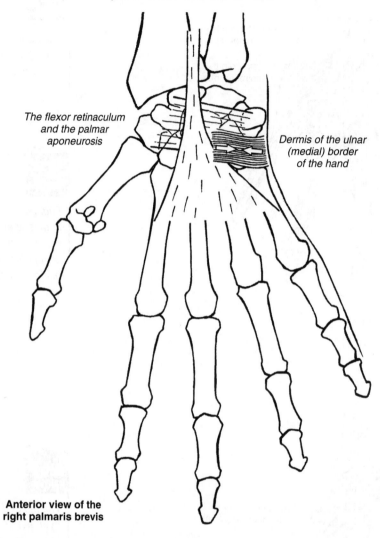

The flexor retinaculum
and the palmar
aponeurosis

Dermis of the ulnar
(medial) border
of the hand

**Anterior view of the
right palmaris brevis**

Action	**Arterial Supply**	**Myofascial Meridians**
Wrinkles the skin of the palm	The ulnar artery and the superficial palmar branch of the radial artery	Deep back arm line
Innervation		
The ulnar nerve		

The palmaris brevis' action of wrinkling the skin of the palm contributes to the strength and security of gripping an object in your hand.

The palmaris brevis overlies the musculature of the hypothenar eminence but is usually not considered to be a member of the hypothenar group.

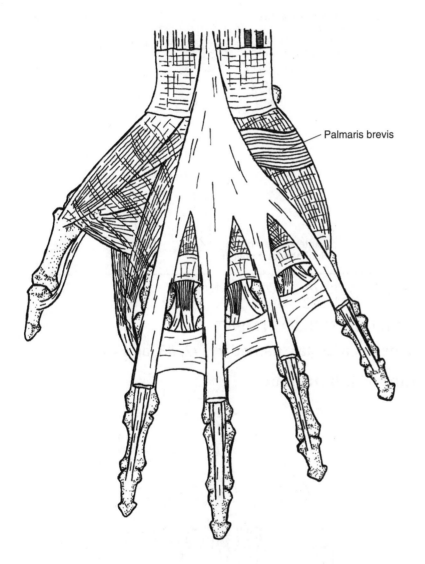

Palmaris brevis

ADDUCTOR POLLICIS
(OF THE CENTRAL COMPARTMENT)

ad-**duk**-tor **pol**-i-sis

Actions
Adduction of the thumb at the carpometa-carpal joint
Flexion of the thumb at the carpometacarpal and metacarpophalangeal joints
Extension of the thumb at the interphalangeal joint

Innervation
The ulnar nerve

Arterial Supply
Branches of the radial artery

Myofascial Meridians
Deep front arm line

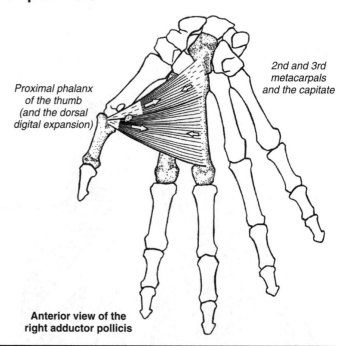

Proximal phalanx of the thumb (and the dorsal digital expansion)

2nd and 3rd metacarpals and the capitate

Anterior view of the right adductor pollicis

LUMBRICALS MANUS
(OF THE CENTRAL COMPARTMENT)
(There are four lumbrical manus muscles, named #1, #2, #3, and #4.)

lum-bri-kuls **man**-us

Actions
Extension of fingers #2-5 at the proximal and distal interphalangeal joints
Flexion of fingers #2-5 at the metacarpopha-langeal joint

Innervation
The median and ulnar nerves

Arterial Supply
Branches of the radial and ulnar arteries

Myofascial Meridians
Superficial front arm line

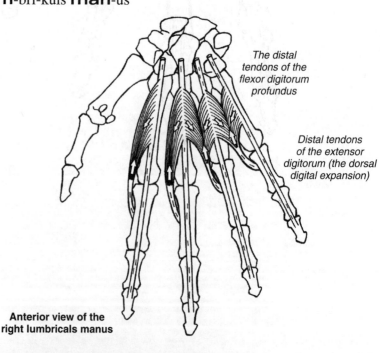

The distal tendons of the flexor digitorum profundus

Distal tendons of the extensor digitorum (the dorsal digital expansion)

Anterior view of the right lumbricals manus

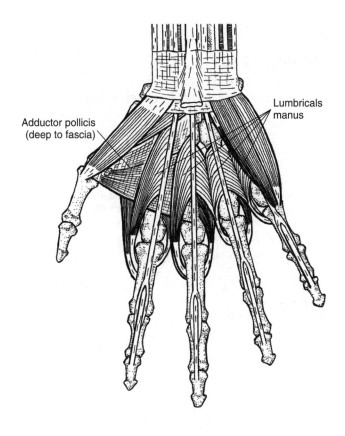

Adductor pollicis
(deep to fascia)

Lumbricals
manus

DID
YOU
KNOW

There is a sesamoid bone in the distal
tendon of the oblique head of the
adductor pollicis.

DID
YOU
KNOW

The adductor pollicis comprises the
majority of the tissue of the thumb web.

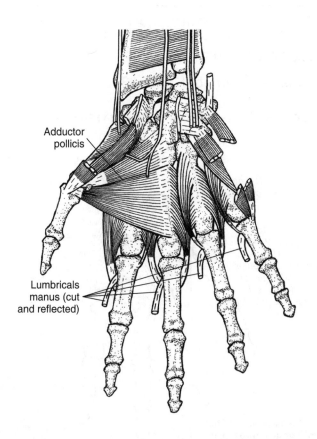

Adductor
pollicis

Lumbricals
manus (cut
and reflected)

DID
YOU
KNOW

The actions of the lumbricals manus
(flexion of the proximal phalanges at
the metacarpophalangeal joints and
extension of the middle and distal
phalanges at the interphalangeal
joints) puts the hand in the shape of the
letter "L", as in Lumbricals ☺.

DID
YOU
KNOW

The lumbricals manus always attach
onto the radial/lateral side of the
fingers.

PALMAR INTEROSSEI
(OF THE CENTRAL COMPARTMENT)

(There are three palmar interossei, named #1, #2, and #3.)

pal-mar **in**-ter-**oss**-ee-i

Actions
Adduction of fingers #2, #4, and #5 at the metacarpophalangeal joint
Flexion of fingers #2, #4, and #5 at the metacarpophalangeal joint
Extension of fingers #2, #4, and #5 at the proximal and distal interphalangeal joints

Innervation
The ulnar nerve

Arterial Supply
Branches of the radial and ulnar arteries

Myofascial Meridians
Superficial back arm line

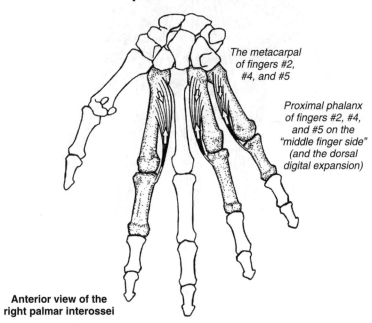

The metacarpal of fingers #2, #4, and #5

Proximal phalanx of fingers #2, #4, and #5 on the "middle finger side" (and the dorsal digital expansion)

Anterior view of the right palmar interossei

DORSAL INTEROSSEI MANUS
(OF THE CENTRAL COMPARTMENT)

(There are four dorsal interossei manus muscles, named #1, #2, #3, and #4.)

dor-sul **in**-ter-**oss**-ee-i **man**-us

Actions
Abduction of fingers #2, #3, and #4 at the metacarpophalangeal joint
Flexion of fingers #2, #3, and #4 at the metacarpophalangeal joint
Extension of fingers #2, #3, and #4 at the proximal and distal interphalangeal joints

Innervation
The ulnar nerve

Arterial Supply
Branches of the radial and ulnar arteries

Myofascial Meridians
Involved: Superficial back arm line

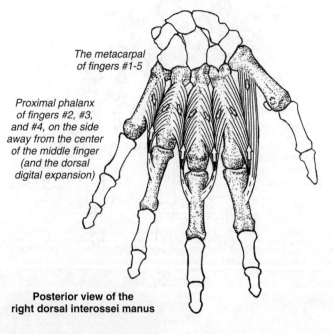

The metacarpal of fingers #1-5

Proximal phalanx of fingers #2, #3, and #4, on the side away from the center of the middle finger (and the dorsal digital expansion)

Posterior view of the right dorsal interossei manus

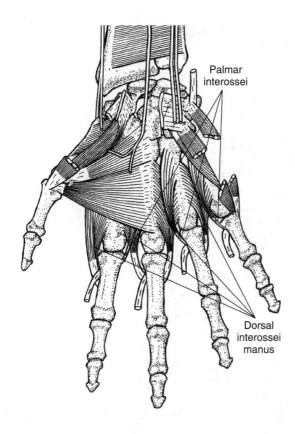

Palmar
interossei

Dorsal
interossei
manus

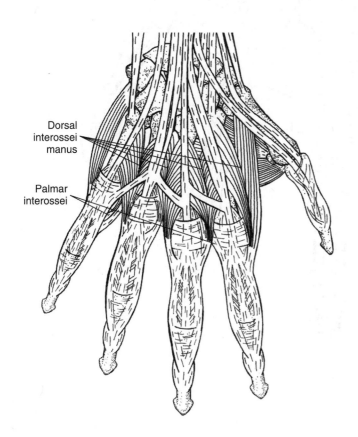

Dorsal
interossei
manus

Palmar
interossei

DID YOU KNOW ?

The main action of the dorsal interossei manus is abduction of the fingers at the metacarpophalangeal joints. The main action of the palmar interossei is adduction of the fingers at the metacarpophalangeal joints. The mnemonic to remember these actions is **DAB PAD**; **D**orsals **AB**duct, **P**almars **AD**duct.

DID YOU KNOW ?

This arrangement is similar to the plantar interossei and dorsal interossei pedis of the foot.

PALMAR VIEW OF THE RIGHT HAND (SUPERFICIAL)

PROXIMAL

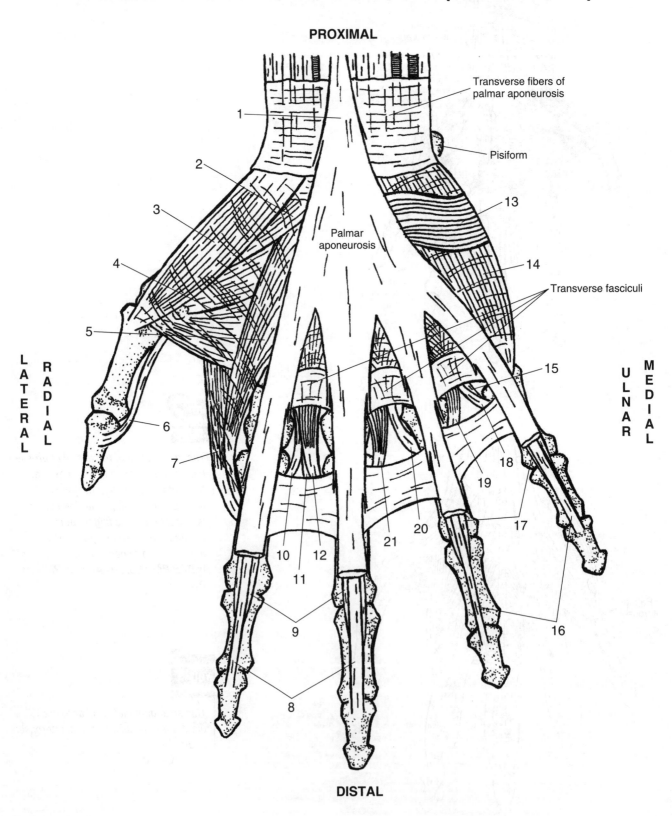

Transverse fibers of
palmar aponeurosis

Pisiform

Palmar
aponeurosis

Transverse fasciculi

LATERAL

RADIAL

ULNAR

MEDIAL

DISTAL

Answers to labeling exercises are on p. 491.

PALMAR VIEW OF THE RIGHT HAND
(SUPERFICIAL MUSCULAR LAYER)

PROXIMAL

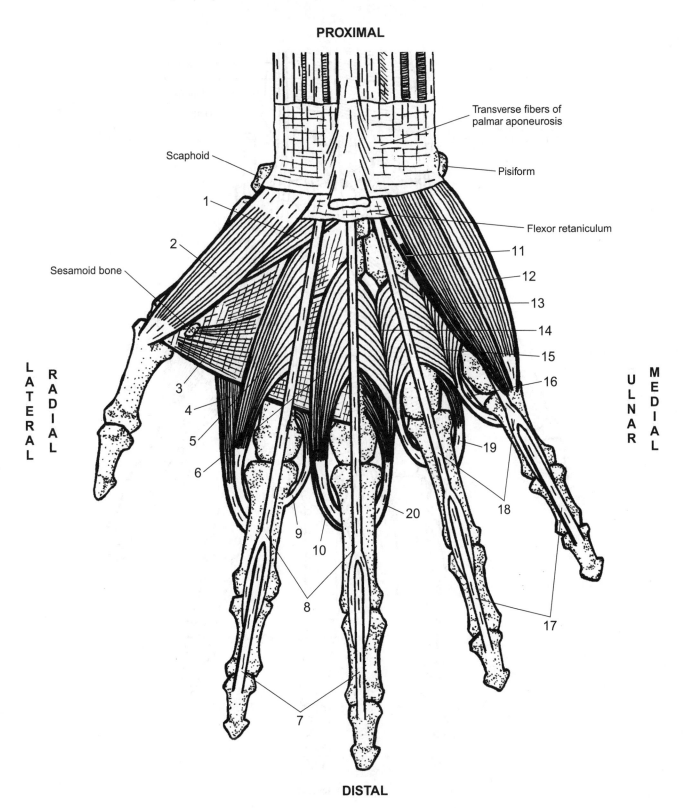

Transverse fibers of
palmar aponeurosis

Scaphoid

Pisiform

1

Flexor retaniculum

2

11

Sesamoid bone

12

13

14

15

3

16

L A T E R A L   R A D I A L

U L N A R   M E D I A L

4

5

19

6

18

20

9

10

8

17

7

DISTAL

PALMAR VIEW OF THE RIGHT HAND
(DEEP MUSCULAR LAYER)

PROXIMAL

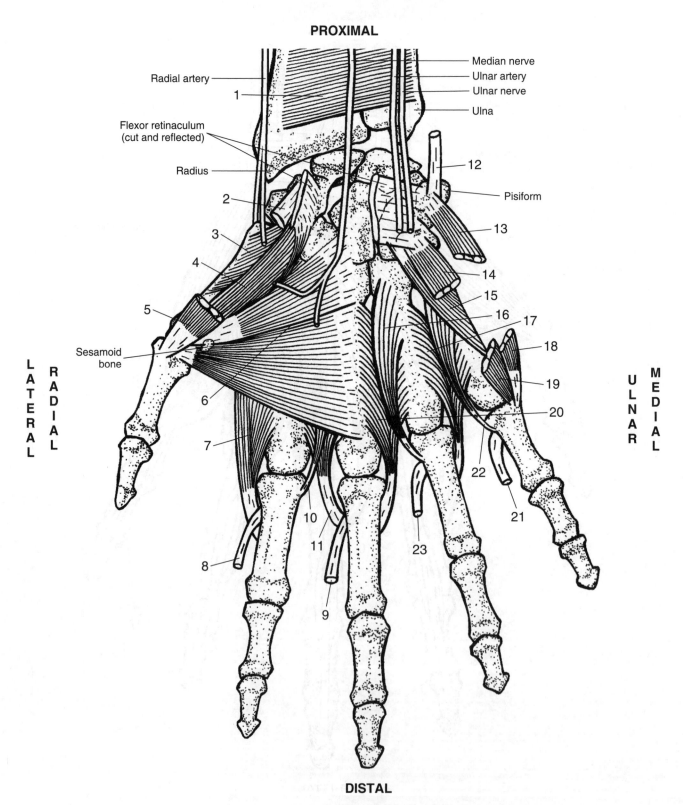

Radial artery

Flexor retinaculum
(cut and reflected)

Radius

Sesamoid
bone

Median nerve
Ulnar artery
Ulnar nerve
Ulna

1

2

3

4

5

6

7

8

9

10

11

12

13

14

15

16

17

18

19

20

21

22

23

Pisiform

LATERAL

RADIAL

ULNAR

MEDIAL

DISTAL

DORSAL VIEW OF THE RIGHT HAND

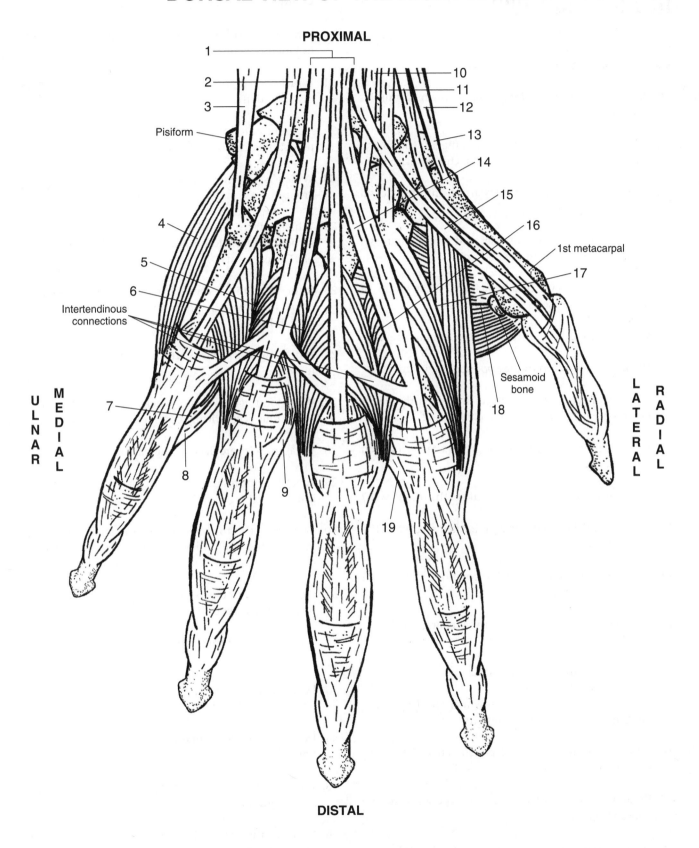

PROXIMAL

1
2
3

Pisiform

4

5

6

Intertendinous
connections

7

8

9

10
11
12

13

14

15

16

1st metacarpal

17

Sesamoid
bone

18

19

U
L
N
A
R

M
E
D
I
A
L

L
A
T
E
R
A
L

R
A
D
I
A
L

DISTAL

Review Questions

Muscles of the Hand
Answers to these questions are found on page 492.

1. What are the three major groups of intrinsic muscles of the hand?

2. What intrinsic hand muscles are antagonistic to the carpometacarpal action of the adductor pollicis?

3. Which intrinsic hand muscles attach into the dorsal digital expansion?

4. How are the palmar interossei and dorsal interossei manus synergistic with each other?

5. The palmaris brevis is superficial to what group of intrinsic hand muscles?

6. What muscle is synergistic with the palmaris brevis?

7. What muscle is deep to the opponens digiti minimi?

8. What joint action(s) is/are occurring when the flexor pollicis brevis is concentrically contracting?

9. All three muscles of the thenar group attach to which carpal bone?

10. What muscle makes up the majority of the thumb web?

11. Where is the flexor retinaculum located relative to the palmaris brevis?

12. What intrinsic hand muscles comprise the central compartment group?

13. What are the three muscles of the thenar group?

14. What intrinsic muscles of the hand do abduction of the thumb at the carpometacarpal joint?

15. From an anterior perspective, which are deeper, the lumbricals manus or the palmar interossei?

16. What is unusual about the attachments of the palmaris brevis?

17. What intrinsic hand muscles are synergistic to the opponens pollicis?

18. How are the opponens digiti minimi and abductor digiti minimi manus antagonistic to each other?

19. During what functional activity does the palmaris brevis usually contract?

20. What joint action occurs when the flexor digiti minimi manus isometrically contracts?

21. Which thenar group muscle has a sesamoid bone in its distal tendon?

22. From an anterior perspective, where is the adductor pollicis relative to the lumbricals manus?

23. Which is the most superficial muscle of the thenar group?

24. Which intrinsic hand muscles flex fingers at the metacarpophalangeal joints and extend fingers at the interphalangeal joints?

25. If the thumb is passively extended at the carpometacarpal joint, what happens to the length of the flexor pollicis brevis?

26. Which two carpals are attached onto by hypothenar muscles?

27. What joint action occurs when the flexor digiti minimi manus eccentrically contracts?

28. What muscles are deep to the palmaris brevis?

29. What type of rotation does the opponens digiti minimi do?

30. What happens to the length of the abductor pollicis brevis when the adductor pollicis is concentrically contracting and moving the carpometacarpal joint?

31. From a posterior perspective, which are deeper, the palmar interossei or the dorsal interossei manus?

32. What are the three intrinsic hand muscles of the hypothenar group?

33. What is similar about the distal attachments of the opponens pollicis and opponens digiti minimi?

34. Do the lumbricals manus flex and/or extend the fingers?

35. What muscle is immediately superficial to the opponens digiti minimi?

36. How are the palmar interossei and dorsal interossei manus antagonistic to each other?

⊖ **More review activities on Evolve at http://evolve.elsevier.com/Muscolino/anatomycoloring/**

Other Skeletal Muscles 13

Answers to labeling exercises are on p. 492.

🔵 More review activities on Evolve at: http://evolve.elsevier.com/Muscolino/anatomycoloring/

ANTERIOR VIEWS OF THE OTHER MUSCLES OF THE ABDOMEN

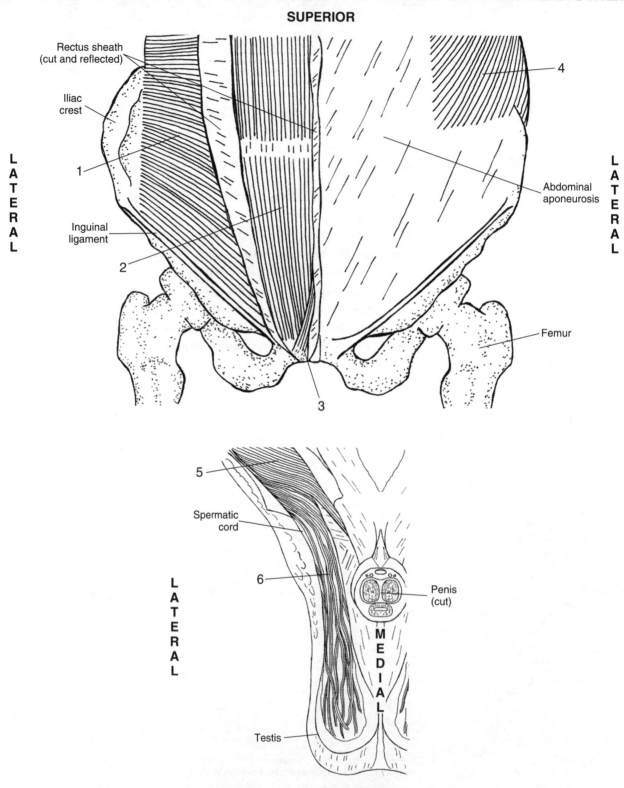

SUPERIOR

Rectus sheath
(cut and reflected)

Iliac
crest

1

Inguinal
ligament

2

4

Abdominal
aponeurosis

Femur

3

LATERAL

LATERAL

5

Spermatic
cord

6

Penis
(cut)

Testis

LATERAL

MEDIAL

INFERIOR

VIEWS OF THE MUSCLES OF THE PERINEUM

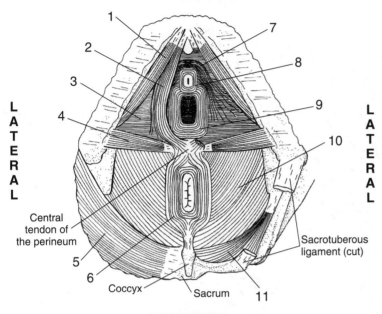

ANTERIOR

1
2
3
4

7
8
9
10

LATERAL

LATERAL

Central
tendon of
the perineum
5
6

Coccyx

Sacrum

11

Sacrotuberous
ligament (cut)

POSTERIOR

**Inferior view of
female perineum**

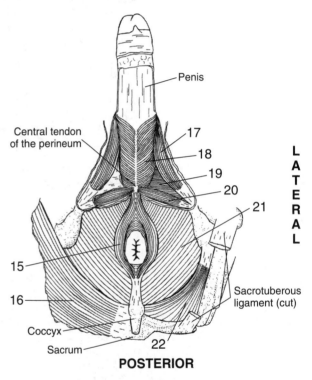

ANTERIOR

Penis

Central tendon
of the perineum

17
18
19
20
21

LATERAL

LATERAL

15

16

Coccyx

Sacrum

22

Sacrotuberous
ligament (cut)

POSTERIOR

**Inferior view of
male perineum (superficial)**

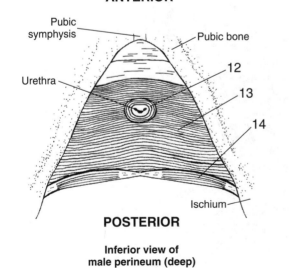

ANTERIOR

Pubic
symphysis

Pubic bone

Urethra

12
13
14

LATERAL

LATERAL

Ischium

POSTERIOR

**Inferior view of
male perineum (deep)**

VIEWS OF THE MUSCLES OF THE TONGUE

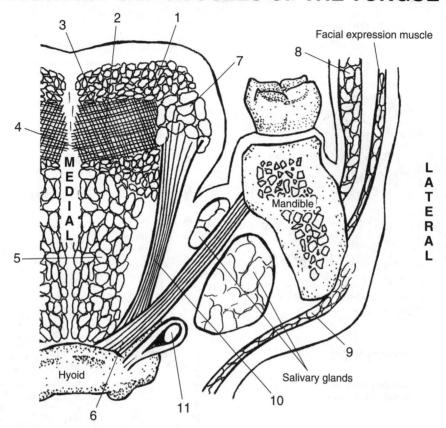

Anterior view (frontal plane section)

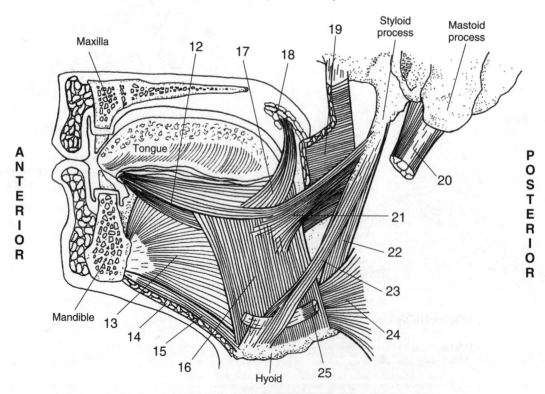

Lateral view (sagittal plane section)

VIEW OF THE MUSCLES OF THE PALATE

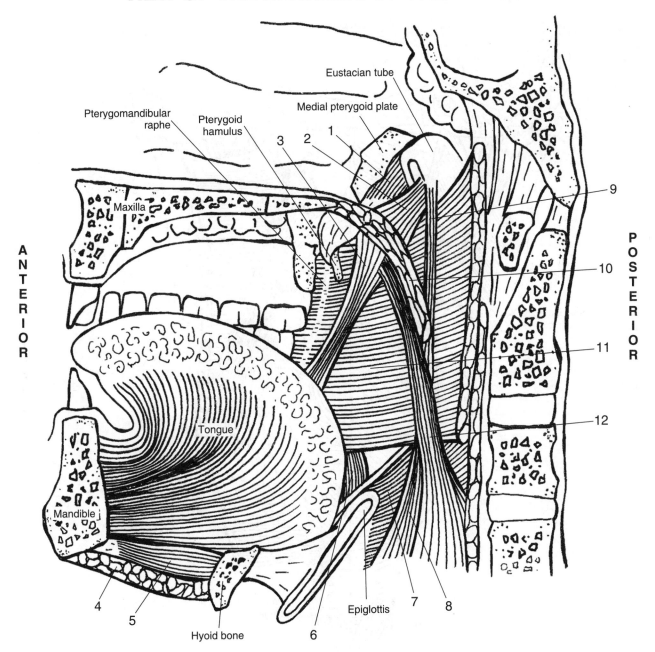

Eustacian tube

Medial pterygoid plate

Pterygomandibular
raphe

Pterygoid
hamulus

3   2   1

Maxilla

Tongue

Mandible

Hyoid bone

Epiglottis

ANTERIOR

POSTERIOR

9

10

11

12

4

5

6

7   8

Medial view (sagittal plane section)

VIEW OF THE MUSCLES OF THE PHARYNX

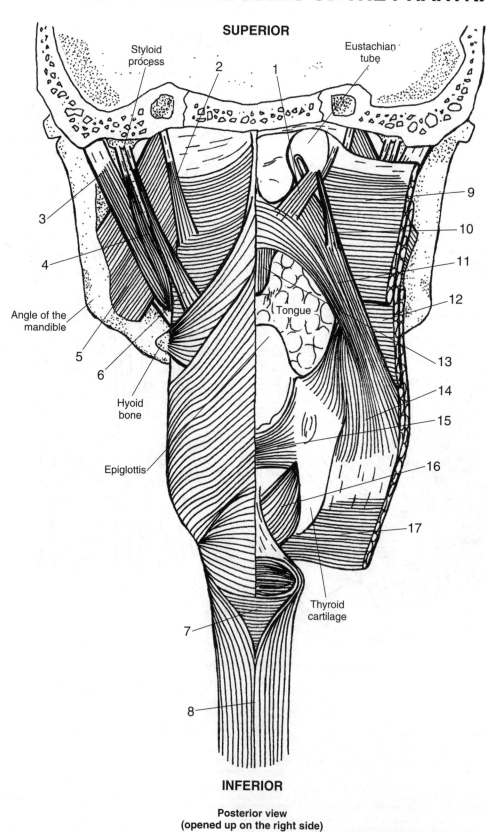

SUPERIOR

Styloid process

Eustachian tube

2

1

3

9

4

10

11

Angle of the mandible

Tongue

12

5

13

6

14

Hyoid bone

15

Epiglottis

16

7

17

Thyroid cartilage

8

INFERIOR

L A T E R A L

L A T E R A L

**Posterior view
(opened up on the right side)**

VIEWS OF THE MUSCLES OF THE LARYNX

SUPERIOR

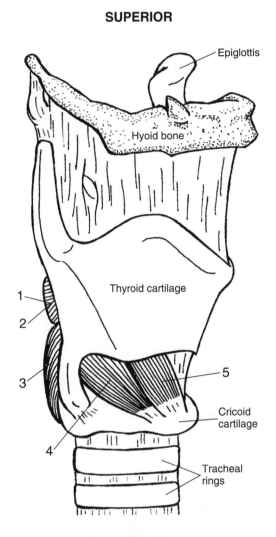

Epiglottis

Hyoid bone

Thyroid cartilage

1

2

3

4

5

Cricoid cartilage

Tracheal rings

INFERIOR

Lateral view

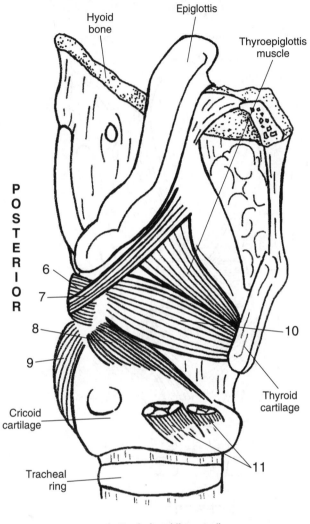

Hyoid bone

Epiglottis

Thyroepiglottis muscle

P O S T E R I O R

A N T E R I O R

6

7

8

9

Cricoid cartilage

Tracheal ring

10

Thyroid cartilage

11

Lateral view (dissected)

VIEWS OF THE MUSCLES OF THE LARYNX

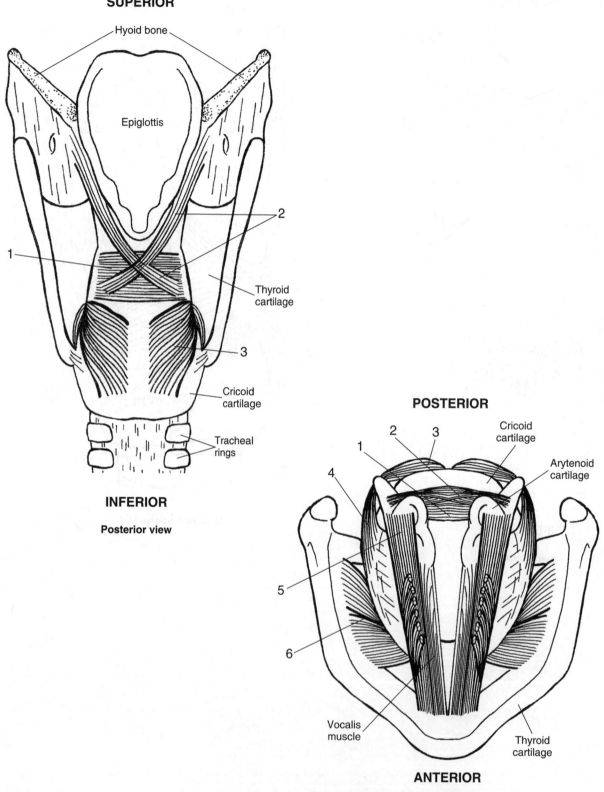

SUPERIOR

Hyoid bone

Epiglottis

2

1

Thyroid
cartilage

3

Cricoid
cartilage

Tracheal
rings

INFERIOR

Posterior view

POSTERIOR

Cricoid
cartilage

2   3

1

Arytenoid
cartilage

4

5

6

Vocalis
muscle

Thyroid
cartilage

ANTERIOR

Superior view

VIEWS OF THE EXTRINSIC MUSCLES OF THE RIGHT EYE

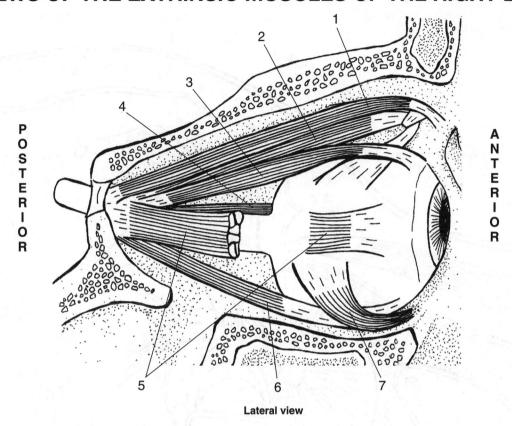

Lateral view

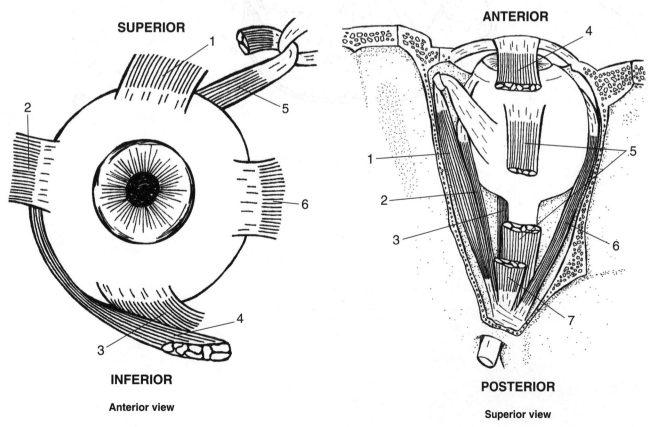

SUPERIOR

INFERIOR

Anterior view

ANTERIOR

POSTERIOR

Superior view

VIEW OF THE MUSCLES OF THE TYMPANIC CAVITY

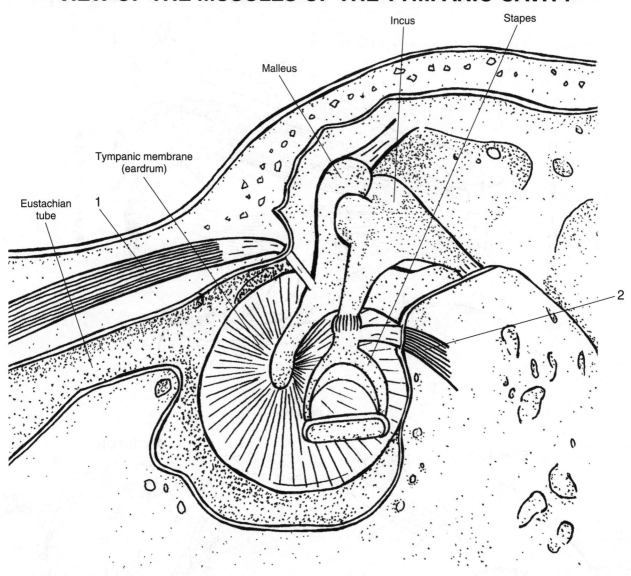

Malleus

Incus

Stapes

Tympanic membrane
(eardrum)

Eustachian
tube

1

2

Medial view (within the temporal bone)

The Nervous System 14

Answers to labeling exercises are on p. 493.

More review activities on Evolve at: http://evolve.elsevier.com/Muscolino/anatomycoloring/

CRANIAL NERVES
ANTERIOR

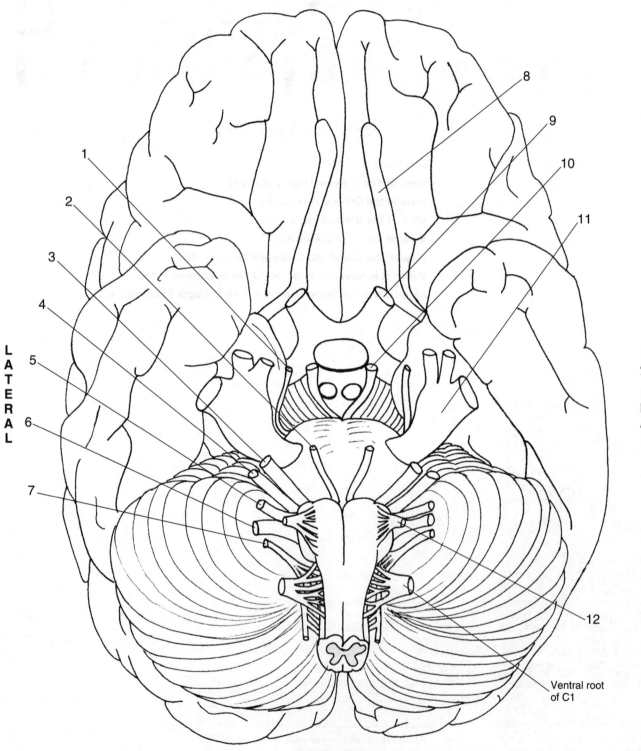

POSTERIOR

Inferior view of the brain

VIEW OF SPINAL NERVE ORGANIZATION

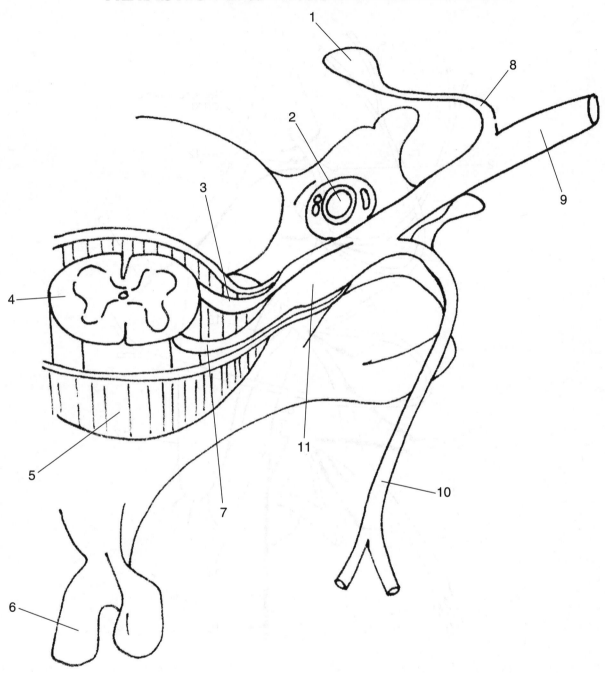

Cross section view of the spinal cord through a cervical vertebra—spinal nerve diagram

VIEW OF THE CERVICAL PLEXUS

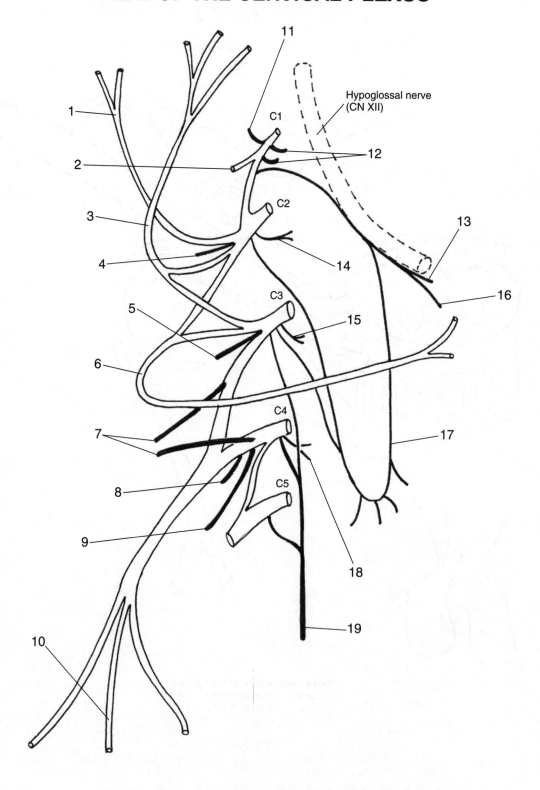

11

Hypoglossal nerve
(CN XII)

C1

1

2

12

C2

3

13

4

14

C3

5

15

6

16

7

C4

17

8

9

C5

18

10

19

VIEW OF THE BRACHIAL PLEXUS

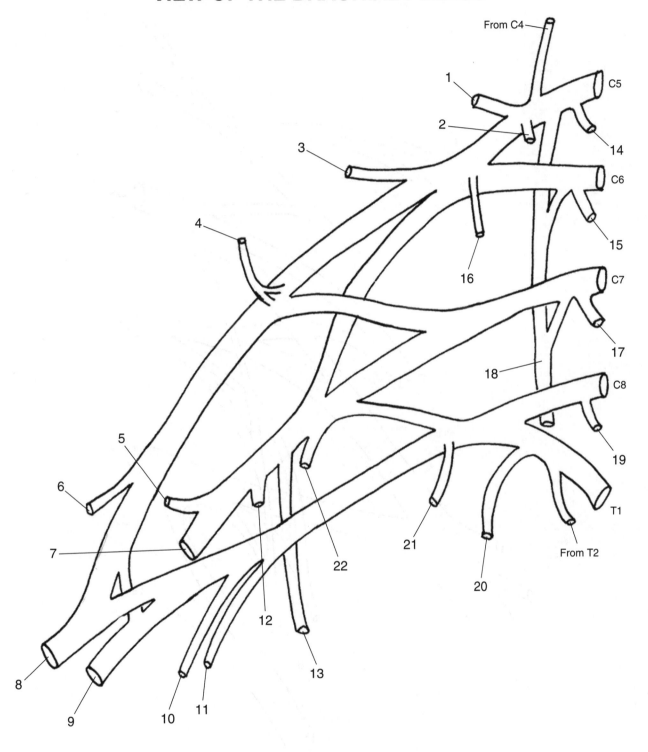

From C4

1

2

3

4

C5

14

C6

15

16

C7

17

18

C8

19

5

6

7

8

9

10

11

12

13

22

21

20

T1

From T2

VIEW OF THE LUMBAR PLEXUS

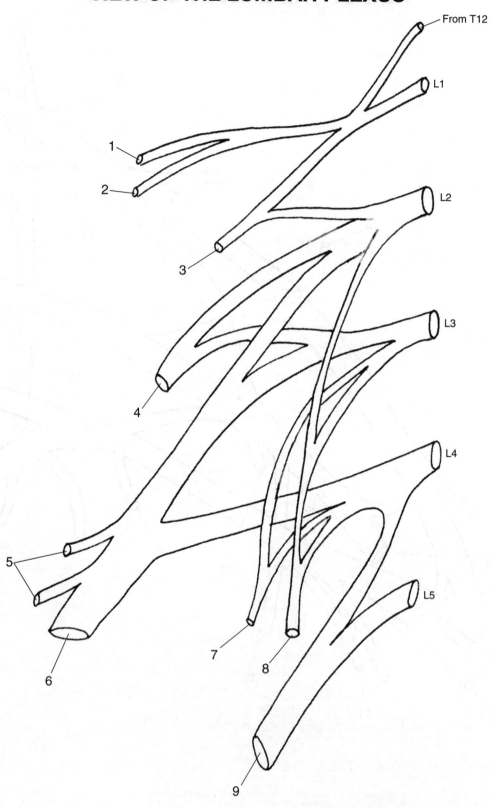

VIEW OF THE SACRAL AND COCCYGEAL PLEXUSES

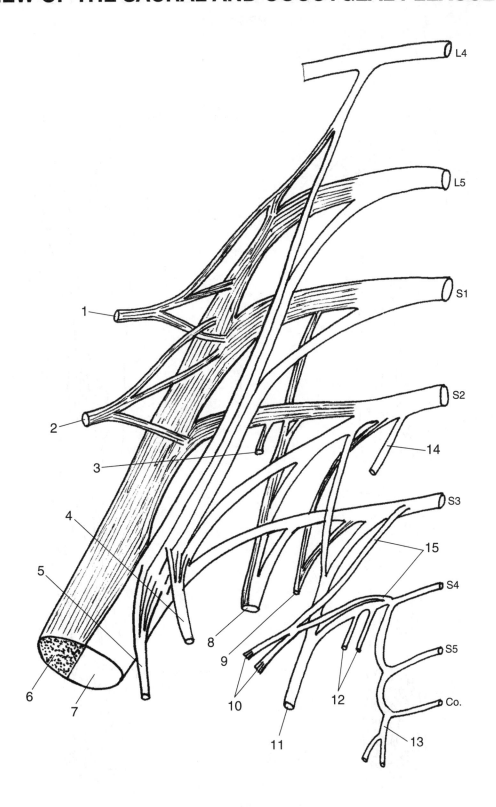

VIEWS OF INNERVATION TO THE RIGHT LOWER EXTREMITY

PROXIMAL

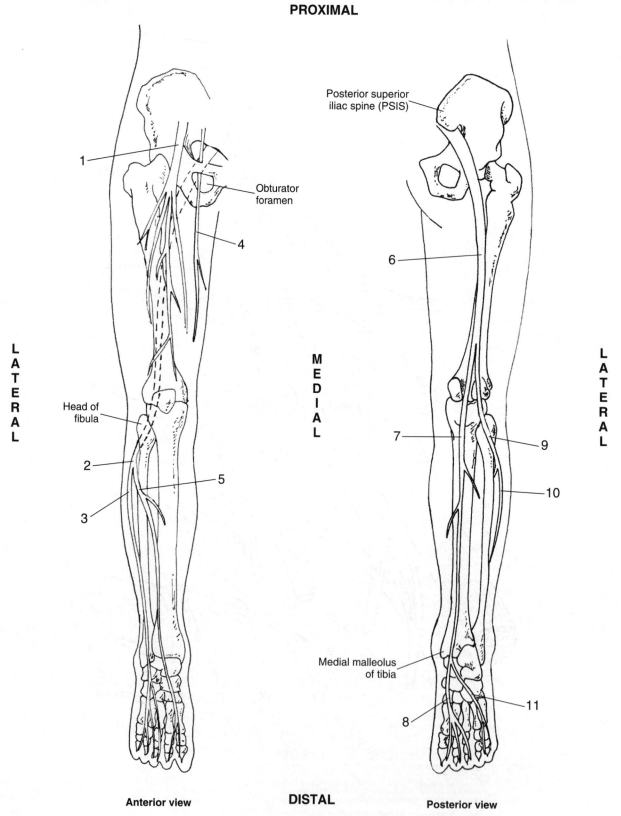

Obturator foramen

Posterior superior iliac spine (PSIS)

Head of fibula

Medial malleolus of tibia

L A T E R A L

M E D I A L

L A T E R A L

Anterior view

DISTAL

Posterior view

ANTERIOR VIEW OF INNERVATION TO THE RIGHT UPPER EXTREMITY

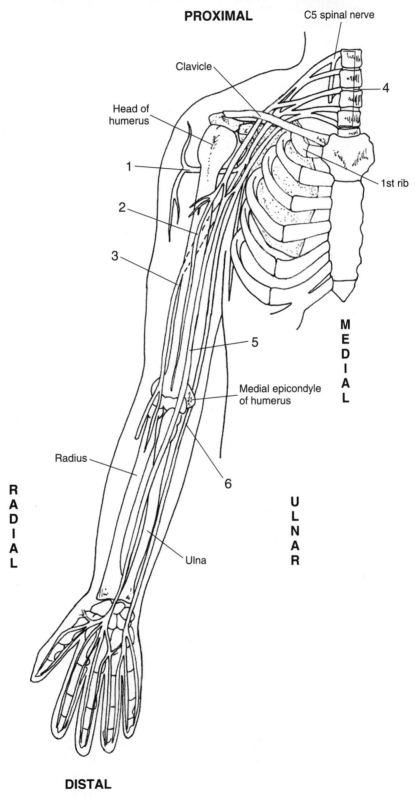

PROXIMAL

C5 spinal nerve

Clavicle

Head of humerus

1st rib

LATERAL

MEDIAL

Medial epicondyle of humerus

Radius

RADIAL

ULNAR

Ulna

DISTAL

The Arterial System 15

Answers to labeling exercises are on p. 494.

ⓔ More review activities on Evolve at: http://evolve.elsevier.com/Muscolino/anatomycoloring/

LATERAL VIEW OF ARTERIAL SUPPLY TO THE HEAD AND NECK

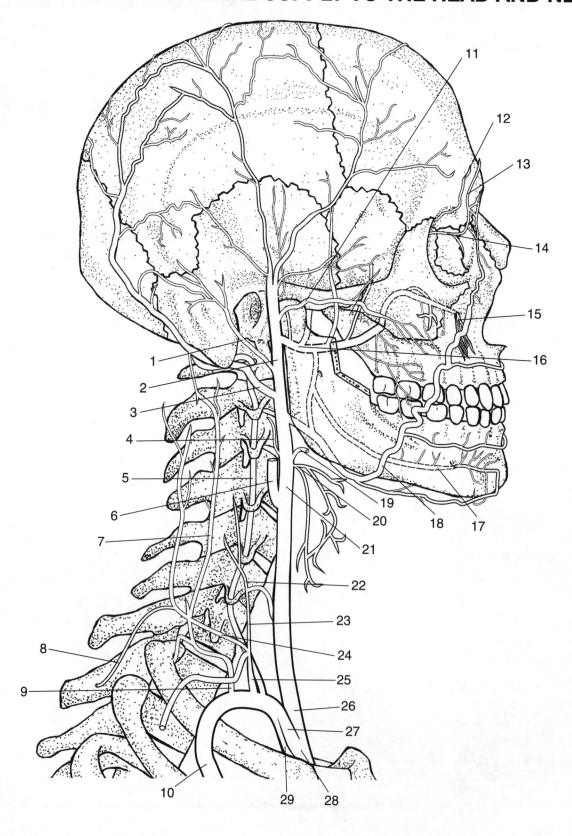

ANTERIOR VIEW OF ARTERIAL SUPPLY TO THE TRUNK AND PELVIS

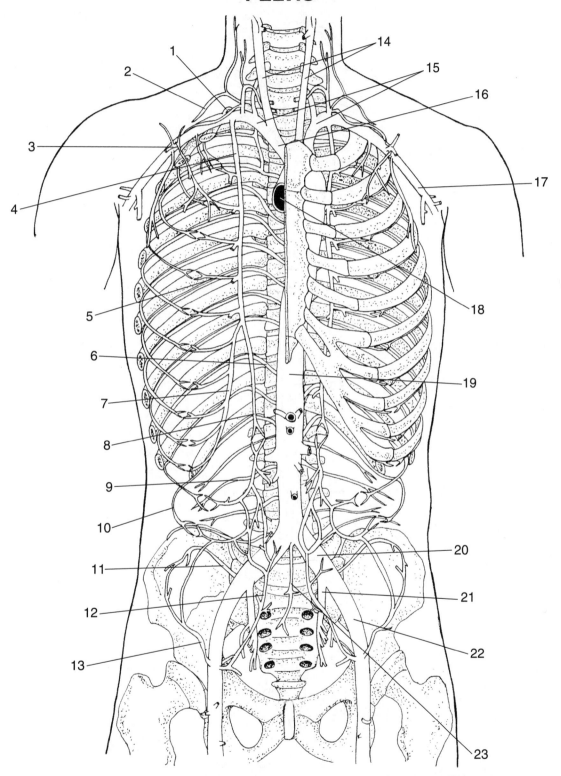

ANTERIOR VIEW OF ARTERIAL SUPPLY TO THE RIGHT LOWER EXTREMITY

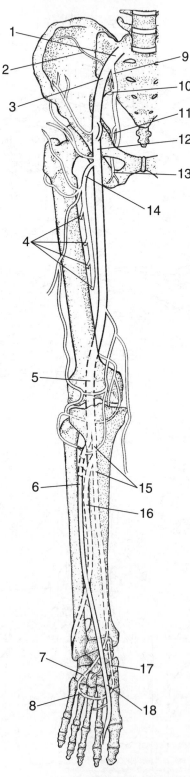

ANTERIOR VIEW OF ARTERIAL SUPPLY TO THE RIGHT UPPER EXTREMITY

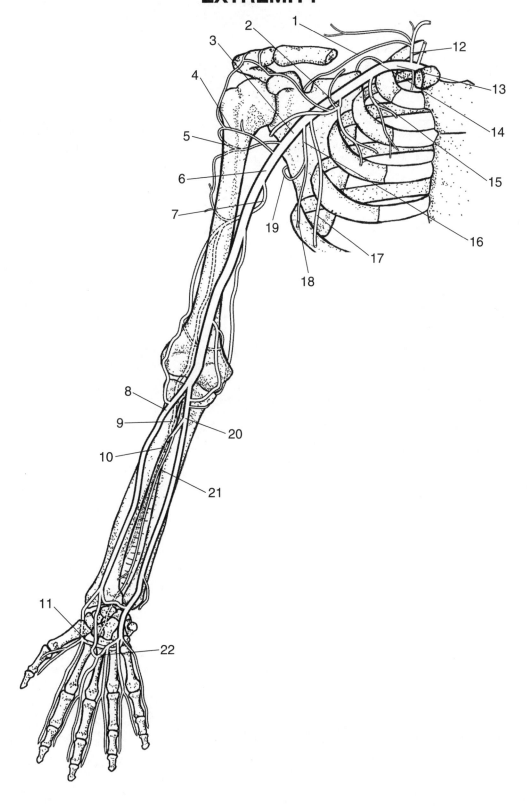

Tissue Structure and Other Systems of the Body

16

Answers to labeling exercises are on p. 494.

More review activities on Evolve at: http://evolve.elsevier.com/Muscolino/anatomycoloring/

BRIEF OVERVIEW OF THE SYSTEMS OF THE BODY

The Cell

The cell is the basic structural and functional building block of the human body. While cells are diverse in structure (and function), there are certain essential elements of most cells. Cells essentially have two parts, an inner nucleus and the surrounding cytoplasmic fluid; both of these two structures have a semipermeable membrane around them. The nucleus contains DNA (the genetic blueprint) and the nucleolus (which makes ribosomes). In the cytoplasm, there are many organelles (small organs), each with a particular function. These organelles are held in place by fine filaments that are found in the cytoplasm; these filaments create a skeletal structure for the cell called the *cytoskeleton*.

The major cytoplasmic organelles are: ribosomes (they function to synthesize proteins), mitochondria (they turn glucose and oxygen into ATP molecules for energy), endoplasmic reticulum (there are two types, "rough" and "smooth"; they function as a transport system within the cell), golgi apparatus (which functions to refine and transport proteins), and lysosomes (which digest and break down intracellular substances).

There are also organelles that can be located on the outside membrane of the cell. These structures are called *cilia* and *flagella*, both of which function to create movement, either of the cell itself, or of substances along the surface of the cell. Usually, a cell has either one long flagellum or numerous shorter cilia.

Integumentary System

An integument is a covering; hence the integumentary system covers the body. The integumentary system is comprised of the cutaneous membrane, (i.e., the skin, and the accessory organs of the skin). The skin has two layers to it: the outer epidermis, which is stratified squamous epithelium, and the deeper dermis, which is fibrous connective tissue. The accessory organs are the hair follicles, arrector pili muscles, sebaceous glands, and eccrine and apocrine sweat glands. The main function of the skin is to provide a barrier between the inside of our body and the outside world. This barrier prevents pathogens (disease-causing microorganisms) from entering the body and keeps moisture and body contents from escaping. The skin also functions to help regulate internal body temperature by two processes: (1) sweating; and (2) dermal blood vessel dilation, which regulates the amount of blood that flows to the skin for exchange of heat with the outside world. Deep to the skin is subcutaneous fascia.

Cardiovascular System

The cardiovascular system is made up of the cardiac system and the vascular system. The cardiac system is comprised of the heart; the vascular system is comprised of blood vessels (i.e., the arteries, capillaries, and the veins).

The heart is essentially a double pump, having a left side and a right side (each side having two chambers: an atrium and a ventricle). The heart's left side pumps oxygen-rich/carbon dioxide–poor blood into vessels that bring the blood out to the cells and tissues of the body; this is called the *systemic circulation*. At the cellular/tissue level, these vessels give their oxygen (and other nutrients) to the cells so that the vital processes of metabolism can occur. These vessels also pick up carbon dioxide (and other waste products) from the cells and transport these substances back to the right side of the heart. The heart's right side then pumps this oxygen-poor/carbon dioxide–rich blood to the lungs, where it is oxygenated and loses much of its carbon dioxide; this is called the *pulmonic circulation*. This oxygen-rich/carbon dioxide–poor blood then returns back to the left side of the heart where it can be pumped out to the cells and tissues of the body once again.

It is the vessels of the cardiovascular system that carry the blood that is pumped by the heart. There are three types of blood vessels: arteries, capillaries, and veins.

Arteries carry blood away from the heart. As they do so, arteries branch and diminish in size, eventually becoming capillaries. Capillaries are thinwalled vessels that do the essential job of exchange of oxygen and carbon dioxide (and other nutrients and waste products) with the intercellular fluid around the cells. Capillaries then converge with each other to form veins, which carry the blood back to the heart. NOTE: Arteries in the systemic circulation carry "oxygenated" blood; arteries in the pulmonic circulation carry "deoxygenated" blood; veins in the systemic circulation carry "deoxygenated" blood; veins in the pulmonic circulation carry "oxygenated" blood. Hence, the cardiovascular system is a double circulation. The systemic circulation is created by the left side of the heart pumping to the cells/tissues of the body and the return of this blood to the right side of the heart; the pulmonic circulation is created by the right side of the heart pumping to the lungs and the return of this blood to the left side of the heart.

Lymphatic System

Not all the fluid of the systemic blood that is pumped out to the tissues of the body by the arteries is returned back to the heart by the veins. A small amount of the fluid that leaves the capillaries at the tissue level is left behind in the tissues. If this extra intercellular tissue fluid is not removed, a build-up of fluid (swelling) will occur in the tissues of the body. It is the job of the lymphatic system to return this fluid back to the heart. The lymphatic system does this by carrying this fluid in lymphatic vessels (where it is termed "lymph") back toward the heart. It actually deposits the lymph into a large vein; from there the venous system returns this fluid back to the right side of the heart. Along the way, the lymph in lymphatic vessels travels through lymph nodes that are high in white blood cells that filter the blood, attacking any foreign disease-causing pathogens. Hence, the lymphatic system has two purposes: to return extra tissue fluid back to the heart and to filter possible pathogens from the blood.

Respiratory System

Oxygen is one of the most important nutrients that the cardiovascular system circulates to the tissues of the body. It is the job of the respiratory system to bring oxygen into the body and place this oxygen into the cardiovascular system. The respiratory system may be divided into the passageways that carry oxygen to the lungs when we breathe in (inspiration), and the lungs themselves. The passageways include: the nose, nasal cavity, mouth, pharynx, larynx, and the trachea. The lungs contain the bronchial tree and the alveolar sacs. It is in the lungs that the blood that comes from the right side of the heart (pulmonic circulation) picks up oxygen to return to the left side of the heart where it can be pumped to the cells and tissues of the body (systemic circulation). The lungs also pick up the waste product carbon dioxide from the blood; this carbon dioxide is then transported out of the lungs to the outside world through the aforementioned passageways when we breathe out (expiration). Hence, the respiratory system has two purposes: to carry oxygen into the body and place it into the blood, and to eliminate carbon dioxide from the blood and carry it out of the body.

Urinary System

As the cardiovascular system circulates blood throughout the body, waste products from cellular metabolism accumulate within the blood. It is the job of the two kidneys of the urinary system to filter these waste products from the blood. The waste products that the kidneys filter from the blood form urine, which leaves each kidney through a long muscular tube called a *ureter*; the two ureters carry the urine to the urinary bladder. The urine is stored in the urinary bladder until a sufficient amount is present. The urine is then expelled from the urinary bladder through the urethra to the outside world. This process of expelling urine is called *urination* or *micturition*.

Gastrointestinal System

As we have said, the cells of the body must be constantly supplied with nutrients by the bloodstream. Other than oxygen that comes from the lungs, these nutrients come from the gastrointestinal system. The gastrointestinal system is comprised of two parts: a long passageway called the *alimentary canal* that begins at the mouth and ends at the anus, and the accessory organs that secrete substances (primarily enzymes) into the alimentary canal. The alimentary canal consists of the mouth, pharynx, esophagus, stomach, small intestine, and large intestine. The accessory organs are the salivary glands, pancreas, liver, and gall bladder. The gastrointestinal system essentially functions as follows: food enters at the mouth; as the food travels through the alimentary canal, whatever is digested and absorbed is taken into the bloodstream for use in the body (i.e., nutrients that the bloodstream carries to the cells); whatever substances are not digested and absorbed continue through the alimentary canal and exit through the anus as feces. The liver also functions to filter unwanted chemicals of the body (both created by metabolism and ingested from external sources) from the blood.

Immune System

"Immunity" means freedom. It is the function of your immune system to keep you free from disease. The immune system does this by fighting foreign microorganisms such as bacteria and viruses (pathogens) that might cause infection and disease. The most important cells of your body that do this are macrophages and a type of white blood cell called *lymphocytes*. There are two main types of lymphocytes, T-lymphocytes and B-lymphocytes (also known as *T cells* and *B cells*); each one of them attacks pathogens in a different manner. T-lymphocytes directly attack the pathogens, engaging in cell to cell contact, secreting substances that are toxic to the pathogen; further, T-lymphocytes help to activate B-lymphocytes. B-lymphocytes secrete antibodies (immunoglobulins) that attack the pathogens. Macrophages destroy pathogens by the process of phagocytosis, in which the pathogens are ingested into the macrophage and broken down by the lysosomes of the macrophage.

Endocrine System

The endocrine system is composed of structures that secrete hormones into the bloodstream. The major endocrine glands are the hypothalamus, pituitary, thyroid, parathyroid, adrenal, pancreas, testes, and ovaries. Other endocrine glands are the pineal and thymus. Generally, the hormones of the hypothalamus control the hormone production of the pituitary and the hormones of the pituitary then control the hormone secretions of other glands such as the thyroid, adrenal, testes, and ovaries. The function of hormones is to act as chemical messengers that regulate the metabolic processes of the body. The endocrine system is also intimately linked to the nervous system of the body; indeed the hypothalamus and pituitary (as well as the pineal gland) are structures of the brain.

Sensory System

The sensory system is the system of receptors in the body that allows us to sense the external world around us as well as sense the internal environment of our body. The senses are usually divided into the somatic senses and special senses. Somatic senses are touch, pressure, temperature, pain, and stretch receptors. Somatic sensory receptors are primarily located in the skin and around the joints. Special senses are smell, taste, vision, hearing, and equilibrium. Special sensory receptors are located in the nasal cavity, mouth, eyes, and ears. All sensory stimuli travel to the central nervous system where they are processed and interpreted. Given these sensory stimuli, the central nervous system determines the appropriate response(s) for our health, enjoyment, and safety.

Nervous System

The nervous system is the master controller of the body. The cells of the nervous system are called *nerve cells* or *neurons*. These neurons carry their messages by the transmission of electrical impulses. There are five types of neuroglial cells that support the neurons in various ways.

Structurally, the nervous system can be divided into the central nervous system (CNS) and the peripheral nervous system (PNS). The central nervous system is in the center of your body; it is comprised of the brain and spinal cord. The brain can be further subdivided into the cerebral hemispheres, cerebellar hemispheres, diencephalon, midbrain, pons, and medulla oblongata. The peripheral nervous system is comprised of all nerves that are located peripheral to the central nervous system; these are the 12 pairs of cranial nerves and the 31 pairs of spinal nerves.

Functionally, the neurons of the nervous system can carry three types of electrical messages: sensory, integrative, and motor. Sensory signals travel through peripheral sensory nerves to the central nervous system. The central nervous system then integrates these sensory stimuli and a response is determined. The order to execute this response, an impulse, then travels through peripheral motor nerves to whatever muscle or gland is being ordered to take action.

The nervous system is a tremendously complex system that controls and coordinates virtually everything in the human body. Further, it is responsible for conscious thought, emotional feeling, memory, and movement, as well as unconscious control of our body.

Reproductive System

The reproductive system has the job of carrying on our species into the future by creating offspring. There are two reproductive systems: the male and female.

The male reproductive system functions to create sperm, maintain them, and then deliver them to the site of fertilization (the reproductive system of the female). The primary structures of the male reproductive system are the testes, which produce the sperm. The accessory organs of the male reproductive system function to maintain and deliver the sperm to the site of fertilization. The accessory reproductive organs can be divided into internal and external structures. The internal accessory reproductive organs are the epididymis, vas deference, seminal vesicle, prostate gland, and the bulbourethral glands. The external accessory reproductive organs are the scrotum and the penis.

The female reproductive system functions to create eggs, maintain and deliver them to the site of fertilization, and, if fertilization occurs, provide a favorable environment for the developing offspring to grow, and then deliver the offspring to the outside world. The primary structures of the female reproductive system are the ovaries, which produce the eggs. The accessory organs of the female reproductive system function to carry on the other activities as listed above. The internal accessory reproductive organs are the fallopian tubes, uterus, and the vagina. The external accessory reproductive organs are the labia majora, labia minora, clitoris, vestibular glands, and the vestibular bulb.

Overview of the Interrelationships of the Organ Systems of the Body—The Big Picture

The preceding was a brief overview of the major visceral organ systems of the body, each one described somewhat independently. However, understanding how each system of the body works without understanding the bigger picture of how these systems interrelate to create the smooth operation of the human body as a whole is like understanding what each piece of a jigsaw puzzle looks like without having any sense of what the bigger picture is that the puzzle creates. Toward that end, the following is a glimpse of the bigger picture of how the organ systems of the human interrelate to operate our body. Admittedly, it is a gross simplification, but is still useful for our purposes.

Our body is composed of trillions of cells, each one a living entity that requires two things: (1) nutrients to carry on its functions and (2) its waste products to be carried away.

These two crucial jobs fall to the cardiovascular system, along with the aid of the lymphatic system (together, these two systems comprise the circulatory system). These two systems circulate fluid (blood and lymph) that carries the nutrients and wastes of the cells of the body. As the circulation of blood occurs, needed nutrients are used up. It is the job of the respiratory system to bring in needed oxygen to the blood, and it is the job of the gastrointestinal system to bring in most every other needed nutrient. As the blood circulates, it also builds up waste products of metabolism and other undesired elements, and needs to be filtered. The blood is filtered by the lungs, lymph nodes, kidney, and liver. The integumentary system provides a covering or barrier between the internal contents and the outside world. This barrier is especially important in preventing foreign microorganisms from entering our body and causing infection and disease. When pathogens do find entry into the body, the immune system functions to attack these foreign invaders. The endocrine system secretes hormones into the bloodstream that function to control the metabolism of the body. Sensory receptors gather sensory stimuli and carry these stimuli to the central nervous system of the body. The brain and spinal cord of the central nervous system then integrate and interpret these sensory stimuli and determine what response(s) the body will have. It is the responsibility of the reproductive system to see that our species is continued into the future by the birth of offspring.

For all movement of the body, the musculoskeletal system is involved. The musculoskeletal system is comprised of the bones of the skeleton, the joints located between the bones, and the muscles that move the bones at the joints of the body.

The Cell

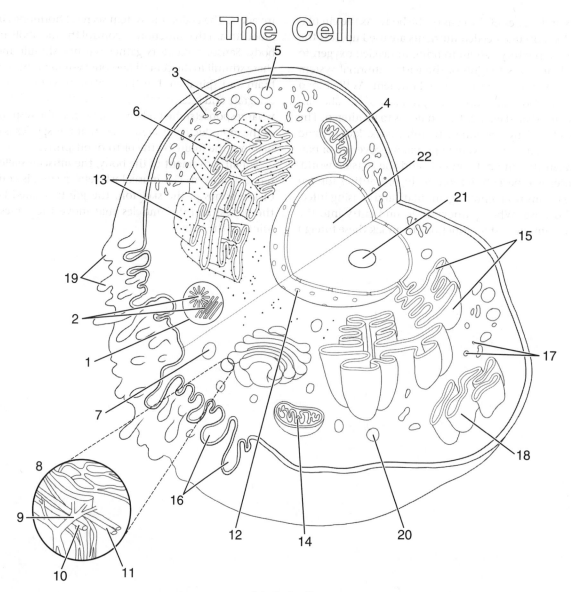

A typical cell.

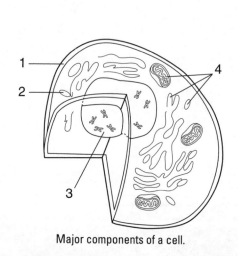

Major components of a cell.

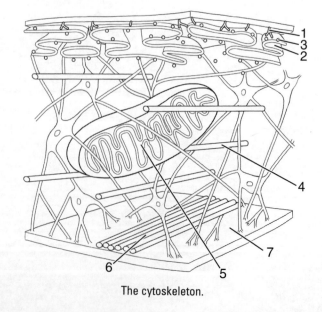

The cytoskeleton.

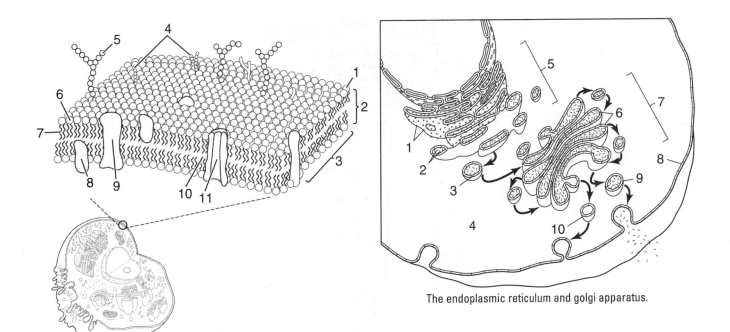

The cell membrane.

The endoplasmic reticulum and golgi apparatus.

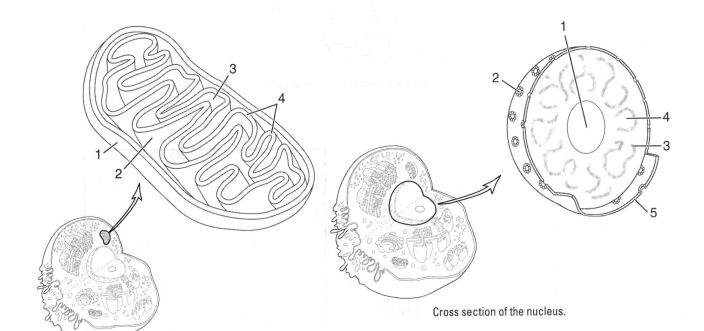

Cross section of a mitochondrion.

Cross section of the nucleus.

Bone Tissue

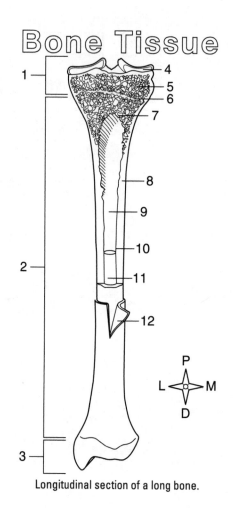

Longitudinal section of a long bone.

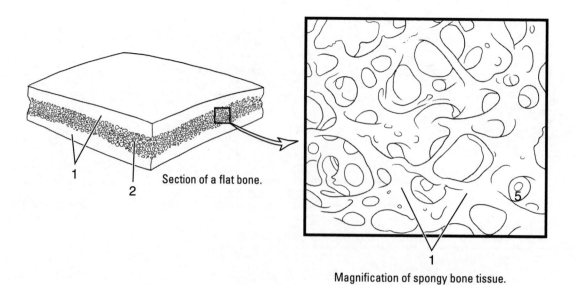

Section of a flat bone.

Magnification of spongy bone tissue.

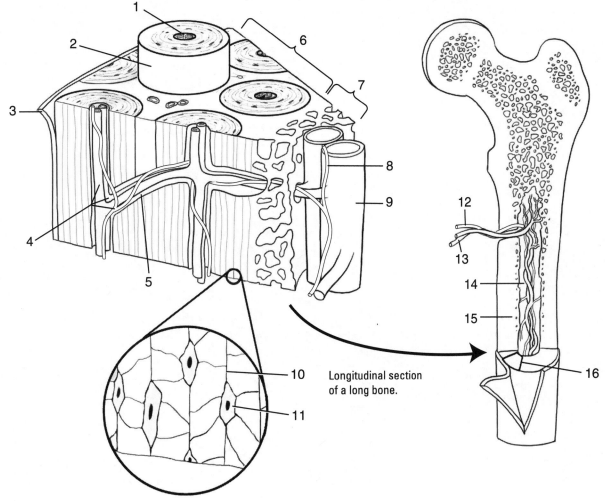

Magnification of compact bone tissue.

Longitudinal section
of a long bone.

Muscle Tissue

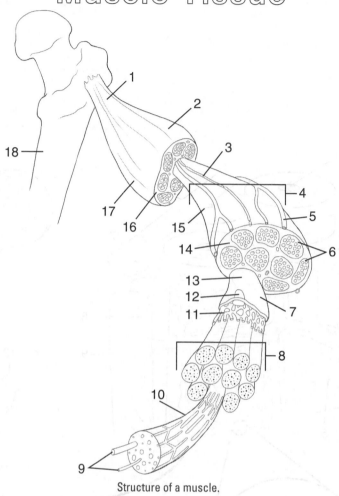

Structure of a muscle.

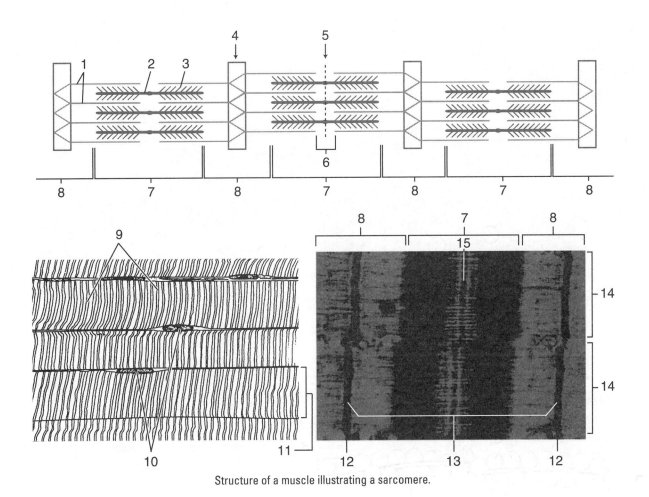

Structure of a muscle illustrating a sarcomere.

Sarcoplasmic reticulum and T tubules of a muscle fiber.

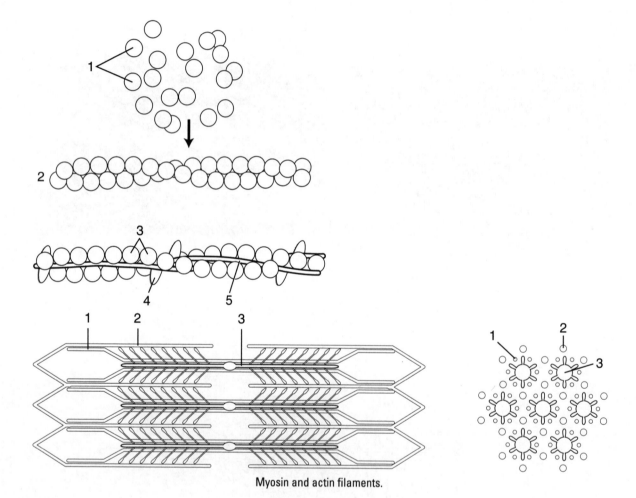

Myosin and actin filaments.

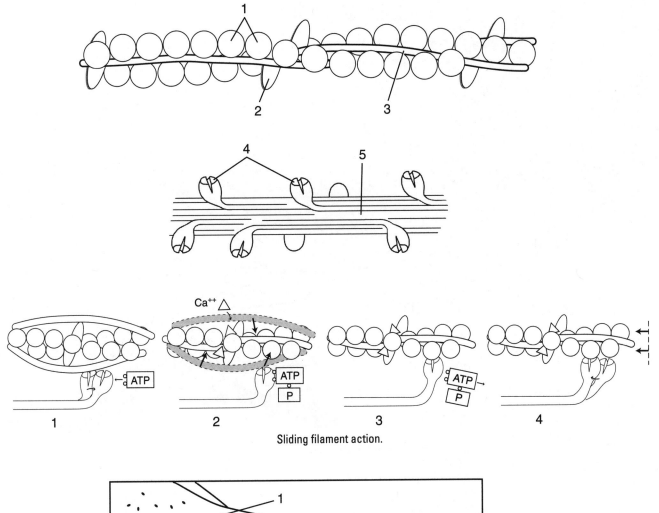

Sliding filament action.

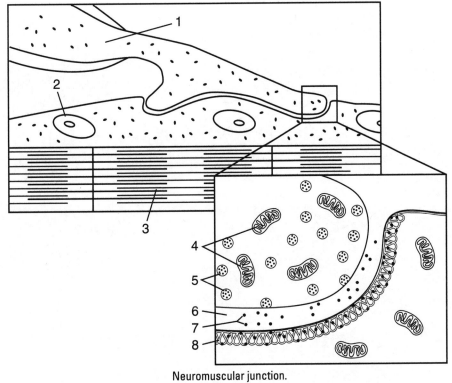

Neuromuscular junction.

Nerve Tissue

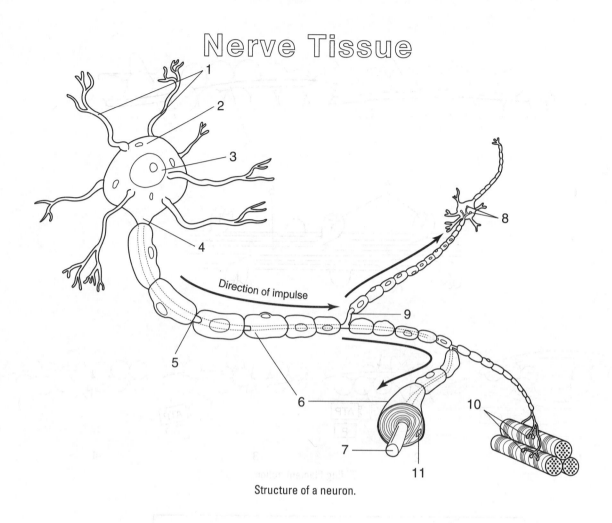

Structure of a neuron.

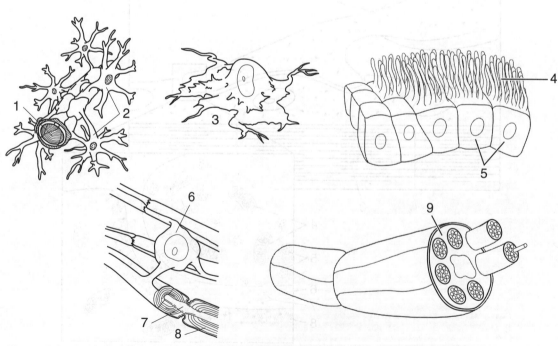

Types of neuroglial cells.

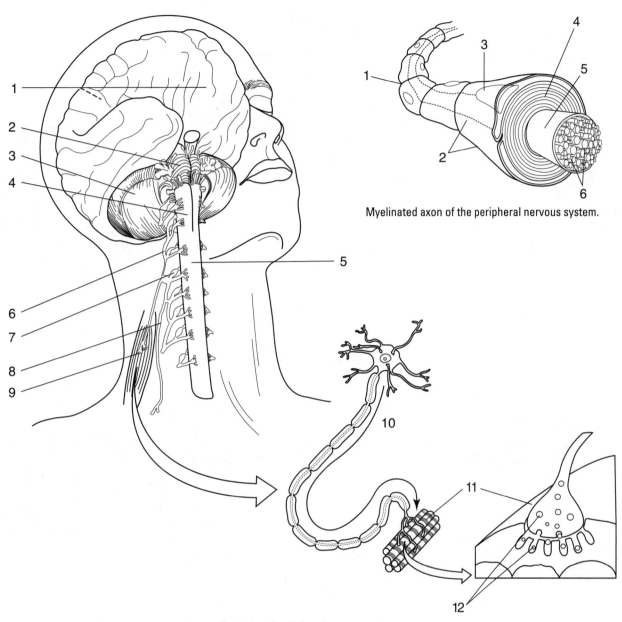

Myelinated axon of the peripheral nervous system.

Central and peripheral nervous systems.

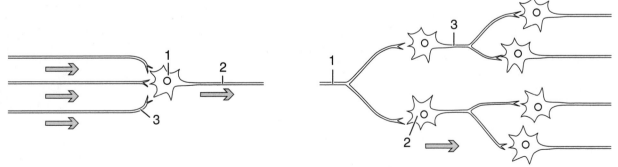

Convergence of neurons. Divergence of neurons.

Joints

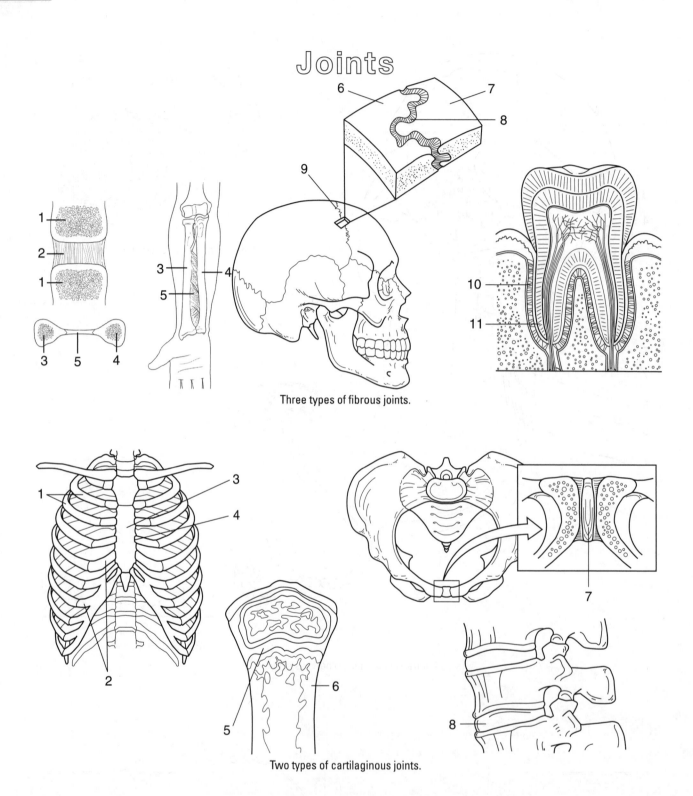

Three types of fibrous joints.

Two types of cartilaginous joints.

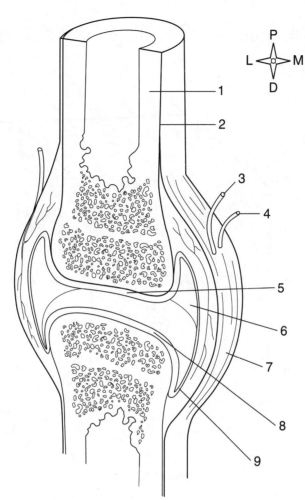

Structure of a typical synovial joint.

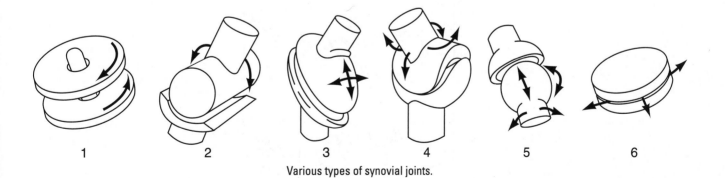

Various types of synovial joints.

Integumentary System

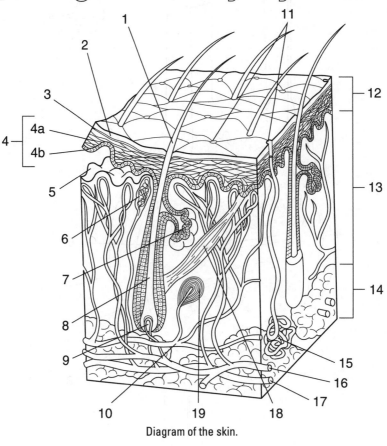

Diagram of the skin.

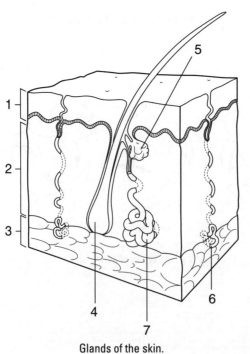

Glands of the skin.

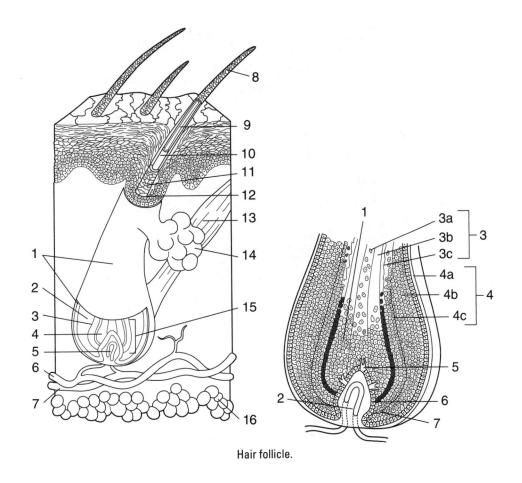

Hair follicle.

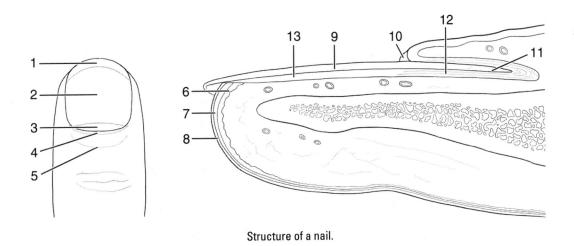

Structure of a nail.

Cardiac System
(THE HEART)

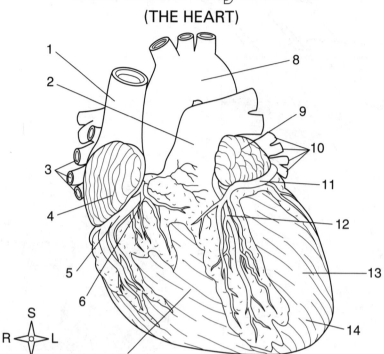

Anterior view of the heart.

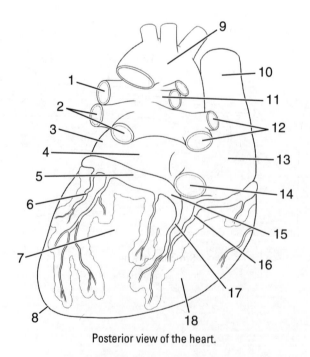

Posterior view of the heart.

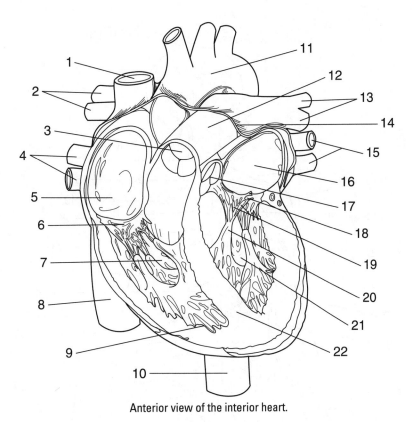

Anterior view of the interior heart.

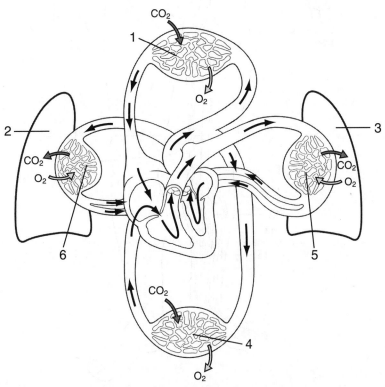

Systemic and pulmonic circulations of the heart.

Venous System

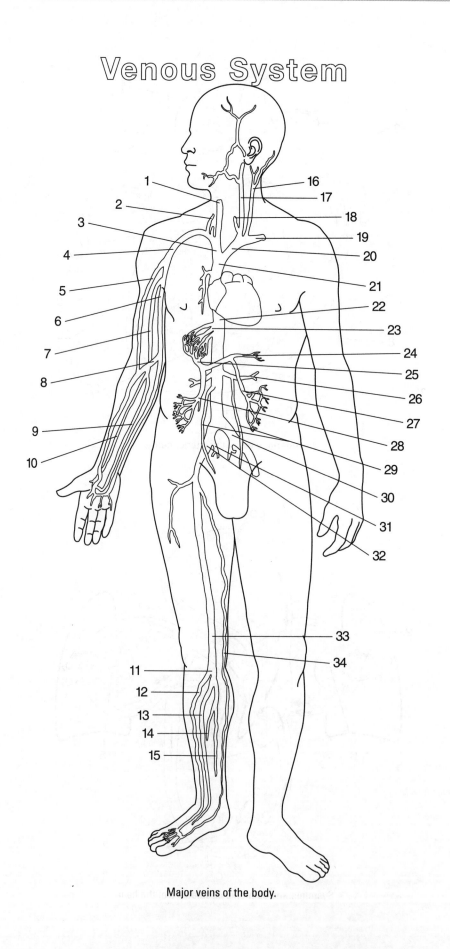

1

2

3

4

5

6

7

8

9

10

11

12

13

14

15

16

17

18

19

20

21

22

23

24

25

26

27

28

29

30

31

32

33

34

Major veins of the body.

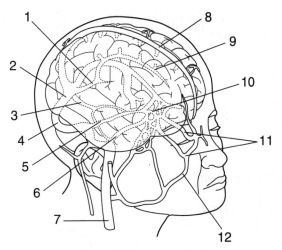

Venous drainage of the brain.

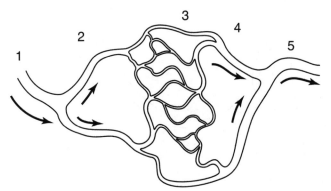

Creation of venous blood flow from capillaries.

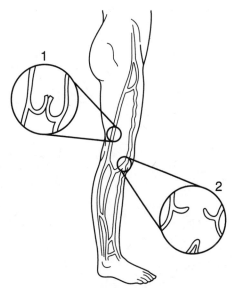

Unidirectional venous valves.

Lymphatic System

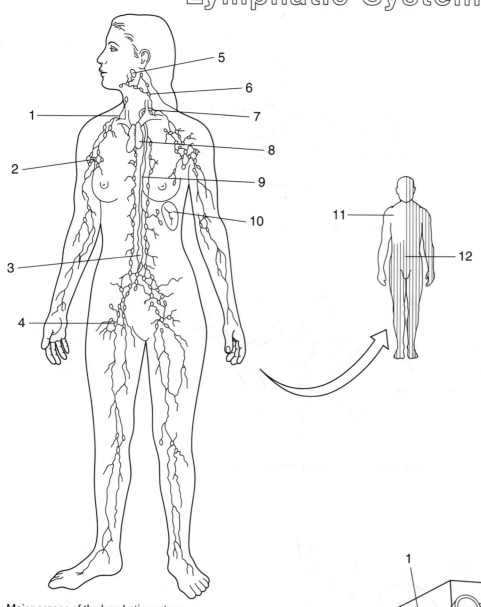

Major organs of the lymphatic system.

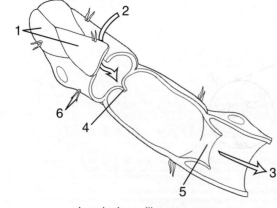

Lymphatic capillary structure.

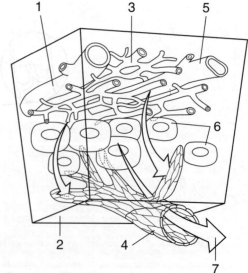

Role of lymphatic capillary in draining intercellular fluid.

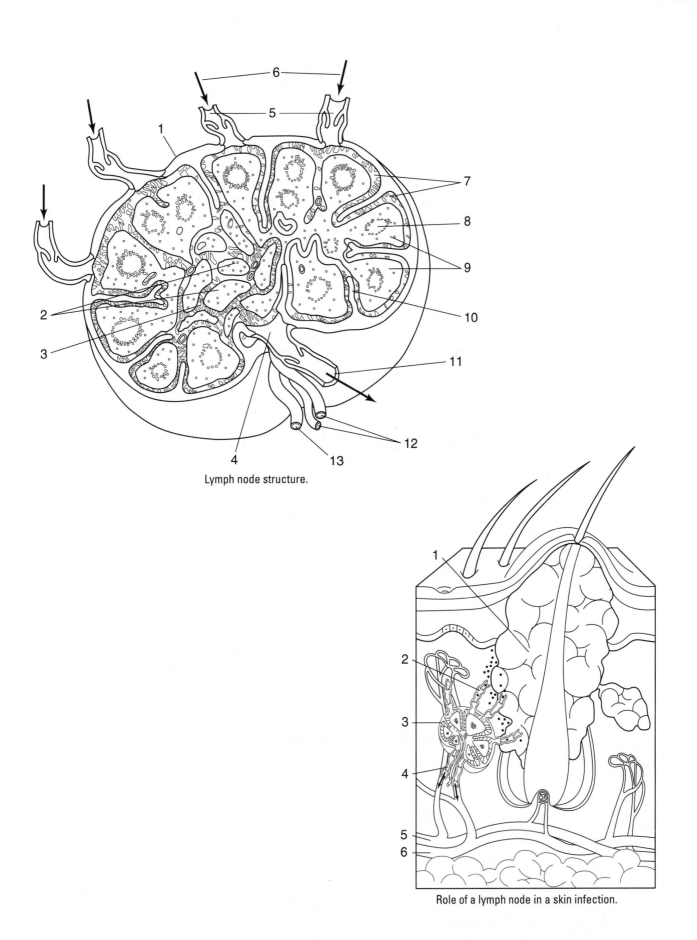

Lymph node structure.

Role of a lymph node in a skin infection.

Respiratory System

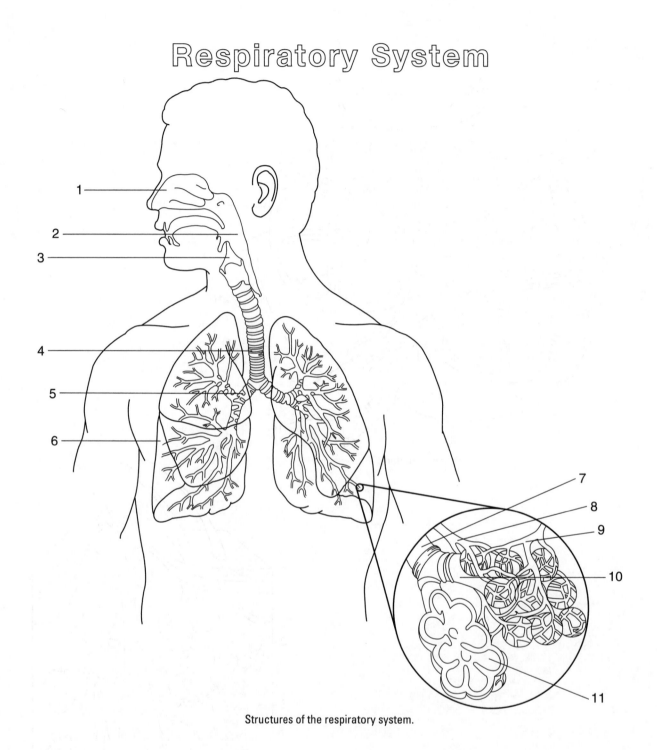

Structures of the respiratory system.

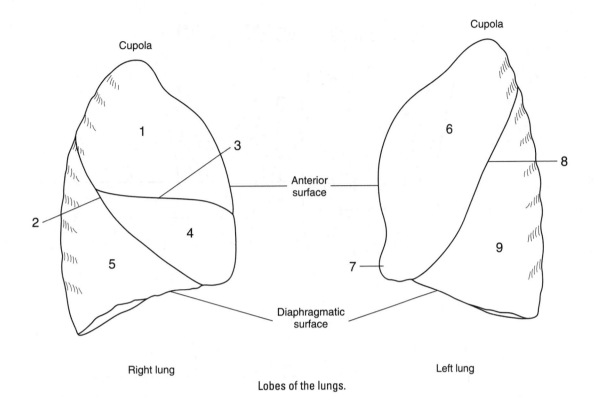

Right lung

Left lung

Lobes of the lungs.

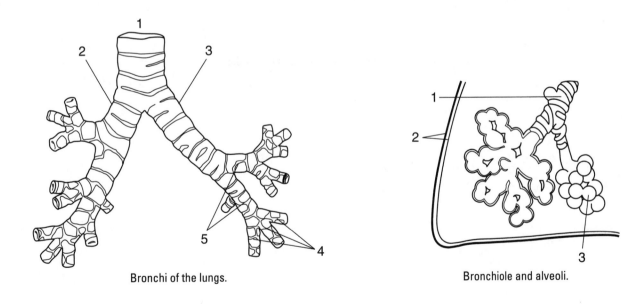

Bronchi of the lungs.

Bronchiole and alveoli.

Urinary System

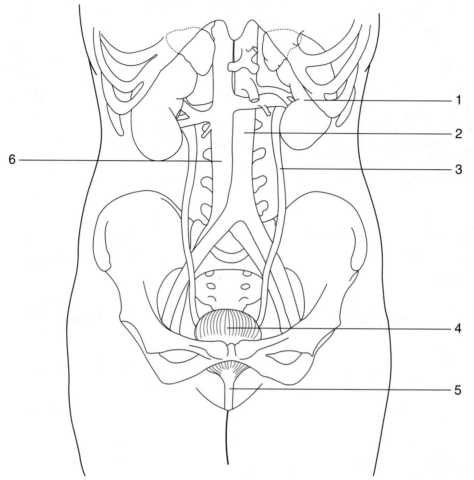

Anterior view of the structures of the urinary system.

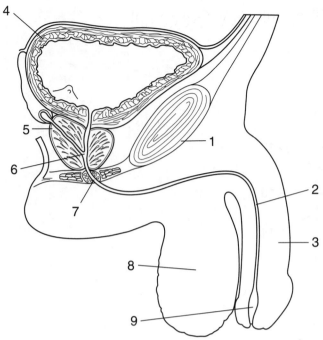

Right lateral view of the bladder and urethra of a male.

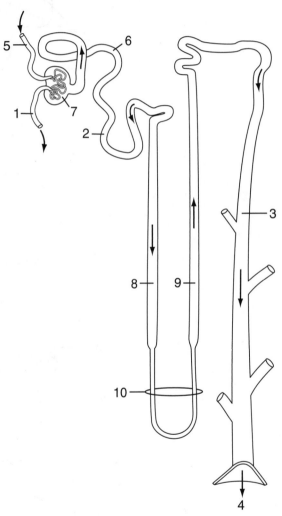

Structures of a nephron.

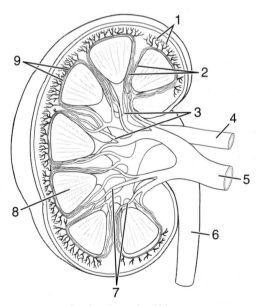

Section through a kidney.

Gastrointestinal System

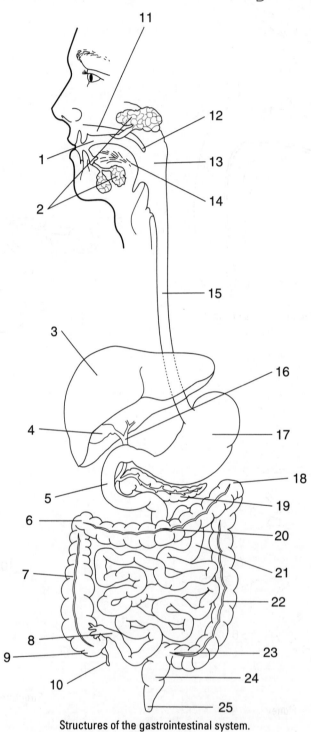

Structures of the gastrointestinal system.

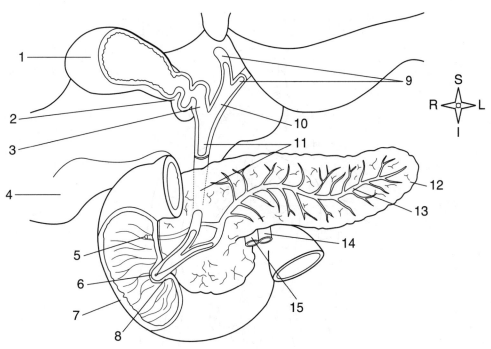

Accessory organs of the gastrointestinal system.

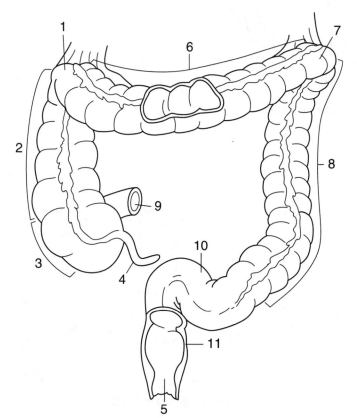

Divisions of the large intestine.

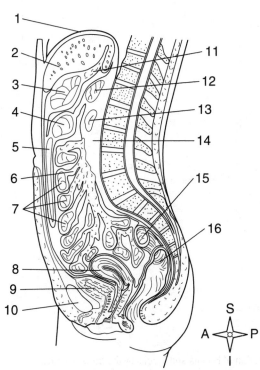

Section through the abdominopelvic cavity.

Immune System

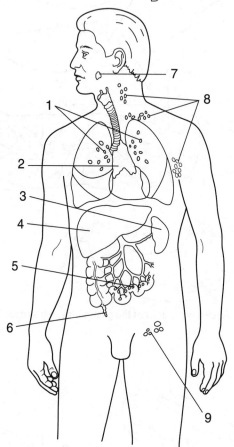

Organization of the immune system.

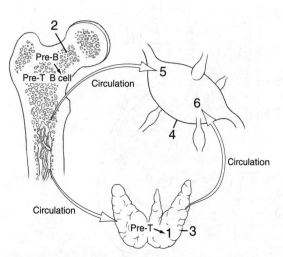

Creation of B cells and T cells by the bone marrow.

Activation and effects of T cells.

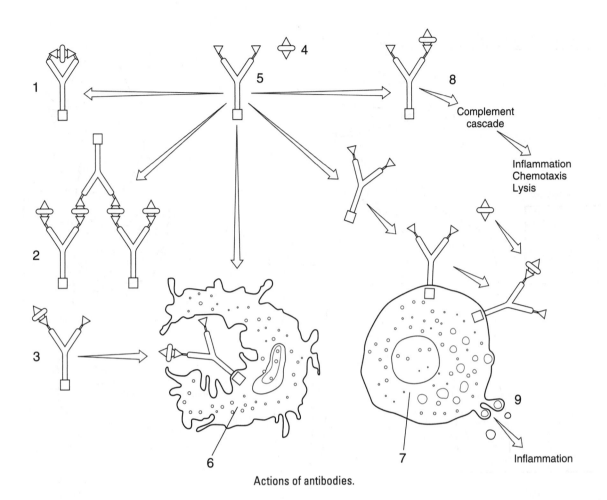

Actions of antibodies.

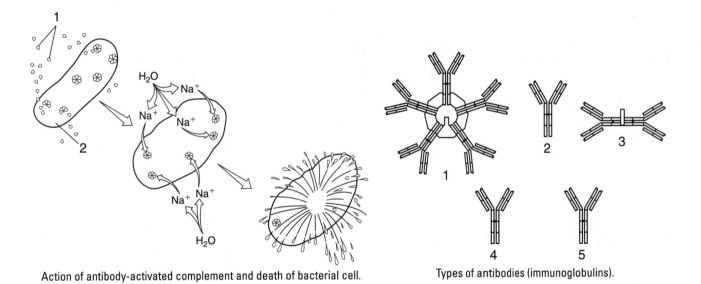

Action of antibody-activated complement and death of bacterial cell.

Types of antibodies (immunoglobulins).

Endocrine System

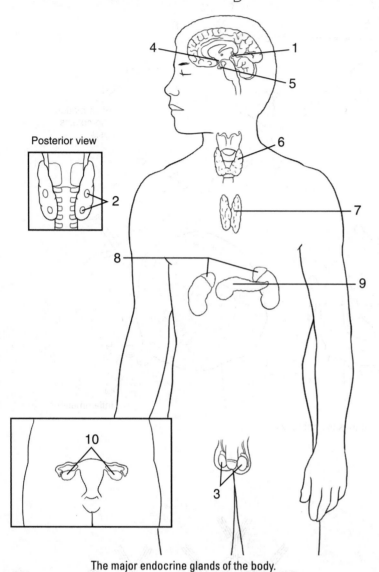

Posterior view

The major endocrine glands of the body.

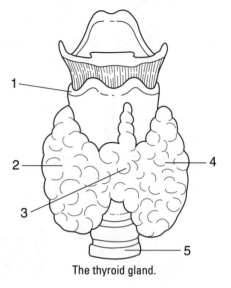

The thyroid gland.

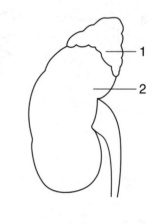

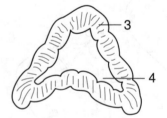

The adrenal gland.

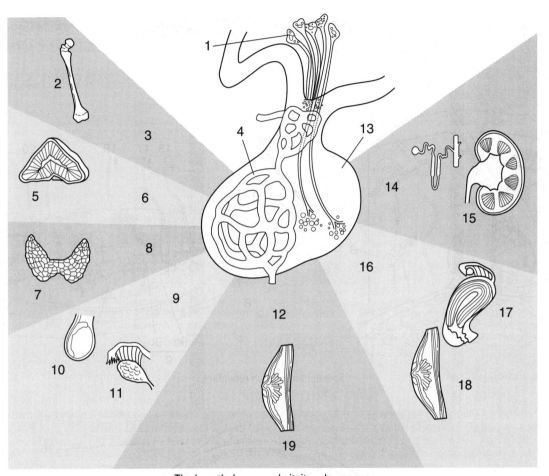

The hypothalamus and pituitary hormones.

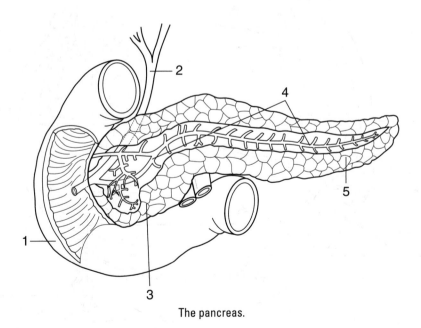

The pancreas.

Sensory System

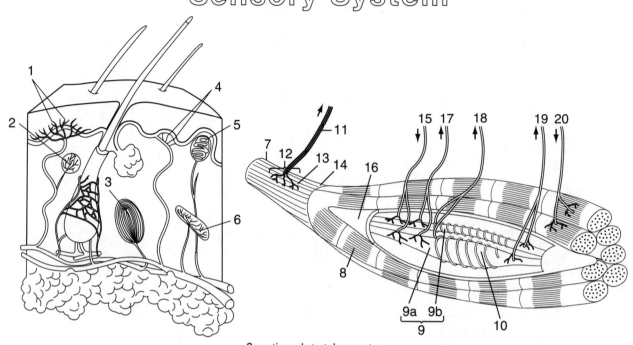

Somatic and stretch receptors.

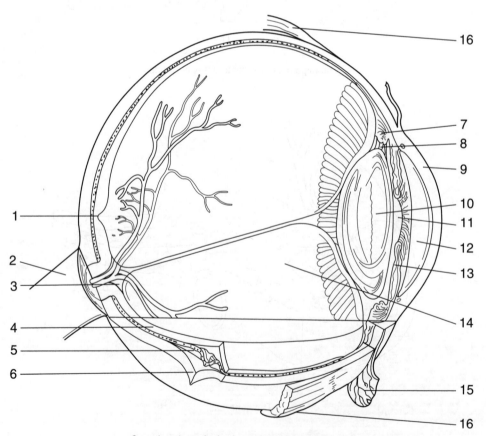

Superior view of a horizontal section of the eye.

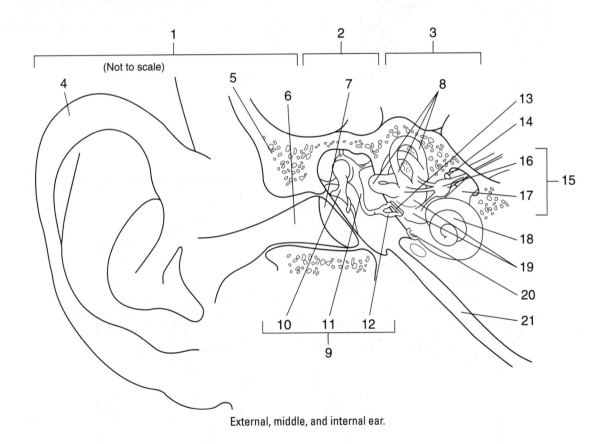

External, middle, and internal ear.

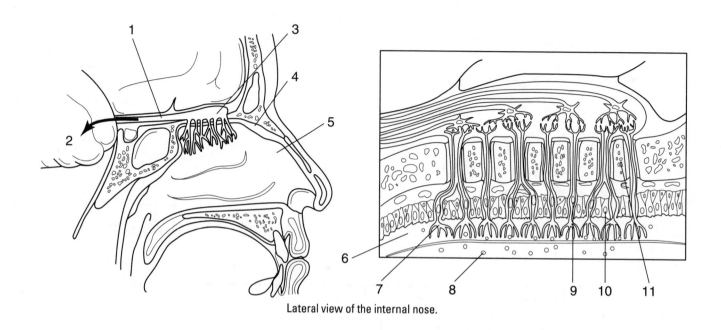

Lateral view of the internal nose.

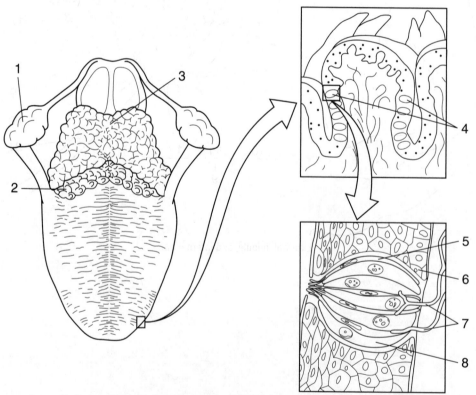

Dorsal surface of a tongue, cross-section through a papilla and a taste bud.

Reproductive System

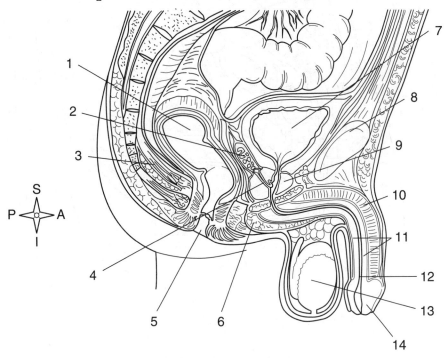

Male reproductive organs.

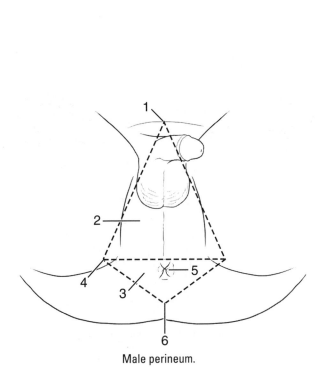

Male perineum.

Tubules of the testis and epididymis.

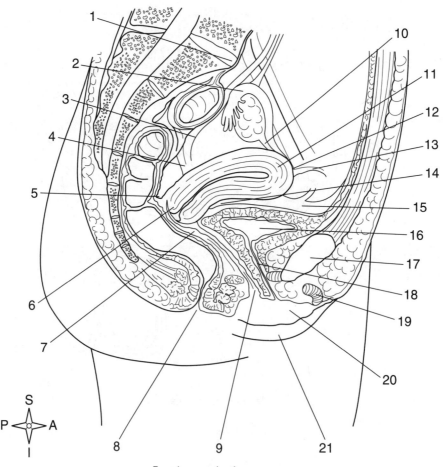

Female reproductive organs.

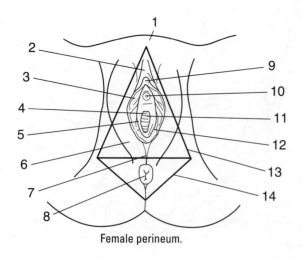

Female perineum.

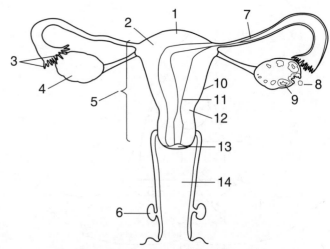

Anterior view of female reproductive organs.

Answer Key

CHAPTER 1 REVIEW QUESTIONS: HOW MUSCLES FUNCTION: THE BIG PICTURE

1. When a muscle contracts, it does not always succeed in shortening. 2. Concentric contraction. 3. One attachment may move, the other attachment may move, or both attachments may move. 4. The muscle attachment that moves is called the mobile attachment; the muscle attachment that does not move is called the fixed attachment. 5. A reverse action occurs when a muscle concentrically contracts and the attachment of the muscle that usually stays fixed does the moving, and the attachment of the muscle that usually moves, stays fixed. An example of a reverse action is when the brachialis concentrically contracts and flexes the elbow joint and the arm is moved toward the forearm instead of the forearm moving toward the arm (for example, when doing a pull-up). Another example of a reverse action is when the quadriceps femoris group concentrically contracts and extends the knee joint, and the thigh moves toward the leg instead of the leg moving toward the thigh (for example, when standing up from a seated position). 6. Step 1: Look at the name of the muscle to see if it gives you any "free information." Step 2: Learn the general location of the muscle well enough to be able to visualize the muscle on your body. Step 3: Use this general knowledge of the muscle's location (from step 2) to figure out the actions of the muscle. Step 4: Go back and learn (memorize, if necessary) the specific attachments of the muscle. Step 5: Now look at the relationship of this muscle to other muscles (and other soft tissue structures) of the body. 7. The questions are: (1) What joint does the muscle cross? (2) Where does the muscle cross the joint? (3) How does the muscle cross the joint (i.e., in what direction are its fibers running?). 8. The action of a muscle is determined by the line of pull of the muscle relative to the joint that it crosses. 9. One action. 10. The oblique plane motion must be broken up into its cardinal plane component actions. 11. Yes. 12. The functional group approach for learning muscles can save time and energy by looking at the larger concepts of the line of pull of all muscles of a particular functional group. In other words, instead of separately memorizing that the biceps brachii, and the brachialis, and the brachioradialis, and the pronator teres (and the flexor carpi radialis, palmaris longus, flexor carpi ulnaris, flexor digitorum superficialis, flexor pollicis longus, extensor carpi radialis longus, and extensor carpi radialis brevis) can each flex the forearm at the elbow joint, it is much more efficient use of time, energy, and brain power to realize that they are all members of a functional group that crosses the elbow joint anteriorly;

therefore, they all can flex the forearm at the elbow joint. 13. Answers include, but are not limited to: gluteus medius, trapezius, deltoid. 14. Sagittal plane. 15. Frontal plane. 16. Transverse plane. 17. The long axis of a bone is a straight line that runs from the center of the articular surface of the bone at one end to the center of the articular surface of the bone at the other end, that is, from the center of the joint at one end to the center of the joint at the other end. 18. Using the off-axis attachment method to determine the rotation action of a muscle necessitates that one visualize the location of the bony attachment of the muscle relative to the long axis of that bone. If a muscle attaches onto the bone on-axis (that is, such that its attachment is directly over the axis), then it has no possible rotation action. However, if it attaches onto the bone off-axis (that is, off the axis to either side), then it can create a rotation action. The specific rotation that the muscle creates is determined by visualizing the muscle pulling the attachment site toward the long axis of the bone. 19. A muscle can create a joint action at a joint that it does not cross if the force of the muscle's contraction is transferred to this other joint that it does not cross. An example of this is lateral rotation of the arm at the shoulder joint with the distal end of the upper extremity fixed. In this scenario, when the lateral rotators of the humerus contract and shorten, the humerus laterally rotates. Because the elbow joint does not allow rotation, this rotation force is transferred to the ulna, which then "rotates laterally" relative to the fixed radius. This motion causes the ulna to cross over the radius. When the ulna and radius cross, this is defined as pronation of the forearm. In this instance, the force for forearm pronation came from lateral rotators of the humerus at the shoulder joint whose force was transferred to the radioulnar joints. Note: adductor musculature of the shoulder joint transferring its force to the elbow joint is another example of this concept. 20. Given that the action of a muscle is determined by the line of pull of the muscle relative to the joint that it crosses, if the joint changes its position, then the relationship of the muscle's line of pull to the joint can change; therefore, its action can change. An example is the clavicular head of the pectoralis major. Above approximately 90 degrees of abduction of the arm at the shoulder joint, the clavicular head of the pectoralis major changes from running inferiorly to the center of the shoulder joint to running superiorly to the center of the shoulder joint. Therefore, its frontal plane action changes from adduction to abduction. Note: the sagittal plane hip joint action of the adductor longus is another example of this concept.

CHAPTER 2 LABELING ANSWERS: THE SKELETAL SYSTEM

Page 21 Anterior View of the Bones and Bony Landmarks of the Head

1. Frontal bone. 2. Nasal bone. 3. Sphenoid bone. 4. Temporal bone. 5. Lacrimal bone. 6. Ethmoid bone. 7. Zygomatic bone. 8. Zygomaticomaxillary suture. 9. Maxilla. 10. Vomer. 11. Alveolar process of the maxilla. 12. Alveolar process of the mandible. 13. Mandible. 14. Superciliary arch of the frontal bone. 15. Parietal bone. 16. Lesser wing of the sphenoid. 17. Greater wing of the sphenoid. 18. Palatine bone. 19. Frontal process of the maxilla. 20. Infraorbital foramen of the maxilla. 21. Canine fossa of the maxilla. 22. Incisive fossa of the maxilla. 23. Ramus of the mandible. 24. Incisive fossa of the mandible. 25. Angle of the mandible. 26. Mental foramen of the mandible. 27. Oblique line of the mandible. 28. Mental tubercle of the mandible. 29. Symphysis menti of the mandible.

Page 22 Lateral View of the Bones and Bony Landmarks of the Head

1. Temporal fossa (within dotted lines). 2. Temporomandibular joint (TMJ). 3. Highest nuchal line of the occipital bone. 4. Temporal bone. 5. Occipital bone. 6. Mastoid process of the temporal bone. 7. Zygomatic arch of the temporal bone. 8. Neck of the mandible. 9. Zygomaticotemporal suture. 10. Coronoid process of the mandible. 11. Zygomaticomaxillary suture. 12. Ramus of the mandible. 13. Angle of the mandible. 14. Mandible. 15. Oblique line of the mandible. 16. Mental foramen of the mandible. 17. Parietal bone. 18. Frontal bone. 19. Sphenoid bone. 20. Superciliary arch of the frontal bone. 21. Lacrimal bone. 22. Nasal bone. 23. Zygomatic bone. 24. Frontal process of the maxilla. 25. Canine fossa of the maxilla. 26. Maxilla. 27. Incisive fossa of the maxilla. 28. Alveolar process of the maxilla. 29. Alveolar process of the mandible. 30. Incisive fossa of the mandible. 31. Mental tubercle of the mandible.

Page 23 Inferior View of the Bones and Bony Landmarks of the Head

1. Maxilla. 2. Palatine bone. 3. Frontal bone. 4. Zygomatic bone. 5. Zygomatic arch (of the temporal & zygomatic bones). 6. Parietal bone. 7. Sphenoid bone. 8. Temporal bone. 9. Parietal bone. 10. Occipital bone. 11. Incisive fossa of the maxilla. 12. Zygomaticomaxillary suture. 13. Tuberosity of the maxilla. 14. Zygomaticotemporal suture. 15. Greater wing of the sphenoid. 16. Medial pterygoid plate of the pterygoid process of the sphenoid bone. 17. Lateral pterygoid plate of the pterygoid process of the sphenoid bone. 18. Vomer. 19. Styloid process of the temporal bone. 20. Mastoid process of the temporal bone. 21. Mastoid notch of the temporal bone. 22. Jugular process of the occipital bone. 23. Foramen magnum. 24. Highest nuchal line of the occipital bone.

Page 24 Anterior View of the Bones and Bony Landmarks of the Neck

1. Temporal bone. 2. Mastoid process of the temporal bone. 3. Styloid process of the temporal bone. 4. Greater cornu of the hyoid bone. 5. Body of the hyoid bone. 6. Hyoid bone. 7. Lamina of the thyroid cartilage. 8. Thyroid cartilage. 9. Sternoclavicular joint. 10. Acromioclavicular joint. 11. Shoulder joint. 12. Clavicle. 13. Scapula. 14. Costal cartilage of the first rib. 15. Manubrium of the sternum. 16. Basilar part of the occiput. 17. Occiput. 18. Anterior arch of the atlas. 19. Atlas (C1). 20. Axis (C2). 21. Vertebral body. 22. Vertebral transverse process (TP). 23. Posterior tubercle of the transverse process. 24. Anterior tubercle of the transverse process. 25. Humerus. 26. Acromion process of the scapula. 27. Superior border of the scapula. 28. Medial border of the scapula.

Page 25 Posterior View of the Bones and Bony Landmarks of the Neck

1. External occipital protuberance (EOP). 2. Occiput. 3. Superior nuchal line of the occiput. 4. Inferior nuchal line of the occiput. 5. Superior angle of the scapula. 6. Clavicle. 7. Acromioclavicular joint. 8. Acromion process of the scapula. 9. Scapula. 10. Spine of the scapula. 11. Tubercle at the root of the spine of the scapula. 12. Medial border of the scapula. 13. Root of the spine of the scapula. 14. Temporal bone. 15. Mastoid process of the temporal bone. 16. Mandible. 17. Atlas (C1). 18. Axis (C2). 19. Vertebral spinous process (SP). 20. Vertebral transverse process (TP). 21. C7. 22. First rib. 23. T3.

Page 26 Anterior View of the Bones and Bony Landmarks of the Trunk

1. Clavicle. 2. Coracoid process of the scapula. 3. Scapula. 4. Medial border of the scapula. 5. Inferior angle of the scapula. 6. Intercostal space. 7. Costal cartilage. 8. Sacroiliac joint. 9. Iliac crest. 10. Pelvic bone. 11. Pubic crest. 12. Pubic tubercle. 13. Pubic symphysis. 14. Sacrum. 15. Cervical transverse process. 16. Body of C7. 17. Humerus. 18. Medial lip of the bicipital groove of the humerus. 19. Lateral lip of the bicipital groove of the humerus. 20. Sternum. 21. Xiphoid process of the sternum. 22. Intervertebral disc (L3-L4). 23. Ilium. 24. Ischium. 25. Pubis.

Page 27 Posterior View of the Bones and Bony Landmarks of the Trunk

1. Clavicle. 2. Spine of the scapula. 3. Root of the spine of the scapula. 4. Medial border of the scapula. 5. Scapula. 6. Inferior angle of the scapula. 7. Vertebral transverse process (TP). 8. Vertebral lamina. 9. Vertebral spinous process (SP). 10. Iliac crest. 11. Posterior superior iliac spine

(PSIS). 12. Pelvic bone. 13. Sacrum. 14. Ischium. 15. Pubis. 16. Pubic symphysis. 17. C7. 18. Tubercle (of the 5th rib). 19. Angle (of the 5th rib). 20. Intercostal space. 21. Inferior articular process (of L1). 22. Superior articular process (of L2). 23. Mamillary process (of L3). 24. Ilium. 25. Sacro-iliac joint. 26. Medial sacral crest. 27. Lateral sacral crest.

Page 28 Anterior View of the Bones and Bony Landmarks of the Right Thigh and Pelvis

1. Vertebral transverse process (TP). 2. Sacral ala. 3. Iliac crest. 4. Iliac fossa. 5. Internal ilium. 6. Ilium. 7. Anterior superior iliac spine (ASIS). 8. Anterior inferior iliac spine (AIIS). 9. Hip joint. 10. Greater trochanter of the femur. 11. Lesser trochanter of the femur. 12. Femur. 13. Fibula. 14. Intervertebral disc. 15. Vertebral body (L3). 16. Sacrum. 17. Iliopectineal eminence (of the ilium and the pubis). 18. Apex of the sacrum. 19. Coccyx. 20. Pectineal line of the pubis on the superior ramus of the pubis. 21. Pubis. 22. Obturator foramen. 23. Inferior ramus of the pubis. 24. Ramus of the ischium. 25. Ischial tuberosity. 26. Ischium. 27. Patella. 28. Knee (tibiofemoral) joint. 29. Medial tibial condyle. 30. Tibial tuberosity. 31. Tibia.

Page 29 Posterior View of the Bones and Bony Landmarks of the Right Thigh and Pelvis

1. Vertebral transverse process (TP) (of L5). 2. Sacrum. 3. Sacrotuberous ligament. 4. Apex of the sacrum. 5. Coccyx. 6. Pectineal line on the superior ramus of the pubis. 7. Pubis. 8. Obturator foramen. 9. Inferior ramus of the pubis. 10. Ramus of the ischium. 11. Ischium. 12. Ischial tuberosity. 13. Trochanteric fossa. 14. Pectineal line of the femur. 15. Medial lip of the linea aspera. 16. Femur. 17. Medial supracondylar line. 18. Adductor tubercle. 19. Medial tibial condyle. 20. Tibia. 21. Iliac crest. 22. Posterior gluteal line of the ilium. 23. Anterior gluteal line of the ilium. 24. Pelvic bone (Ilium). 25. Anterior superior iliac spine (ASIS). 26. Inferior gluteal line of the ilium. 27. Anterior inferior iliac spine (AIIS). 28. Ischial spine. 29. Head of the femur. 30. Hip (femoroacetabular) joint. 31. Greater trochanter. 32. Intertrochanteric crest. 33. Lesser trochanter. 34. Gluteal tuberosity. 35. Lateral lip of the linea aspera. 36. Linea aspera. 37. Lateral supracondylar line. 38. Knee (tibiofemoral) joint. 39. Lateral tibial condyle. 40. Head of the fibula. 41. Fibula.

Page 30 Anterior View of the Bones and Bony Landmarks of the Right Leg

1. Lateral supracondylar line of the femur. 2. Lateral condyle of the femur. 3. Knee joint. 4. Lateral condyle of the tibia. 5. Head of the fibula. 6. Fibula. 7. Lateral malleolus of the fibula. 8. Calcaneus. 9. Cuboid. 10. Base of (5th) metatarsal. 11. Proximal phalanx of (5th) toe. 12. Middle phalanx of (5th) toe. 13. Distal phalanx of (5th) toe. 14. Femur. 15. Medial condyle of the femur. 16. Tibia.

17. Interosseus membrane. 18. Ankle joint. 19. Medial malleolus of the tibia. 20. Talus. 21. Navicular. 22. 1st cuneiform. 23. 2nd cuneiform. 24. 3rd cuneiform. 25. Metatarsals #1-5. 26. Proximal phalanx of the big toe. 27. Distal phalanx of the big toe.

Page 31 Posterior View of the Bones and Bony Landmarks of the Right Leg

1. Femur. 2. Medial condyle of the femur. 3. Knee joint. 4. Soleal line of the tibia. 5. Tibia. 6. Calcaneus. 7. Medial malleolus of the tibia. 8. Tuberosity of the calcaneus. 9. Talus. 10. Navicular. 11. 3rd cuneiform. 12. 2nd cuneiform. 13. 1st cuneiform. 14. Metatarsals #1-5. 15. Proximal phalanx of the big toe. 16. Distal phalanx of the big toe. 17. Lateral supracondylar line of the femur. 18. Lateral condyle of the femur. 19. Lateral condyle of the tibia. 20. Head of the fibula. 21. Fibula. 22. Interosseus membrane. 23. Lateral malleolus of the fibula. 24. Cuboid. 25. Base of (5th) metatarsal. 26. Proximal phalanx of (5th) toe. 27. Middle phalanx of (5th) toe. 28. Distal phalanx of (5th) toe.

Page 32 Dorsal View of the Bones and Bony Landmarks of the Right Foot

1. Cuboid. 2. Metatarsals #1-5 (Numbering begins with the big toe as toe #1 and ends with the little toe as toe #5.). 3. Metatarsophalangeal joint (MTP joint). 4. Proximal phalanx of a toe. 5. Proximal interphalangeal joint (PIP joint). 6. Middle phalanx of a toe. 7. Distal interphalangeal joint (DIP joint). 8. Distal phalanx of a toe. 9. Calcaneus. 10. Talus. 11. Navicular. 12. 1st cuneiform. 13. 2nd cuneiform. 14. 3rd cuneiform. 15. Base of a metatarsal. 16. Head of a metatarsal. 17. Base of a phalanx. 18. Proximal phalanx of the big toe. 19. Head of a phalanx. 20. Interphalangeal joint (IP joint). 21. Distal phalanx of the big toe.

Page 33 Plantar View of the Bones and Bony Landmarks of the Right Foot

1. Talus. 2. Navicular. 3. 3rd cuneiform. 4. 2nd cuneiform. 5. 1st cuneiform. 6. Base of a metatarsal. 7. Sesamoid bones. 8. Base of a phalanx. 9. Proximal phalanx of the big toe. 10. Interphalangeal joint (IP joint). 11. Distal phalanx of the big toe. 12. Calcaneal tuberosity. 13. Calcaneus. 14. Cuboid. 15. Metatarsals #1-5 (Numbering begins with the big toe as toe #1 and ends with the little toe as toe #5.). 16. Metatarsophalangeal joint (MTP joint). 17. Proximal phalanx of a toe. 18. Proximal interphalangeal joint (PIP joint). 19. Middle phalanx of a toe. 20. Distal interphalangeal joint (DIP joint). 21. Distal phalanx of a toe. 22. Base of a phalanx. 23. Head of a phalanx.

Page 34 Anterior View of the Bones and Bony Landmarks of the Right Scapula/Arm

1. Acromion process of the scapula. 2. Supraglenoid tubercle of the scapula. 3. Superior facet of the greater

tubercle of the humerus. 4. Greater tubercle of the humerus. 5. Bicipital groove of the humerus. 6. Lesser tubercle of the humerus. 7. Deltoid tuberosity of the humerus. 8. Humerus. 9. Shaft of the humerus. 10. Elbow joint. 11. Radius. 12. Radial tuberosity. 13. Clavicle. 14. Coracoid process of the scapula. 15. Shoulder joint. 16. Scapula. 17. Subscapular fossa of the scapula. 18. Infraglenoid tubercle of the scapula. 19. Lateral border of the scapula. 20. Coronoid process of the ulna. 21. Ulna. 22. Ulnar tuberosity.

Page 35 Posterior View of the Bones and Bony Landmarks of the Right Scapula/Arm

1. Clavicle. 2. Supraspinous fossa of the scapula. 3. Shoulder joint. 4. Spine of the scapula. 5. Scapula. 6. Infraspinous fossa of the scapula. 7. Lateral border of the scapula. 8. Infraglenoid tubercle of the scapula. 9. Olecranon process of the ulna. 10. Ulna. 11. Acromion process of the scapula. 12. Supraglenoid tubercle of the scapula. 13. Superior facet of the greater tubercle of the humerus. 14. Middle facet of the greater tubercle of the humerus. 15. Greater tubercle of the humerus. 16. Inferior facet of the greater tubercle of the humerus. 17. Deltoid tuberosity of the humerus. 18. Humerus. 19. Shaft of the humerus. 20. Head of the radius. 21. Radius. 22. Radial tuberosity.

Page 36 Anterior View of the Bones and Bony Landmarks of the Right Forearm

1. Lateral supracondylar ridge of the humerus. 2. Lateral epicondyle of the humerus. 3. Head of the radius. 4. Radial tuberosity. 5. Radial shaft. 6. Radius. 7. Interosseus membrane. 8. Wrist joint. 9. Styloid process of the radius. 10. Metacarpals #1-5. 11. Proximal phalanx of the thumb. 12. Distal phalanx of the thumb. 13. Humerus. 14. Medial supracondylar ridge of the humerus. 15. Medial epicondyle of the humerus. 16. Elbow joint. 17. Coronoid process of the ulna. 18. Supinator crest of the ulna. 19. Ulna. 20. Pisiform. 21. Hook of hamate. 22. Base of a metacarpal. 23. Base of a phalanx. 24. Proximal phalanx of a finger (the little finger). 25. Middle phalanx of a finger (the little finger). 26. Distal phalanx of a finger (the little finger).

Page 37 Posterior View of the Bones and Bony Landmarks of the Right Forearm

1. Medial supracondylar ridge of the humerus. 2. Medial epicondyle of the humerus. 3. Coronoid process of the ulna. 4. Supinator crest of the ulna. 5. Ulna. 6. Interosseus membrane. 7. Styloid process of the ulna. 8. Pisiform. 9. Base of a metacarpal. 10. Base of a phalanx. 11. Proximal phalanx of a finger (the little finger). 12. Middle phalanx of a finger (the little finger). 13. Distal phalanx of a finger (the little finger). 14. Humerus. 15. Lateral supracondylar ridge of the humerus. 16. Lateral epicondyle of the humerus. 17. Olecranon process of the ulna. 18. Head of the radius. 19. Radial tuberosity. 20. Radial shaft. 21. Radius. 22. Styloid process of the radius.

23. Metacarpals #1-5. 24. Proximal phalanx of the thumb. 25. Distal phalanx of the thumb.

Page 38 Palmar View of the Bones and Bony Landmarks of the Right Hand

1. Scaphoid. 2. Scaphoid tubercle. 3. Trapezium. 4. Tubercle of trapezium. 5. Trapezoid. 6. Interphalangeal joint (IP joint). 7. Sesamoid bones. 8. Proximal phalanx of the thumb. 9. Distal phalanx of the thumb. 10. Proximal phalanx of a finger (index finger). 11. Middle phalanx of a finger (index finger). 12. Distal phalanx of a finger (index finger). 13. Capitate. 14. Lunate. 15. Triquetrum. 16. Pisiform. 17. Hamate. 18. Hook of hamate. 19. Base of a metacarpal. 20. Metacarpals #1-5 (Numbering begins with the thumb as finger #1 and ends with the little finger as finger #5.). 21. Head of a metacarpal. 22. Base of a phalanx. 23. Head of a phalanx. 24. Proximal interphalangeal joint (PIP joint). 25. Distal interphalangeal joint (DIP joint). 26. Metacarpophalangeal joint (MCP joint).

Page 39 Dorsal View of the Bones and Bony Landmarks of the Right Hand

1. Lunate. 2. Pisiform. 3. Triquetrum. 4. Hamate. 5. Base of a metacarpal. 6. Metacarpals #1-5 (Numbering begins with the thumb as finger #1 and ends with the little finger as finger #5.). 7. Head of a metacarpal. 8. Metacarpophalangeal joint (MCP joint). 9. Base of a phalanx. 10. Head of a phalanx. 11. Proximal interphalangeal joint (PIP joint). 12. Distal interphalangeal joint (DIP joint). 13. Capitate. 14. Scaphoid. 15. Trapezium. 16. Trapezoid. 17. Proximal phalanx of the thumb. 18. Interphalangeal joint (IP joint). 19. Sesamoid bone. 20. Distal phalanx of the thumb. 21. Proximal phalanx of a finger. 22. Middle phalanx of a finger. 23. Distal phalanx of a finger.

CHAPTER 3 LABELING ANSWERS: MUSCLES OF THE HEAD

Page 70 Anterior View of the Head

1. Occipitofrontalis. 2. Temporoparietalis. 3. Orbicularis oculi. 4. Procerus. 5. Levator labii superioris alaeque nasi. 6. Nasalis. 7. Zygomaticus minor. 8. Levator labii superioris. 9. Zygomaticus major. 10. Levator anguli oris. 11. Masseter. 12. Risorius. 13. Depressor anguli oris. 14. Depressor labii inferioris. 15. Mentalis. 16. Platysma. 17. Occipitofrontalis (frontalis belly, cut). 18. Corrugator supercillii. 19. Orbicularis oculi (partially cut away). 20. Levator palpebrae superioris. 21. Levator labii superioris alaeque nasi (cut). 22. Levator labii superioris (cut). 23. Zygomaticus minor (cut). 24. Zygomaticus major (cut). 25. Levator anguli oris (cut). 26. Depressor septi nasi. 27. Buccinator. 28. Orbicularis oris. 29. Depressor anguli oris (cut). 30. Depressor labii inferioris (cut).

Page 71 Lateral View of the Head
1. Temporoparietalis. 2. Occipitofrontalis (occipitalis belly). 3. Auricularis muscles. 4. Splenius capitis. 5. Sterno-cleidomastoid. 6. Levator scapulae. 7. Trapezius. 8. Occipi-tofrontalis (frontalis belly). 9. Temporalis (deep to facia). 10. Corrugator supercilii. 11. Procerus. 12. Orbicularis oculi (partially cut). 13. Levator labii superioris alaeque nasi. 14. Nasalis. 15. Levator labii superioris. 16. Lateral pterygoid. 17. Depressor septi nasi. 18. Zygomaticus minor. 19. Leva-tor anguli oris. 20. Zygomaticus major. 21. Orbicularis oris. 22. Mentalis. 23. Depressor labii inferioris. 24. Depressor anguli oris. 25. Risorius. 26. Buccinator. 27. Platysma.

Muscles of the Head: Answers to Review Questions (pp 72–73)
1. Lateral pterygoid. 2. Deep. 3. Mentalis. 4. Occipito-frontalis and temporoparietalis. 5. 2. 6. Depressor labii inferioris. 7. Levator labii superioris alaeque nasi. 8. The depressor labii inferioris depresses the lower lip; the men-talis elevates it. 9. Levator labii superioris alaeque nasi. 10. Depressor labii inferioris and mentalis. 11. 3. 12. Occip-itofrontalis. 13. It shortens. 14. Depressor labii inferioris. 15. Temporalis, masseter, medial pterygoid. 16. They both elevate the angle of the mouth. 17. Levator labii superioris alaeque nasi. 18. Masseter. 19. Orbicularis oris. 20. Occipita-lis and frontalis. 21. They both contralaterally deviate and protract the mandible at the temporomandibular joints. 22. Trapezius. 23. The temporalis elevates the mandible at the temporomandibular joints; the digastric depresses it. 24. Depressor septi nasi and nasalis. 25. Procerus. 26. They both draw laterally the angle of the mouth. 27. Levator labii superioris alaeque nasi and zygomaticus minor. 28. Nasalis. 29. Galea aponeurotica. 30. Auricularis poste-rior. 31. Corrugator supercilii frontalis (occipitofrontalis). 32. Frontalis (occipitofrontalis). 33. Zygomaticus minor. 34. Levator anguli oris. 35. Levator anguli oris. 36. Masseter. 37. Depressor anguli oris. 38. They both evert the lower lip. 39. Risorius and buccinator. 40. Mandible. 41. Pro-cerus. 42. Levator labii superioris alaeque nasi. 43. Leva-tor labii superioris, levator labii superioris alaeque nasi, zygomaticus minor. 44. Temporalis. 45. Orbicularis oculi. 46. Mentalis. 47. Zygomaticus minor. 48. Orbicularis oris. 49. It shortens. 50. Transverse and alar parts. 51. Risorius and zygomaticus major. 52. Orbicularis oculi. 53. Auricu-laris, superior, temporoparietalis. 54. Levator labii supe-rioris. 55. Temporalis, masseter, lateral pterygoid, medial pterygoid. 56. Their fibers run in the same direction, but the masseter is superficial to the mandible and the medial pterygoid is deep to it. 57. Levator labii superioris alae-que nasi. 58. Frontalis. 59. Procerus. 60. Anterior, supe-rior, posterior auricularis. 61. Depressor labii inferioris. 62. Depressor septi nasi. 63. Orbicularis oculi. 64. Buccinator. 65. Orbicularis oris. 66. Auricularis superior. 67. Leva-tor labii superioris. 68. Medial pterygoid. 69. Laughing. 70. Orbicularis oculi. 71. It raises it. 72. The temporalis

is deep. 73. Depressor anguli oris, depressor labii inferi-oris. mentalis, buccinator, platysma. 74. It lengthens. 75. Procerus. 76. It lengthens. 77. Levator labii superioris alaeque nasi. 78. 3.

CHAPTER 4 LABELING ANSWERS: MUSCLES OF THE NECK

Page 112 Anterior View of the Neck (Superficial)
1. Omohyoid. 2. Platysma. 3. Sternothyroid. 4. Digastric (anterior belly). 5. Mylohyoid. 6. Stylohyoid. 7. Digastric (posterior belly). 8. Thyrohyoid. 9. Sternocleidomastoid (sternal head). 10. Sternocleidomastoid (clavicular head). 11. Levator scapulae. 12. Sternohyoid. 13. Middle scalene. 14. Posterior scalene. 15. Omohyoid (inferior belly). 16. Trapezius. 17. Anterior scalene. 18. Deltoid. 19. Pecto-ralis major.

Page 113 Anterior View of the Neck (Intermediate)
1. Mylohyoid. 2. Sternocleidomastoid (cut). 3. Omohyoid (superior belly). 4. Omohyoid (inferior belly). 5. Sterno-cleidomastoid (cut). 6. Sternohyoid. 7. Digastric (anterior belly). 8. Stylohyoid. 9. Digastric (posterior belly). 10. Ster-nocleidomastoid (cut). 11. Thyrohyoid. 12. Levator scapu-lae. 13. Omohyoid (cut and reflected). 14. Sternothyroid. 15. Middle scalene. 16. Posterior scalene. 17. Trapezius. 18. Anterior scalene. 19. Deltoid. 20. Pectoralis major. 21. Sternohyoid (cut and reflected).

Page 114 Anterior View of the Neck (Deep)
1. Rectus capitis lateralis. 2. Rectus capitis anterior. 3. Longus capitis. 4. Longus colli. 5. Middle scalene. 6. Anterior scalene. 7. Posterior scalene. 8. Longus capitis (cut). 9. Rectus capitis anterior. 10. Rectus capitis lateralis. 11. Longus colli. 12. Mid-dle scalene. 13. Anterior scalene (cut). 14. Posterior scalene.

Page 115 Lateral View of the Neck
1. Stylohyoid. 2. Digastric (posterior belly). 3. Splenius capitis. 4. Longus capitis. 5. Sternocleidomastoid. 6. Levator scapulae. 7. Anterior scalene. 8. Middle scalene. 9. Posterior scalene. 10. Trapezius. 11. Omohyoid (infe-rior belly). 12. Deltoid. 13. Masseter (cut). 14. Mylohyoid. 15. Digastric (anterior belly). 16. Thyrohyoid. 17. Omo-hyoid (superior belly). 18. Sternohyoid. 19. Sternothyroid. 20. Sternocleidomastoid (sternal head). 21. Sternocleido-mastoid (clavicular head). 22. Pectoralis major.

Page 116 Posterior View of the Neck (Superficial and Intermediate)
1. Sternocleidomastoid. 2. Splenius capitis. 3. Leva-tor scapulae. 4. Trapezius. 5. Deltoid. 6. Triceps brachii. 7. Latissimus dorsi. 8. Semispinalis capitis (of transverso-spinalis group). 9. Splenius capitis. 10. Splenius cervicis.

11. Levator scapulae. 12. Rhomboid minor. 13. Supraspinatus. 14. Infraspinatus. 15. Teres minor. 16. Rhomboid major. 17. Teres major. 18. Erector spinae. 19. Latissimus dorsi.

Page 117 Posterior View of the Neck (Intermediate and Deep)
1. Semispinalis capitis (of transversospinalis group). 2. Longissimus capitis (of erector spinae group). 3. Splenius capitis. 4. Splenius cervicis. 5. Iliocostalis cervicis (of erector spinae group). 6. Serratus posterior superior. 7. Iliocostalis and longissimus (of erector spinae group). 8. Splenius cervicis. 9. Rectus capitis posterior minor. 10. Rectus capitis posterior major. 11. Obliquus capitis superior. 12. Obliquus capitis inferior. 13. Interspinales. 14. Rotatores (of transversospinalis group). 15. Levatores costarum. 16. External intercostals.

Muscles of the Neck: Answers to Review Questions (pp 118–121)
1. Left rotation. 2. Semispinalis capitis. 3. Trapezius. 4. Depression of the mandible at the temporomandibular joints. 5. Two bellies. 6. Digastric. 7. Elevation of the hyoid bone. 8. Thyrohyoid. 9. The right one does right rotation and the left one does left rotation of the atlas at the atlantoaxial joint. 10. Inferior and superior bellies. 11. Right lateral flexion of the neck at the spinal joints. 12. Rhomboids. 13. Platysma. 14. The sternohyoid depresses the hyoid; the stylohyoid elevates the hyoid. 15. It would lengthen and stretch it. 16. Rectus capitis posterior major and minor. 17. Sternothyroid. 18. Digastric [anterior belly]. 19. Elevation of the hyoid bone. 20. Extension, right lateral flexion, and right rotation of the head and neck at the spinal joints. 21. Obliquus capitis inferior. 22. Levator scapulae, serratus anterior and rhomboids major and minor. 23. Geniohyoid. 24. Serratus anterior and the upper and lower trapezius. 25. Digastric, stylohyoid, mylohyoid, geniohyoid. 26. It lengthens. 27. They both left laterally flex the neck at the spinal joints. 28. Anterior, middle, and posterior scalenes. 29. Levator scapulae. 30. Middle scalene. 31. They lengthen. 32. Flexion of the neck at the spinal joint. 33. They both flex the neck at the spinal joints. 34. Longus capitis. 35. The scalenes. 36. C1-C5. 37. Left lateral flexion of the head at the atlanto-occipital joint. 38. Longus colli and capitis and rectus capitis anterior and lateralis. 39. Flexion of the neck at the spinal joints. 40. The transverse process of the atlas (C1). 41. Longus capitis. 42. The occiput. 43. Thyroid cartilage. 44. They both do left lateral flexion and right rotation of the head and neck at the spinal joints. 45. The digastric depresses the mandible at the temporomandibular joints; the masseter elevates the mandible. 46. Flexion, left lateral flexion, and left rotation of the neck at the spinal joints. 47. Rectus capitis posterior major and minor, obliquus capitis inferior and superior. 48. It would shorten and slacken it. 49. Right lateral flexion. 50. Lateral flexion of the neck at the spinal joints. 51. Flexion of the head at the atlanto-occipital joint. 52. Sternohyoid, sternothyroid, thyrohyoid, omohyoid. 53. Middle scalene. 54. Trapezius and deltoid. 55. Flexion of the neck at the spinal joints [the lateral flexion and rotation components would cancel each other out]. 56. Obliquus capitis inferior and superior. 57. Stylohyoid, mylohyoid, geniohyoid. 58. Trapezius. 59. It would lengthen and stretch it. 60. Depression of the hyoid bone. 61. Levator scapulae. 62. They both do left rotation and right lateral flexion of the head and neck at the spinal joints. 63. It lengthens. 64. Anterior scalene and omohyoid. 65. Elevation and protraction of the mandible at the temporomandibular joints and depression of the hyoid bone. 66. Depression of the hyoid bone. 67. Sternocleidomastoid, longissimus capitis. 68. Omohyoid. 69. Upper trapezius. 70. Posterior scalene. 71. It lengthens. 72. Right lateral flexion. 73. Left rotation. 74. 3. 75. Obliquus capitis inferior and rectus capitis posterior major. 76. Obliquus capitis inferior. 77. Omohyoid. 78. Elevation and protraction [abduction] of the left scapula at the scapulocostal joint. 79. Retraction [adduction] of the scapula at the scapulocostal joint. 80. The *golf tee* muscles. 81. They both depress the hyoid bone. 82. Right rotation of the head at the atlantooccipital joint. 83. Sternocleidomastoid. 84. Between the anterior and middle scalenes.

CHAPTER 5 LABELING ANSWERS: MUSCLES OF THE TRUNK

Page 172 Posterior View of the Trunk (Superficial and Intermediate)
1. Splenius capitis. 2. Sternocleidomastoid. 3. Rhomboid minor (cut). 4. Rhomboid major (cut). 5. Deltoid. 6. Trapezius. 7. Teres major. 8. Triceps brachii. 9. Latissimus dorsi. 10. External abdominal oblique. 11. Gluteus medius. 12. Gluteus maximus. 13. Semispinalis capitis (of transversospinalis group). 14. Splenius capitis. 15. Splenius cervicis. 16. Levator scapulae. 17. Supraspinatus. 18. Serratus posterior superior. 19. Infraspinatus. 20. Teres minor. 21. Teres major. 22. Longissimus (of erector spinae group). 23. Latissimus dorsi (cut). 24. Spinalis (of erector spinae group). 25. Triceps brachii. 26. Iliocostalis (of erector spinae group). 27. Serratus anterior. 28. Serratus posterior inferior. 29. External abdominal oblique. 30. Latissimus dorsi (cut and reflected). 31. Internal abdominal oblique. 32. Gluteus medius. 33. Gluteus maximus.

Page 173 Posterior View of the Trunk (Deep Layers)
1. Semispinalis capitis (of transversospinalis group). 2. Longissimus (of erector spinae group). 3. Splenius capitis. 4. Splenius cervicis. 5. Iliocostalis (of erector spinae group). 6. Spinalis (of erector spinae group). 7. Longissimus (of erector spinae group). 8. Transversus abdominis. 9. Internal abdominal oblique. 10. External abdominal oblique (cut).

11. Iliocostalis (of erector spinae group). 12. Rectus capitis posterior minor. 13. Rectus capitis posterior major. 14. Obliquus capitis superior. 15. Obliquus capitis inferior. 16. Interspinales. 17. Rotatores (of transversospinalis group). 18. Semispinalis (of transversospinalis group). 19. External intercostals. 20. Levatores costarum. 21. Quadratus lumborum. 22. Multifidus (of transversospinalis group). 23. Intertransversarii. 24. Sacrum.

Page 174 Anterior View of the Trunk (Superficial and Intermediate)

1. Platysma. 2. Deltoid. 3. Pectoralis major. 4. Triceps brachii. 5. Biceps brachii. 6. Latissimus dorsi. 7. Serratus anterior. 8. External abdominal oblique. 9. Iliopsoas. 10. Sartorius. 11. Rectus femoris (of quadriceps femoris group). 12. Pectineus. 13. Adductor longus. 14. Sternocleidomastoid. 15. Trapezius. 16. Subclavius. 17. External intercostals. 18. Pectoralis minor. 19. Coracobrachialis. 20. Internal intercostals. 21. Biceps brachii. 22. External intercostals. 23. Rectus abdominis. 24. External abdominal oblique (cut). 25. Internal abdominal oblique. 26. Gluteus medius. 27. Tensor fasciae latae. 28. Gracilis.

Page 175 Anterior View of the Trunk (Intermediate and Deep)

1. Sternocleidomastoid. 2. Trapezius. 3. Subclavius. 4. External intercostals. 5. Pectoralis minor. 6. Coracobrachialis. 7. Internal intercostals. 8. Biceps brachii. 9. External intercostals. 10. Rectus abdominis. 11. External abdominal oblique (cut). 12. Internal abdominal oblique. 13. Gracilis. 14. Internal intercostals. 15. Rectus abdominis. 16. External abdominal oblique (cut). 17. Transversus abdominis. 18. Internal abdominal oblique (cut). 19. Gluteus medius. 20. Iliopsoas. 21. Tensor fasciae latae. 22. Sartorius. 23. Rectus femoris (of quadriceps femoris group). 24. Pectineus. 25. Adductor longus.

Page 176 Lateral View of the Trunk

1. Trapezius. 2. Supraspinatus (cut). 3. Biceps brachii (cut). 4. Subscapularis (cut). 5. Infraspinatus (cut). 6. Teres minor (cut). 7. Triceps brachii (cut). 8. Teres major (cut). 9. Serratus anterior. 10. Erector spinae. 11. External intercostals. 12. Serratus posterior inferior. 13. Internal abdominal oblique. 14. Gluteus medius. 15. Gluteus maximus. 16. Vastus lateralis (of quadriceps femoris group). 17. Sternocleidomastoid. 18. Subclavius. 19. External intercostals. 20. Internal intercostals. 21. Pectoralis minor. 22. External abdominal oblique. 23. Tensor fasciae latae. 24. Sartorius. 25. Rectus femoris (of quadriceps femoris group). 26. Vastus lateralis (of quadriceps femoris group).

Page 177 Cross Section Views of the Trunk (Thoracic)

1. Transversus thoracis. 2. Internal intercostals. 3. Erector spinae and transversospinalis groups. 4. Rhomboid major. 5. Trapezius. 6. Infraspinatus. 7. Teres major.

8. Subscapularis. 9. Latissimus dorsi. 10. Serratus anterior. 11. External intercostals.

Page 177 Cross Section Views of the Trunk (Lumbar)

1. Diaphragm. 2. Psoas major. 3. Quadratus lumborum. 4. Transversus abdominis. 5. Erector spinae and transversospinalis groups. 6. Serratus posterior inferior. 7. Latissimus dorsi. 8. Internal abdominal oblique. 9. External abdominal oblique.

Muscles of the Trunk: Answers to Review Questions (pp 178–181)

1. Multifidus. 2. Pectoralis major. 3. Rotatores. 4. Clavicular and sternocostal heads. 5. External and internal abdominal obliques. 6. Left lateral flexion of the neck and trunk at the spinal joints. 7. Protraction and depression of the scapula at the scapulocostal joint. 8. Pectoralis major. 9. True. 10. Opposite, i.e., perpendicular. 11. Latissimus dorsi and teres major. 12. Brachial plexus of nerves, subclavian artery and vein. 13. Flexion of the neck and trunk at the spinal joints. 14. It is shortening. 15. Psoas major and quadratus lumborum. 16. Subclavius. 17. Lengthen. 18. Spinalis. 19. External abdominal oblique. 20. Erector spinae group. 21. Pectoralis major and minor. 22. The lower rib will elevate at the sternocostal and costospinal joints. 23. External abdominal obliques. 24. It is lengthening. 25. Internal abdominal oblique and transversus abdominis. 26. They lengthen. 27. The rhomboids. 28. Transversus thoracis. 29. The upper rib will depress at the sternocostal and costospinal joints. 30. Serratus anterior and trapezius (upper and lower fibers). 31. They both depress the twelfth rib at the costospinal and sternocostal joints. 32. Trapezius. 33. It lengthens. 34. Latissimus dorsi. 35. Left rotation. 36. Between costal cartilages. 37. Retracting. 38. Iliocostalis. 39. Multifidus. 40. External abdominal oblique on that side of the body. 41. They are synergistic because they both do flexion and right lateral flexion of the trunk at the spinal joints; they are antagonistic because the right external abdominal oblique does left rotation and the right internal abdominal oblique does right rotation of the trunk. 42. Longissimus. 43. It shortens. 44. Posterior tilt and/or depression of the pelvis at the lumbosacral joint. 45. External and internal abdominal obliques and the transversus abdominis. 46. It shortens. 47. They lengthen. 48. Quadratus lumborum. 49. Rotatores. 50. Right rotation. 51. Spinalis. 52. Iliocostalis. 53. Semispinalis. 54. It is shortening. 55. Trapezius. 56. Transverse processes inferiorly to spinous processes superiorly. 57. Internal abdominal oblique. 58. They both elevate upper ribs (ribs #1-2) at the costospinal and sternocostal joints. 59. Transversus abdominis. 60. It lengthens. 61. It drops. 62. The low back. 63. Serratus posterior superior. 64. Quadratus lumborum. 65. Rectus sheath (abdominal aponeurosis). 66. Spinalis. 67. Serratus anterior, pectoralis major. 68. It lengthens.

69. Internal abdominal oblique. 70. Erector spine group. 71. Costoclavicular syndrome, a type of thoracic outlet syndrome. 72. Rotatores, because they are oriented most horizontally. 73. Lamina of the vertebrae (spinous processes of the vertebrae). 74. Subcostales. 75. Internal intercostals. 76. They both retract (adduct) the scapula at the scapulocostal joint. 77. Upper trapezius. 78. Elevation of ribs #9-12 at the costospinal and sternocostal joints. 79. Left rotation. 80. The neck. 81. It is lengthening. 82. Erector spinae group. 83. Its central tendon/dome. 84. Clavicular head. 85. Antagonistic; they laterally flex the spine to opposite sides. 86. Teres major. 87. Transversospinalis group. 88. Transversus abdominis. 89. Biceps brachii (long head proximal attachment). 90. It lengthens. 91. Internal abdominal oblique on that side of the body. 92. Thoracic. 93. Extension. 94. External intercostals. 95. The levatores costarum elevate ribs; the subcostales depress ribs.

CHAPTER 6 LABELING ANSWERS: MUSCLES OF THE PELVIS

Page 206 Anterior View of the Right Pelvis
1. Transversus abdominis (cut). 2. Quadratus lumborum. 3. Psoas major. 4. Iliacus. 5. Psoas minor.

Page 207 Lateral View of the Right Pelvis
1. Gluteus medius. 2. Gluteus maximus. 3. Vastus lateralis. 4. Biceps femoris. 5. Semimembranosus. 6. Plantaris. 7. Gastrocnemius (lateral head). 8. Soleus. 9. Fibularis longus. 10. Tensor fasciae latae. 11. Sartorius. 12. Rectus femoris. 13. Vastus lateralis. 14. Tibialis anterior. 15. Extensor digitorum longus.

Page 208 Posterior View of the Right Pelvis (Superficial)
1. Gluteus maximus. 2. Adductor magnus. 3. Semitendinosus. 4. Gracilis. 5. Semimembranosus. 6. Sartorius. 7. Gluteus medius. 8. Tensor fasciae latae. 9. Biceps femoris.

Page 209 Posterior View of the Right Pelvis (Deep)
1. Piriformis. 2. Superior gemellus. 3. Obturator internus. 4. Inferior gemellus. 5. Semitendinosus (cut). 6. Biceps femoris (long head, cut). 7. Gracilis. 8. Adductor magnus. 9. Semimembranosus. 10. Gluteus medius (cut). 11. Gluteus minimus. 12. Tensor fasciae latae. 13. Gluteus medius (cut and reflected). 14. Quadratus femoris. 15. Gluteus maximus (cut and reflected). 16. Pectineus. 17. Adductor magnus.

Muscles of the Pelvis: Answers to Review Questions (pp 210–211)
1. Obturator internus. 2. Piriformis. 3. Medial rotation and/or abduction. 4. Piriformis and quadratus femoris, respectively. 5. Obturator internus and externus. 6. Lengthen and stretch it. 7. Gluteus maximus, medius, minimus. 8. Gluteus maximus. 9. Superior gemellus and inferior gemellus. 10. Tensor fasciae latae, anterior fibers of the gluteus medius and minimus (they are medial rotators). 11. Synergistic. 12. Psoas major. 13. It lengthens. 14. Left rotation of the pelvis. 15. Tensor fasciae latae. 16. Both: the upper and lower fibers both extend and laterally rotate the thigh and posteriorly tilt and contralaterally rotate the pelvis at the hip joint, hence they are synergistic; however, the upper fibers abduct the thigh, but the lower fibers adduct the thigh, hence they are antagonistic. 17. Psoas major and iliacus. 18. Depression of the pelvis at the hip joint. 19. Adduction of the thigh at the hip joint. 20. Deep. 21. Deep lateral rotators of the thigh. 22. Inferior to it. 23. They are synergistic for every action. 24. It shortens. 25. Either lateral rotation or abduction (horizontal abduction or horizontal extension of the thigh). 26. Gluteus maximus. 27. Superior gemellus. 28. They share the same spinal joint actions. 29. The posterior fibers do extension and lateral rotation of the thigh and posterior tilt and contralateral rotation of the pelvis at the hip joint; the anterior fibers do flexion and medial rotation of the thigh and anterior tilt and ipsilateral rotation of the pelvis at the hip joint. 30. The right quadratus femoris does left rotation of the pelvis; the left quadratus femoris does right rotation of the pelvis. 31. Gluteus maximus. 32. Extension of the right thigh at the hip joint. 33. Lateral rotation and adduction of the thigh at the hip joint. 34. Synergistic, they both flex and laterally rotate the thigh and anteriorly tilt the pelvis at the hip joint. 35. Gluteus maximus and tensor fasciae latae. 36. Lengthen. 37. Either medial rotation or adduction (horizontal adduction or horizontal flexion) of the thigh. 38. All three hamstrings and the adductor magnus also attach to the ischial tuberosity. 39. It lengthens. 40. Lengthen and stretch. 41. Flexion or left lateral flexion of the trunk at the spinal joints or posterior tilt of the pelvis at the lumbosacral joint. 42. Quadratus femoris. 43. Psoas major and minor. 44. It shortens. 45. Inferior gemellus. 46. Piriformis, superior and inferior gemelli, obturator internus and externus, quadratus femoris. 47. Inferior gemellus. 48. Psoas minor. 49. Left rotation of the pelvis at the right hip joint. 50. Psoas major. 51. Sartorius. 52. Gluteus minimus. 53. Medial rotation of the thigh at the hip joint. 54. Obturator externus.

CHAPTER 7 LABELING ANSWERS: MUSCLES OF THE THIGH

Page 242 Anterior View of the Right Thigh (Superficial)
1. Iliacus. 2. Gluteus medius. 3. Tensor fasciae latae. 4. Rectus femoris. 5. Vastus lateralis. 6. Tibialis anterior. 7. Gastrocnemius. 8. Fibularis longus. 9. Psoas major. 10. Pectineus. 11. Adductor longus. 12. Gracilis.

13. Adductor magnus. 14. Sartorius. 15. Vastus medialis. 16. Gastrocnemius.

Page 243 Anterior View of the Right Thigh (Deep)

1. Iliopsoas (cut). 2. Quadratus femoris. 3. Pectineus (cut and reflected). 4. Vastus intermedius. 5. Adductor longus (cut and reflected). 6. Vastus lateralis (cut). 7. Rectus femoris (cut). 8. Vastus medialis (cut). 9. Pectineus (cut and reflected). 10. Adductor longus (cut and reflected). 11. Obturator externus. 12. Gracilis (cut). 13. Adductor brevis. 14. Adductor magnus. 15. Gracilis (cut). 16. Sartorius (cut). 17. Semitendinosus.

Page 244 Posterior View of the Right Thigh (Superficial)

1. Gluteus maximus. 2. Adductor magnus. 3. Gracilis. 4. Semitendinosus. 5. Semimembranosus. 6. Sartorius. 7. Gastrocnemius (medial head). 8. Soleus. 9. Gluteus medius. 10. Tensor fasciae latae. 11. Biceps femoris (long head). 12. Biceps femoris (short head). 13. Plantaris. 14. Gastrocnemius (lateral head). 15. Soleus.

Page 245 Posterior View of the Right Thigh (Deep)

1. Semitendinosus (cut and reflected). 2. Biceps femoris (long head, cut and reflected). 3. Semimembranosus. 4. Semitendinosus (cut and reflected). 5. Biceps femoris (short head). 6. Biceps femoris (long head, cut and reflected).

Page 246 Lateral View of the Right Thigh

1. Gluteus medius. 2. Gluteus maximus. 3. Vastus lateralis. 4. Biceps femoris. 5. Semimembranosus. 6. Plantaris. 7. Gastrocnemius (lateral head). 8. Soleus. 9. Fibularis longus. 10. Tensor fasciae latae. 11. Sartorius. 12. Rectus femoris. 13. Vastus lateralis. 14. Tibialis anterior. 15. Extensor digitorum longus.

Page 247 Medial View of the Right Thigh

1. Iliacus. 2. Adductor longus. 3. Gracilis. 4. Adductor magnus. 5. Rectus femoris. 6. Sartorius. 7. Vastus medialis. 8. Sartorius. 9. Gracilis. 10. Semitendinosus. 11. Tibialis anterior. 12. Piriformis. 13. Obturator internus. 14. Gluteus maximus. 15. Semitendinosus. 16. Semimembranosus. 17. Gastrocnemius (medial head). 18. Soleus.

Muscles of the Thigh: Answers to Review Questions (pp 248–249)

1. Tensor fasciae latae and sartorius. 2. Gluteus maximus. 3. 3. 4. Semitendinosus. 5. Flexion of the leg at the knee joint. 6. Gluteus maximus, posterior fibers of the gluteus medius and minimus. 7. Adductor magnus. 8. It lengthens. 9. Short head of the biceps femoris. 10. Sartorius. 11. Articularis genu. 12. Posterior tilt of the pelvis at the hip joint. 13. Vastus lateralis, medialis, and intermedius; and the tensor fasciae latae and gluteus maximus. 14. 4. 15. The biceps femoris laterally rotates the thigh and leg; the semitendinosus medially rotates the thigh and leg. 16. They all extend the leg at the knee joint. 17. The TFL flexes the thigh and

anteriorly tilts the pelvis at the hip joint; the hamstrings extend the thigh and posteriorly tilts the pelvis at the hip joint. 18. Short head of the biceps femoris. 19. Tibial tuberosity. 20. Tensor fasciae latae and gluteus maximus. 21. Sartorius, gracilis, semitendinosus. 22. It lengthens. 23. Iliopsoas. 24. They both flex the thigh and anteriorly tilt the pelvis at the hip joint. 25. Posterior tilt and depression of the same-side pelvis at the hip joint. 26. Extension. 27. Posterior tilt and depression of the pelvis same-side at the hip joint. 28. Semitendinosus, gracilis, and sartorius. 29. Adductor magnus. 30. Articularis genu. 31. Adductor magnus. 32. Biceps femoris, semitendinosus, semimembranosus. 33. It shortens. 34. Flexion of the thigh at the hip joint. 35. Vastus lateralis. 36. It shortens. 37. Gracilis. 38. Biceps femoris. 39. It shortens. 40. The sartorius flexes the thigh and anteriorly tilts the pelvis at the hip joint; the semitendinosus extends the thigh and posteriorly tilts the pelvis at the hip joint. 41. Gluteus medius, anterior fibers. 42. It is extending. 43. Adductor longus. 44. Vastus lateralis. 45. Iliopsoas. 46. Adductor brevis. 47. They both posteriorly tilt the pelvis. 48. 3. 49. Sartorius. 50. Adductor longus. 51. Vastus intermedius. 52. It lengthens. 53. All three vastus muscles of the quadriceps femoris group, all three 'adductor' muscles of the adductor group, and the biceps femoris of the hamstring group. 54. It shortens. 55. Pectineus, gracilis, adductors longus, brevis, and magnus. 56. It lengthens. 57. Rectus femoris. 58. Rectus femoris, vastus lateralis, medialis, and intermedius. 59. Vastus lateralis or medialis, rectus femoris, tensor fasciae latae and gluteus maximus.

CHAPTER 8 LABELING ANSWERS: MUSCLES OF THE LEG

Page 276 Anterior View of the Right Leg

1. Vastus lateralis. 2. Rectus femoris. 3. Biceps femoris. 4. Fibularis longus. 5. Tibialis anterior. 6. Extensor digitorum longus. 7. Fibularis brevis. 8. Fibularis tertius. 9. Fibularis tertius tendon. 10. Extensor digitorum brevis. 11. Vastus medialis. 12. Sartorius. 13. Gracilis. 14. Semitendinosus. 15. Gastrocnemius. 16. Soleus. 17. Extensor hallucis longus. 18. Extensor hallucis brevis.

Page 277 Posterior View of the Right Leg (Superficial)

1. Semimembranosus. 2. Gracilis. 3. Sartorius. 4. Semitendinosus. 5. Gastrocnemius (medial head). 6. Soleus. 7. Plantaris (tendon). 8. Tibialis posterior. 9. Flexor digitorum longus. 10. Flexor hallucis longus. 11. Biceps femoris. 12. Plantaris. 13. Gastrocnemius (lateral head). 14. Soleus. 15. Fibularis longus. 16. Fibularis brevis.

Page 278 Posterior View of the Right Leg (Intermediate)

1. Gastrocnemius (medial head, cut). 2. Semimembranosus (cut). 3. Popliteus. 4. Soleus. 5. Gastrocnemius (medial

head, cut). 6. Tibialis posterior. 7. Flexor digitorum longus. 8. Flexor hallucis longus. 9. Plantaris. 10. Gastrocnemius (lateral head, cut). 11. Biceps femoris (cut). 12. Fibularis longus. 13. Gastrocnemius (lateral head, cut). 14. Fibularis brevis.

Page 279 Posterior View of the Right Leg (Deep)
1. Gastrocnemius (cut). 2. Semimembranosus. 3. Popliteus. 4. Tibialis posterior. 5. Flexor digitorum longus. 6. Biceps femoris. 7. Gastrocnemius (lateral head, cut). 8. Plantaris (cut and reflected). 9. Soleus (cut and reflected). 10. Fibularis longus. 11. Flexor hallucis longus. 12. Fibularis brevis.

Page 280 Lateral View of the Right Leg
1. Biceps femoris. 2. Plantaris. 3. Fibularis longus. 4. Gastrocnemius. 5. Soleus. 6. Fibularis brevis. 7. Fibularis tertius. 8. Extensor digitorum brevis & extensor hallucis brevis. 9. Vastus lateralis. 10. Rectus femoris. 11. Tibialis anterior. 12. Extensor digitorum longus. 13. Extensor hallucis longus.

Page 281 Medial View of the Right Leg
1. Gracilis. 2. Rectus femoris. 3. Sartorius. 4. Vastus medialis. 5. Sartorius (pes anserine tendon). 6. Gracilis (pes anserine tendon). 7. Semitendinosus (pes anserine tendon). 8. Tibialis anterior. 9. Extensor hallucis longus. 10. Extensor digitorum longus. 11. Adductor magnus. 12. Semitendinosus. 13. Semimembranosus. 14. Gastrocnemius. 15. Soleus. 16. Plantaris. 17. Flexor digitorum longus. 18. Tibialis posterior. 19. Flexor hallucis longus.

Muscles of the Leg: Answers to Review Questions (pp 282–283)
1. They both evert the foot at the subtalar joint. 2. In the distal medial leg. 3. Popliteus. 4. The fibula. 5. The fibularis tertius dorsiflexes the foot at the ankle joint; the fibularis brevis plantarflexes it. 6. Extensor digitorum longus. 7. Dorsiflexion and inversion of the foot at the ankle and subtalar joints, respectively. 8. Fibularis longus. 9. They both dorsiflex the foot at the ankle joint. 10. Gastrocnemius, soleus, plantaris. 11. Fibularis brevis and tertius. 12. Nothing; the flexor digitorum longus does not cross the knee joint. 13. Medial and lateral gastrocnemius and the soleus. 14. Distal. 15. Gastrocnemius and soleus. 16. Tom is tibialis posterior; Dick is the flexor digitorum longus; Harry is the flexor hallucis longus. 17. Extensor hallucis longus. 18. Gastrocnemius. 19. Soleus. 20. Tibialis anterior, extensors digitorum and hallucis longus, fibularis tertius. 21. Dorsiflexion and/or inversion of the foot at the ankle and subtalar joints, respectively. 22. Plantaris and lateral head of the gastrocnemius. 23. It lengthens. 24. Tibialis posterior. 25. Flexor digitorum longus. 26. Soleus. 27. Tibialis anterior and fibularis longus. 28. Both synergistic and antagonistic. 29. Fibularis brevis. 30. The popliteus. 31. It medially rotates the leg at the knee joint; it laterally rotates the thigh at the knee joint. 32. Plantarflexion and inversion of the foot at the ankle and subtalar joints, respectively. 33. Tibialis anterior and fibularis longus. 34. Fibularis longus and brevis. 35. Soleus. 36. Extensor digitorum longus and fibularis tertius. 37. Talus. 38. Flexor digitorum longus. 39. Inversion and/or dorsiflexion of the foot at the subtalar and ankle joints, respectively. 40. Soleus. 41. It shortens. 42. Popliteus, flexors digitorum and hallucis longus, tibialis posterior.

CHAPTER 9 LABELING ANSWERS: INTRINSIC MUSCLES OF THE FOOT

Page 304 Dorsal View of the Right Foot
1. Fibularis longus tendon. 2. Fibularis brevis. 3. Extensor digitorum longus. 4. Fibularis brevis tendon. 5. Fibularis tertius tendon. 6. Extensor digitorum brevis. 7. Abductor digiti minimi pedis. 8. Dorsal interossei pedis. 9. Extensor hallucis longus. 10. Tibialis anterior. 11. Soleus. 12. Extensor hallucis brevis. 13. Abductor hallucis. 14. Dorsal interossei pedis.

Page 305 Plantar View of the Right Foot (Superficial Muscular Layer)
1. Flexor digitorum longus tendons. 2. Flexor digitorum brevis tendons. 3. Adductor hallucis (transverse head). 4. Lumbricals pedis. 5. Flexor digiti minimi pedis. 6. Abductor digiti minimi pedis. 7. Flexor hallucis longus tendon. 8. Flexor hallucis brevis. 9. Flexor digitorum brevis. 10. Abductor hallucis.

Page 306 Plantar View of the Right Foot (Intermediate Muscular Layer)
1. Flexor digitorum longus tendons. 2. Flexor digitorum brevis tendons (cut). 3. Adductor hallucis (transverse head). 4. Lumbricals pedis. 5. Flexor digiti minimi pedis. 6. Plantar interossei. 7. Abductor digiti minimi pedis (partially cut). 8. Quadratus plantae. 9. Flexor digitorum brevis (cut). 10. Flexor hallucis longus tendon. 11. Flexor hallucis brevis. 12. Abductor hallucis (cut). 13. Tibialis posterior tendon. 14. Flexor digitorum longus tendon. 15. Flexor hallucis longus tendon. 16. Abductor hallucis (cut).

Page 307 Plantar View of the Right Foot (Deep Muscular Layer)
1. Flexor digitorum longus tendons (cut). 2. Flexor digitorum brevis tendons (cut). 3. Lumbricals pedis (cut). 4. Adductor hallucis (transverse head). 5. Flexor digiti minimi pedis. 6. Abductor digiti minimi pedis (cut). 7. Plantar interossei. 8. Fibularis brevis tendon. 9. Fibularis longus tendon. 10. Quadratus plantae (cut). 11. Flexor digitorum brevis (cut). 12. Abductor digiti minimi pedis (cut). 13. Flexor hallucis longus tendon (cut). 14. Flexor hallucis brevis. 15. Adductor hallucis (oblique head). 16. Abductor hallucis (cut). 17. Tibialis posterior tendon. 18. Flexor

digitorum longus tendon (cut and reflected). 19. Flexor hallucis longus tendon (cut). 20. Abductor hallucis (cut).

Intrinsic Muscles of the Foot: Answers to Review Questions (pp 308–309)

1. Flexor digitorum accessorius. 2. Extensor digitorum longus. 3. Flexion of toes #2–5 at the metatarsophalangeal and proximal interphalangeal joints. 4. Extensors hallucis brevis and longus. 5. Adduction or flexion of the big toe at the metatarsophalangeal joint. 6. Abductor hallucis. 7. It shortens. 8. The 2nd dorsal interosseus pedis muscle. 9. Flexor hallucis brevis, flexor digiti minimi pedis, adductor hallucis. 10. Flexor hallucis brevis. 11. Flexor hallucis brevis. 12. 2; the extensors hallucis and digitorum brevis; the dorsal interossei pedis are technically plantar muscles. 13. Plantar interossei. 14. Abductor hallucis, abductor digiti minimi pedis, flexor digitorum brevis. 15. The lumbricals pedis are superficial. 16. DAB and PAD; Dorsals Abduct. Plantars ADDuct. 17. Quadratus plantae. 18. Calcaneus. 19. 3rd plantar interosseus. 20. Extensor digitorum longus and fibularis tertius. 21. Quadratus plantae and lumbricals pedis. 22. Dorsal interossei pedis. 23. Flexor digitorum longus. 24. Tuberosity of the calcaneus. 25. Oblique and transverse heads. 26. The 1st and 2ND DIP; the 1st DIP tibially abducts the 2nd toe; the 2nd DIP fibularly abducts the 2nd toe. 27. Flexor digitorum brevis. 28. Abductor digiti minimi pedis. 29. Abductor hallucis, abductor digiti minimi pedis, flexor digitorum brevis. 30. Fibularis longus. 31. Extensor hallucis longus. 32. Flexor digitorum brevis. 33. Extension of toes #2–5 at the metatarsophalangeal and/or proximal interphalangeal joints. 34. Abductor digiti minimi pedis. 35. Adductor hallucis. 36. Adduction of the big toe at the metatarsophalangeal joint. 37. Flexor digitorum longus. 38. The distal tendons of the flexor digitorum longus. 39. Plantar interossei and dorsal interossei pedis. 40. The flexor hallucis brevis. 41. It lengthens. 42. Both; they flex the toes at the metatarsophalangeal joints and extend the toes at the interphalangeal joints.

CHAPTER 10 LABELING ANSWERS: MUSCLES OF THE SCAPULA/ARM

Page 334 Anterior View of the Right Shoulder

1. Anterior scalene. 2. Middle scalene. 3. Levator scapulae. 4. Omohyoid. 5. Posterior scalene. 6. Trapezius. 7. Deltoid. 8. Biceps brachii. 9. Triceps brachii. 10. Latissimus dorsi. 11. Serratus anterior. 12. External abdominal oblique. 13. Sternocleidomastoid. 14. Pectoralis major.

Page 335 Posterior View of the Shoulders (Superficial and Intermediate)

1. Sternocleidomastoid. 2. Splenius capitis. 3. Levator scapulae. 4. Trapezius. 5. Deltoid. 6. Triceps brachii. 7. Latissimus

dorsi. 8. Semispinalis capitis (of transversospinalis group). 9. Splenius capitis. 10. Splenius cervicis. 11. Levator scapulae. 12. Rhomboid minor. 13. Supraspinatus. 14. Infraspinatus. 15. Rhomboid major. 16. Teres minor. 17. Teres major. 18. Triceps brachii. 19. Erector spinae.

Page 336 Anterior View of the Right Arm (Superficial)

1. Deltoid. 2. Pectoralis major (cut and reflected). 3. Biceps brachii (long head). 4. Biceps brachii (short head). 5. Biceps brachii. 6. Brachialis. 7. Brachioradialis. 8. Pectoralis minor (cut). 9. Coracobrachialis. 10. Subscapularis. 11. Teres major. 12. Latissimus dorsi. 13. Triceps brachii. 14. Pronator teres. 15. Flexor carpi radialis. 16. Palmaris longus. 17. Flexor carpi ulnaris.

Page 337 Anterior View of the Right Arm (Deep)

1. Supraspinatus. 2. Biceps brachii (cut). 3. Deltoid (cut). 4. Biceps brachii (cut). 5. Pectoralis minor (cut). 6. Subscapularis. 7. Teres major. 8. Latissimus dorsi. 9. Coracobrachialis. 10. Brachialis.

Page 338 Medial View of the Right Arm

1. Biceps brachii (long head, cut). 2. Subscapularis (cut). 3. Pectoralis major (cut). 4. Biceps brachii (short head, cut). 5. Coracobrachialis (cut). 6. Biceps brachii. 7. Bicipital aponeurosis of the biceps brachii. 8. Brachioradialis. 9. Flexor carpi radialis. 10. Supraspinatus (cut). 11. Infraspinatus (cut). 12. Teres minor (cut). 13. Deltoid (cut). 14. Teres major (cut). 15. Latissimus dorsi (cut). 16. Triceps brachii (long head). 17. Triceps brachii (medial head). 18. Brachialis. 19. Pronator teres. 20. Palmaris longus. 21. Flexor carpi ulnaris.

Page 339 Lateral View of the Right Arm

1. Deltoid. 2. Triceps brachii. 3. Anconeus. 4. Extensor carpi ulnaris. 5. Extensor digitorum. 6. Extensor digiti minimi. 7. Biceps brachii. 8. Brachialis. 9. Brachioradialis. 10. Extensor carpi radialis longus. 11. Extensor carpi radialis brevis.

Page 340 Posterior View of the Right Arm

1. Supraspinatus. 2. Infraspinatus. 3. Teres minor. 4. Teres major. 5. Triceps brachii (medial head). 6. Flexor carpi ulnaris. 7. Deltoid (cut and reflected). 8. Triceps brachii (lateral head). 9. Triceps brachii (long head). 10. Brachioradialis. 11. Extensor carpi radialis longus. 12. Anconeus. 13. Extensor carpi radialis brevis. 14. Extensor digitorum. 15. Extensor digiti minimi. 16. Extensor carpi ulnaris.

Page 341 Anterior View of the Right Glenohumeral Joint

1. Supraspinatus. 2. Coracobrachialis (cut). 3. Biceps brachii (short head, cut). 4. Biceps brachii (long head, cut). 5. Triceps brachii. 6. Coracobrachialis (cut). 7. Biceps brachii (cut). 8. Supraspinatus. 9. Pectoralis minor (cut). 10. Subscapularis. 11. Teres major. 12. Latissimus dorsi.

Page 341 **Posterior View of the Right Glenohumeral Joint**
1. Supraspinatus (cut). 2. Infraspinatus (cut and reflected). 3. Teres major. 4. Teres minor. 5. Supraspinatus (cut). 6. Infraspinatus (cut and reflected). 7. Deltoid (cut and reflected). 8. Triceps brachii (medial head). 9. Triceps brachii (long head). 10. Triceps brachii (lateral head).

Muscles of the Scapula/Arm: Answers to Review Questions (pp 342–343)
1. Triceps brachii, anconeus, extensor carpi ulnaris. 2. Synergistic; they both flex and adduct the arm at the shoulder joint. 3. Superficial. 4. Medial rotation of the arm at the shoulder joint. 5. They both do abduction of the arm at the shoulder joint. 6. Teres major and teres minor. 7. Deep; anterior. 8. Medial head. 9. Anterior fibers flex while the posterior fibers extend; anterior fibers medially rotate while the posterior fibers laterally rotate. 10. Anterior. 11. Deltoid. 12. Coracobrachialis, pectoralis minor, and biceps brachii, short head. 13. Subscapularis; they both do medial rotation of the arm at the shoulder joint. 14. Long head. 15. Inferior. 16. Antagonistic; the pronator teres flexes the elbow joint; the triceps brachii extends it. 17. Brachialis. 18. Shorten. 19. Neither; pronation and supination have no effect upon the length of the brachialis. 20. Shortened. 21. Deep. 22. Brachialis. 23. Synergistic; they both flex the elbow joint. 24. Lateral rotation, abduction, and flexion of the arm at the shoulder joint. 25. Latissimus dorsi. 26. Supraspinatus. 27. Lateral. 28. 3; The elbow, radioulnar, and shoulder joints. 29. Supraspinatus and teres minor. 30. Shortened. 31. Supraspinatus, infraspinatus, teres minor, subscapularis. 32. Antagonistic; minor does lateral rotation; major does medial rotation. 33. Infraspinatus. 34. They both do abduction of the arm at the shoulder joint. 35. Supraspinatus, infraspinatus, teres minor. 36. Clavicular head. 37. Extension and abduction. 38. Inferior. 39. Superior. 40. Latissimus dorsi. 41. Trapezius and deltoid. 42. Deltoid.

CHAPTER 11 LABELING ANSWERS: MUSCLES OF THE FOREARM

Page 380 **Anterior View of the Right Forearm (Superficial)**
1. Biceps brachii. 2. Brachialis. 3. Brachioradialis. 4. Extensor carpi radialis longus. 5. Extensor carpi radialis brevis. 6. Flexor pollicis longus. 7. Pronator quadratus. 8. Abductor pollicis longus. 9. Triceps brachii (medial head). 10. Brachialis (deep to median nerve and brachial artery from this view). 11. Bicipital aponeurosis of the biceps brachii. 12. Pronator teres. 13. Flexor carpi radialis. 14. Palmaris longus. 15. Flexor carpi ulnaris. 16. Flexor digitorum superficialis. 17. Flexor digitorum profundus.

Page 381 **Anterior View of the Right Forearm (Intermediate)**
1. Biceps brachii. 2. Brachialis. 3. Brachialis (tendon). 4. Biceps brachii (tendon). 5. Supinator. 6. Brachioradialis. 7. Pronator teres (cut). 8. Flexor pollicis longus. 9. Abductor pollicis longus. 10. Pronator quadratus. 11. Flexor carpi radialis (cut). 12. Triceps brachii (medial head). 13. Pronator teres (humeral head, cut and reflected). 14. Brachialis. 15. Flexor carpi radialis (cut). 16. Palmaris longus (cut). 17. Pronator teres (ulnar head, cut and reflected). 18. Flexor digitorum profundus. 19. Flexor carpi ulnaris. 20. Flexor digitorum superficialis. 21. Flexor digitorum profundus.

Page 382 **Anterior View of the Right Forearm (Deep)**
1. Brachialis. 2. Biceps brachii (tendon). 3. Supinator. 4. Flexor digitorum superficialis (cut). 5. Pronator teres (cut and reflected). 6. Flexor pollicis longus (cut). 7. Pronator quadratus. 8. Brachioradialis (cut). 9. Flexor carpi radialis (cut). 10. Flexor pollicis longus (cut). 11. Triceps brachii (medial head). 12. Pronator teres (humeral head, cut and reflected). 13. Flexor carpi radialis (cut). 14. Palmaris longus (cut). 15. Flexor carpi ulnaris (cut and reflected). 16. Flexor digitorum superficialis (cut). 17. Pronator teres (ulnar head, cut). 18. Flexor digitorum profundus (cut). 19. Flexor carpi ulnaris (cut).

Page 383 **Anterior Views of the Pronators and Supinator of the Right Radius**
1. Supinator: ulnar head. 1. Supinator: humeral head. 2. Pronator quadratus. 3. Pronator teres: humeral head. 3. Pronator teres: ulnar head.

Page 384 **Posterior View of the Right Forearm (Superficial)**
1. Triceps brachii. 2. Flexor carpi ulnaris. 3. Extensor carpi ulnaris. 4. Extensor digiti minimi. 5. Abductor digiti minimi manus. 6. Dorsal interossei manus. 7. Brachioradialis. 8. Anconeus. 9. Extensor carpi radialis longus. 10. Extensor carpi radialis brevis. 11. Extensor digitorum. 12. Abductor pollicis longus. 13. Extensor pollicis brevis. 14. Extensor pollicis longus. 15. Dorsal interossei manus. 16. Extensor indicis tendon.

Page 385 **Posterior View of the Right Forearm (Deep)**
1. Flexor carpi ulnaris. 2. Extensor digitorum tendons (cut). 3. Extensor indicis. 4. Extensor digiti minimi (cut). 5. Extensor carpi ulnaris (cut). 6. Abductor digiti minimi manus. 7. Dorsal interossei manus. 8. Triceps brachii tendon (cut). 9. Brachioradialis. 10. Anconeus. 11. Extensor carpi radialis longus. 12. Extensor carpi radialis brevis. 13. Supinator. 14. Pronator teres. 15. Abductor pollicis longus. 16. Extensor pollicis longus. 17. Extensor pollicis brevis. 18. Dorsal interossei manus. 19. Extensor indicis tendon.

Page 386 Posterior View of the Right Forearm and Hand (Superficial)

1. Extensor digiti minimi. 2. Extensor carpi ulnaris. 3. Extensor carpi radialis longus. 4. Extensor carpi radialis brevis. 5. Extensor digitorum. 6. Abductor pollicis longus. 7. Extensor pollicis brevis. 8. Extensor pollicis longus. 9. Extensor indicis (tendon).

Page 387 Posterior View of the Right Forearm and Hand (Deep)

1. Extensor digiti minimi (cut). 2. Extensor carpi ulnaris (cut). 3. Extensor pollicis longus. 4. Extensor indicis. 5. Extensor carpi ulnaris tendon (cut). 6. Extensor carpi radialis longus. 7. Extensor carpi radialis brevis. 8. Extensor digitorum (cut). 9. Abductor pollicis longus. 10. Extensor pollicis brevis.

Muscles of the Forearm: Answers to Review Questions (pp 388–390)

1. Flexor digitorum superficialis. 2. Deep. 3. Extensor carpi ulnaris. 4. Palmaris longus and flexor carpi radialis. 5. Brachioradialis. 6. Extension and/or ulnar deviation of the hand at the wrist joint. 7. Anconeus, extensor carpi radialis brevis, extensors digitorum and digiti minimi, extensor carpi ulnaris, and supinator. 8. Metacarpals 2, 3, and 5, respectively. 9. Extension and ulnar deviation of the hand at the wrist joint. 10. Extensor digitorum. 11. The anconeus extends the forearm at the elbow joint; the flexor carpi radialis flexes it. 12. Both muscles can supinate the forearm at the radioulnar joints. 13. Extensor carpi ulnaris. 14. Flexor pollicis longus. 15. Brachioradialis and extensor carpi radialis longus. 16. Extension of the elbow joint. 17. Flexor digitorum profundus. 18. Median nerve. 19. The common flexor tendon. 20. Flexor pollicis longus. 21. Extensor carpi radialis longus. 22. Both do flexion of the hand at the wrist joint and flexion of the forearm at the elbow joint. 23. Extensors carpi radialis longus and brevis, extensor carpi ulnaris. 24. Extensor digiti minimi. 25. Supinator and anconeus. 26. Abductor pollicis longus. 27. Extensor digiti minimi and extensor indicis. 28. Abductor pollicis longus and extensor pollicis brevis laterally; extensor pollicis longus medially. 29. Extensor carpi radialis brevis and extensor digitorum. 30. The extensor pollicis brevis radially deviates the hand at the wrist joint; the extensor carpi ulnaris ulnar deviates it. 31. Extensors carpi radialis brevis and longus and the brachioradialis. 32. Radial deviation. 33. Anconeus. 34. Extensor pollicis brevis. 35. Abductor pollicis longus, extensors pollicis brevis and longus, extensor indicis. 36. Flexor digitorum profundus. 37. Extensors carpi radialis longus and brevis. 38. It lengthens. 39. Extensor pollicis brevis. 40. Flexor digitorum profundus. 41. Brachioradialis, extensors carpi radialis longus and brevis. 42. Triceps brachii. 43. Flexor carpi ulnaris. 44. The FCR radially deviates the hand at the wrist joint;

the FCU ulnar deviates the hand at the wrist joint. 45. Pronator teres. 46. Pronators teres and quadratus. 47. The radius. 48. They shorten. 49. It shortens. 50. Flexor pollicis longus and brevis, opponens and adductor pollicis. 51. Common flexor tendon at the medial epicondyle of the humerus. 52. Triceps brachii. 53. Flexors carpi radialis and ulnaris, palmaris longus. 54. Pronator teres. 55. They both flex the hand at the wrist joint and flex the forearm at the elbow joint. 56. Supinator, abductor pollicis longus, extensors pollicis longus and brevis, extensor indicis. 57. Extensor carpi ulnaris. 58. Flexor digitorum profundus. 59. Extensor digitorum. 60. Brachioradialis, abductor or extensor pollicis longus, extensor indicis. 61. Brachialis, biceps brachii, pronator teres. 62. Flexor carpi radialis. 63. Pronator quadratus. 64. Flexors digitorum superficialis and profundus. 65. Pronation of the forearm at the radioulnar joints. 66. Extensors digitorum, digiti minimi, carpi ulnaris and carpi radialis brevis. 67. Flexor digitorum superficialis. 68. It shortens. 69. Extensor carpi radialis longus. 70. Extension and/or radial deviation of the hand at the wrist joint. 71. It lengthens. 72. Extensor digitorum. 73. They lengthen. 74. It lengthens. 75. Extension of the elbow joint. 76. It shortens. 77. Extension of the fingers at the metacarpophalangeal and/or proximal interphalangeal joints, and/or extension of the hand at the wrist joint and the forearm at the elbow joint. 78. Flexor digitorum profundus.

CHAPTER 12 LABELING ANSWERS: MUSCLES OF THE HAND

Page 408 Palmar View of the Right Hand (Superficial)

1. Palmaris longus. 2. Flexor pollicis brevis (deep to fascia). 3. Abductor pollicis brevis (deep to fascia). 4. Adductor pollicis (deep to fascia). 5. Lumbricals manus (partially deep to fascia). 6. Flexor pollicis longus. 7. Dorsal interossei manus. 8. Flexor digitorum profundus. 9. Flexor digitorum superficialis. 10. Palmar interossei. 11. Dorsal interossei manus. 12. Lumbricals manus. 13. Palmaris brevis. 14. Hypothenar muscle group (deep to fascia). 15. Palmar interossei. 16. Flexor digitorum profundus. 17. Flexor digitorum superficialis. 18. Lumbricals manus. 19. Dorsal interossei manus. 20. Lumbricals manus. 21. Dorsal interossei manus.

Page 409 Palmar View of the Right Hand (Superficial Muscular Layer)

1. Flexor pollicis brevis. 2. Abductor pollicis brevis. 3. Adductor pollicis (deep to fascia). 4. Dorsal interossei manus. 5. Lumbricals manus. 6. Lumbricals manus. 7. Flexor digitorum profundus. 8. Flexor digitorum superficialis. 9. Palmar interossei. 10. Dorsal interossei manus. 11. Opponens digiti minimi. 12. Abductor digiti minimi manus. 13. Flexor digiti minimi manus. 14. Lumbricals manus. 15. Lumbricals

manus. 16. Palmar interossei. 17. Flexor digitorum profundus. 18. Flexor digitorum superficialis. 19. Dorsal interossei manus. 20. Dorsal interossei manus.

Page 410 Palmar View of the Right Hand (Deep Muscular Layer)

1. Pronator quadratus. 2. Abductor pollicis brevis (cut). 3. Opponens pollicis. 4. Flexor pollicis brevis. 5. Abductor pollicis brevis (cut). 6. Adductor pollicis. 7. Dorsal interossei manus. 8. Lumbricals manus (cut and reflected). 9. Lumbricals manus (cut and reflected). 10. Palmar interossei. 11. Dorsal interossei manus. 12. Flexor carpi ulnaris. 13. Abductor digiti minimi manus (cut). 14. Flexor digiti minimi manus (cut). 15. Opponens digiti minimi. 16. Palmar interossei. 17. Dorsal interossei manus. 18. Abductor digiti minimi manus (cut). 19. Flexor digiti minimi manus (cut). 20. Dorsal interossei manus. 21. Lumbricals manus (cut and reflected). 22. Palmar interossei. 23. Lumbricals manus (cut and reflected).

Page 411 Dorsal View of the Right Hand

1. Extensor digitorum. 2. Extensor digiti minimi. 3. Extensor carpi ulnaris. 4. Abductor digiti minimi manus. 5. Dorsal interossei manus. 6. Dorsal interossei manus. 7. Palmar interossei. 8. Lumbricals manus. 9. Lumbricals manus. 10. Extensor carpi radialis brevis. 11. Extensor carpi radialis longus. 12. Extensor pollicis brevis. 13. Abductor pollicis longus. 14. Extensor indicis. 15. Extensor pollicis longus. 16. Dorsal interossei manus. 17. Dorsal interossei manus. 18. Adductor pollicis. 19. Palmar interossei.

Muscles of the Hand: Answers to Review Questions (pp 412–413)

1. Thenar, hypothenar, central compartment. 2. Abductor and flexor pollicis brevis. 3. Lumbricals manus, palmar interossei, dorsal interossei manus, adductor pollicis. 4. They both flex fingers at the metacarpophalangeal joints and extend fingers at the interphalangeal joints. 5. Hypothenar group. 6. Palmaris longus. 7. 3rd palmar interosseus. 8. Flexion of the thumb at the carpometacarpal and/or metacarpophalangeal joints and/or abduction of the thumb at the carpometacarpal joint. 9. Trapezium. 10. Adductor pollicis. 11. Deep. 12. Adductor pollicis, lumbricals manus, palmar interossei, dorsal interossei manus. 13. Abductor and flexor pollicis brevis, opponens pollicis. 14. Abductor and flexor pollicis brevis, opponens pollicis. 15. Palmar interossei. 16. It has no bony attachments; it attaches only into soft tissues. 17. Abductor and flexor pollicis brevis; adductor pollicis. 18. The abductor digiti minimi manus abducts the little finger at the metacarpophalangeal joint; the opponens digiti minimi adducts it. 19. When objects are being gripped in the hand. 20. No joint action occurs when any muscle isometrically contracts. 21. Flexor pollicis brevis. 22. Deep. 23. Abductor pollicis brevis. 24. Lumbricals manus, palmar interossei, dorsal interossei manus,

adductor pollicis. 25. It lengthens. 26. Pisiform and hamate. 27. Extension of the little finger at the metacarpophalangeal joint. 28. Abductor and flexor digiti minimi manus and opponens digiti minimi. 29. Lateral rotation of the little finger. 30. It lengthens. 31. Palmar interossei. 32. Abductor and flexor digiti minimi manus, opponens digiti minimi. 33. Their distal attachments are onto metacarpals. 34. Both; the metacarpophalangeal joints are flexed; the interphalangeal joints are extended. 35. Flexor digiti minimi manus. 36. The palmar interossei adduct fingers at the metacarpophalangeal joints; the dorsal interossei manus abduct fingers at the metacarpophalangeal joints.

CHAPTER 13 LABELING ANSWERS: OTHER SKELETAL MUSCLES

Page 414 Anterior Views of the Other Muscles of the Abdomen

1. External abdominal oblique. 2. Rectus abdominis. 3. Pyramidalis. 4. External abdominal oblique. 5. Internal abdominal oblique. 6. Cremaster.

Page 415 Views of the Muscles of the Perineum

1. Ischiocavernosus. 2. Bulbospongiosus. 3. Deep transverse perineal. 4. Superficial transverse perineal. 5. Gluteus maximus. 6. External anal sphincter. 7. Compressor urethrae. 8. Sphincter urethrae. 9. Sphincter urethrovaginalis. 10. Levator ani. 11. Coccygeus. 12. Sphincter urethrae. 13. Deep transverse perineal. 14. Superficial transverse perineal. 15. External anal sphincter. 16. Gluteus maximus. 17. Ischiocavernosus. 18. Bulbospongiosus. 19. Deep transverse perineal. 20. Superficial transverse perineal. 21. Levator ani. 22. Coccygeus.

Page 416 Views of the Muscles of the Tongue

1. Superior longitudinal muscle. 2. Vertical muscle. 3. Transverse muscle. 4. Inferior longitudinal muscle. 5. Genioglossus. 6. Stylohyoid. 7. Styloglossus. 8. Buccinator. 9. Platysma. 10. Hyoglossus. 11. Digastric. 12. Inferior longitudinal muscle. 13. Genioglossus. 14. Mylohyoid. 15. Geniohyoid. 16. Hyoglossus. 17. Palatoglossus. 18. Palatopharyngeus. 19. Superior pharyngeal constrictor (partially cut). 20. Digastric (cut). 21. Styloglossus. 22. Stylopharyngeus. 23. Stylohyoid. 24. Middle pharyngeal constrictor. 25. Digastric (cut).

Page 417 Views of the Muscles of the Palate

1. Tensor veli palatini. 2. Levator veli palatini. 3. Palatoglossus. 4. Mylohyoid. 5. Geniohyoid. 6. Hyoglossus. 7. Middle pharyngeal constrictor. 8. Stylopharyngeus. 9. Salpingopharyngeus. 10. Musculus uvulae. 11. Superior pharyngeal constrictor. 12. Palatopharyngeus.

Page 418 Views of the Muscles of the Pharynx

1. Levator veli palatini. 2. Accessory muscle bundle from temporal bone. 3. Digastric. 4. Stylohyoid. 5. Medial

pterygoid. 6. Stylopharyngeus. 7. Circular esophageal muscle. 8. Longitudinal esophageal muscle. 9. Superior pharyngeal constrictor. 10. Salpingopharyngeus. 11. Palatopharyngeus. 12. Middle pharyngeal constrictor. 13. Musculus uvulae. 14. Longitudinal pharyngeal muscle. 15. Transverse and oblique arytenoids. 16. Posterior cricoarytenoid. 17. Inferior pharyngeal constrictor.

Page 419 Views of the Muscles of the Larynx

1. Transverse arytenoid. 2. Oblique arytenoid. 3. Posterior cricoarytenoid. 4. Cricothyroid. 5. Cricothyroid. 6. Transverse arytenoid. 7. Oblique arytenoid. 8. Lateral cricoarytenoid. 9. Posterior cricoarytenoid. 10. Thyroarytenoid. 11. Cricothyroid (cut).

Page 420 Views of the Muscles of the Larynx: Superior/Inferior View

1. Transverse arytenoid. 2. Oblique arytenoid. 3. Posterior cricoarytenoid.

Page 420 Views of the Muscles of the Larynx: Posterior/Anterior View

1. Posterior cricoarytenoid. 2. Transverse arytenoid. 3. Oblique arytenoid. 4. Lateral cricoarytenoid. 5. Thyroarytenoid. 6. Cricothyroid.

Page 421 Views of the Extrinsic Muscles of the Right Eye: Top Illustration

1. Levator palpebrae superioris. 2. Superior oblique. 3. Superior rectus. 4. Medial rectus. 5. Lateral rectus (cut). 6. Inferior rectus. 7. Inferior oblique.

Bottom Left Illustration

1. Superior rectus (cut). 2. Lateral rectus (cut). 3. Inferior rectus (cut). 4. Inferior oblique (cut). 5. Superior oblique (cut). 6. Medial rectus (cut).

Bottom Right Illustration

1. Superior oblique. 2. Medial rectus. 3. Inferior rectus. 4. Levator palpebrae superioris. 5. Superior rectus. 6. Lateral rectus. 7. Levator palpebrae superioris.

Page 422 Views of the Muscles of the Tympanic Cavity

1. Tensor tympani. 2. Stapedius.

CHAPTER 14 LABELING ANSWERS: THE NERVOUS SYSTEM

Page 424 Cranial Nerves

1. CN IV (trochlear nerve). 2. CN VI (adbucens nerve). 3. CN VII (facial nerve). 4. CN VIII (acoustic nerve, also known as vestibulocochlear nerve). 5. CN IX (glossopharyngeal nerve). 6. CN X (vagus nerve). 7. CN XI (spinal accessory nerve). 8. CN I (olfactory nerve). 9. CN II (optic nerve). 10. CN III (occulomotor nerve). 11. CN V (trigeminal nerve). 12. CN XII (hypoglossal nerve).

Page 425 Cross Section View of the Spinal Cord Through a Cervical Vertebra—Spinal Nerve Diagram

1. Sympathetic ganglion. 2. Vertebral artery. 3. Ventral nerve root. 4. Spinal cord. 5. Dura mater. 6. Vertebral spinous process (SP). 7. Dorsal nerve root. 8. Gray ramus communicans of a spinal nerve. 9. Ventral ramus of a spinal nerve. 10. Dorsal ramus of a spinal nerve. 11. Dorsal root ganglion.

Page 426 View of the Cervical Plexus

1. Lesser occipital nerve. 2. to the vagus nerve. 3. Greater auricular nerve. 4. to sternocleidomastoid. 5. to levator scapulae. 6. Transverse cutaneous nerve of the neck. 7. to trapezius. 8. to levator scapulae. 9. to middle scalene. 10. Supraclavicular nerve. 11. to rectus lateralis. 12. to rectus capitis anterior and longus capitis. 13. to geniohyoid. 14. to longus capitis and longus colli. 15. to longus capitis, longus colli, and middle scalene. 16. to thyrohyoid. 17. Ansa cervicalis. 18. to longus colli. 19. Phrenic nerve.

Page 427 View of the Brachial Plexus

1. Dorsal scapular nerve. 2. to the phrenic nerve. 3. Suprascapular nerve. 4. Lateral pectoral nerve. 5. Axillary nerve. 6. Musculocutaneous nerve. 7. Radial nerve. 8. Median nerve. 9. Ulnar nerve. 10. Medial antebrachial cutaneous nerve. 11. Medial brachial cutaneous nerve. 12. Lower subscapular nerve. 13. Thoracodorsal nerve. 14. Nerve to scalenes. 15. Nerve to scalenes. 16. Nerve to subclavius. 17. Nerve to scalenes. 18. Long thoracic nerve. 19. Nerve to scalenes. 20. First intercostal nerve. 21. Medial pectoral nerve. 22. Upper subscapular nerve.

Page 428 View of the Lumbar Plexus

1. Iliohypogastric nerve. 2. Ilio-inguinal. 3. Genitofemoral. 4. Lateral cutaneous nerve of the thigh. 5. to psoas and iliacus (iliopsoas). 6. Femoral nerve. 7. Accessory obturator nerve. 8. Obturator nerve. 9. Lumbosacral trunk.

Page 429 View of the Sacral and Coccygeal Plexuses

1. Superior gluteal nerve. 2. Inferior gluteal nerve. 3. to piriformis. 4. to superior gemellus and obturator internus. 5. to inferior gemellus and quadratus femoris. 6. Common fibular nerve of the sciatic nerve. 7. Tibial nerve of the sciatic nerve. 8. Posterior femoral cutaneous nerve. 9. Perforating cutaneous nerve. 10. Pelvic splanchnic nerves. 11. Pudendal nerve. 12. to levator ani, coccygeous, and external anal sphincter. 13. Anococcygeal nerves. 14. Visceral branches. 15. Visceral branches.

Page 430 **Views of Innervation to the Right Lower Extremity**
1. Femoral nerve. 2. Common fibular nerve of the sciatic nerve. 3. Superficial fibular nerve. 4. Obturator nerve. 5. Deep fibular nerve. 6. Sciatic nerve. 7. Tibial nerve of the sciatic nerve. 8. Medial plantar nerve. 9. Common fibular nerve of the sciatic nerve. 10. Superficial fibular nerve. 11. Lateral plantar nerve.

Page 431 **Anterior View of Innervation to the Right Upper Extremity**
1. Axillary nerve. 2. Musculocutaneous nerve. 3. Radial nerve. 4. Brachial plexus. 5. Median nerve. 6. Ulnar nerve.

CHAPTER 15 LABELING ANSWERS: THE ARTERIAL SYSTEM

Page 434 **Lateral View of Arterial Supply to the Head and Neck**
1. Posterior auricular artery. 2. Superficial temporal artery. 3. Occipital artery. 4. Ascending pharyngeal artery. 5. Vertebral artery. 6. Internal carotid artery. 7. Deep cervical artery. 8. Dorsal scapular artery. 9. Costocervical trunk. 10. Axillary artery. 11. Transverse facial artery. 12. Supraorbital artery. 13. Supratrochlear artery. 14. Ophthalmic artery. 15. Infraorbital artery. 16. Maxillary artery. 17. Inferior alveolar artery. 18. Facial artery. 19. Lingual artery. 20. Superior thyroid artery. 21. External carotid artery. 22. Ascending cervical artery. 23. Inferior thyroid artery. 24. Transverse cervical artery. 25. Thyrocervical trunk. 26. Common carotid artery. 27. Subclavian artery. 28. Brachiocephalic trunk. 29. Internal thoracic artery.

Page 435 **Anterior View of Arterial Supply to the Trunk and Pelvis**
1. Costocervical trunk. 2. Dorsal scapular artery. 3. Thoracoacromial trunk. 4. Internal thoracic artery. 5. Anterior intercostal artery. 6. Posterior intercostal artery. 7. Musculophrenic artery. 8. Superior epigastric artery. 9. Lumbar artery. 10. Subcostal artery. 11. Iliolumbar artery. 12. Inferior epigastric artery. 13. Deep circumflex iliac artery. 14. Common carotid artery. 15. Subclavian artery. 16. Brachiocephalic trunk. 17. Axillary artery. 18. Ascending aorta. 19. Descending aorta. 20. Common iliac artery. 21. Internal iliac artery. 22. External iliac artery. 23. Median sacral artery.

Page 436 **Anterior View of Arterial Supply to the Right Lower Extremity**
1. Common iliac artery. 2. Iliolumbar artery. 3. External iliac artery. 4. Perforating branches of the deep femoral artery. 5. Popliteal artery. 6. Anterior tibial artery. 7. Lateral plantar artery. 8. Plantar arch. 9. Internal iliac artery.
10. Superior gluteal artery. 11. Inferior gluteal artery. 12. Femoral artery. 13. Obturator artery. 14. Deep femoral artery. 15. Posterior tibial artery. 16. Fibular artery. 17. Medial plantar artery. 18. Dorsalis pedis artery.

Page 437 **Anterior View of Arterial Supply to the Right Upper Extremity**
1. Suprascapular artery. 2. Thoracoacromial trunk. 3. Axillary artery. 4. Anterior circumflex humeral artery. 5. Posterior circumflex humeral artery (posterior to the humerus). 6. Brachial artery. 7. Deep brachial artery. 8. Radial artery. 9. Interosseus recurrent artery (posterior to the radius and humerus). 10. Posterior interosseus artery. 11. Deep palmar arterial arch. 12. Thyrocervical trunk. 13. Subclavian artery. 14. Dorsal scapular artery. 15. Superior thoracic artery. 16. Subscapular artery. 17. Lateral thoracic artery. 18. Thoracodorsal artery. 19. Circumflex scapular artery. 20. Ulnar artery. 21. Anterior interosseus artery. 22. Superficial palmar arterial arch.

CHAPTER 16 LABELING ANSWERS: OTHER STRUCTURES AND SYSTEMS OF THE BODY

Page 444 **A Typical Cell**
1. Centrosome. 2. Centrioles. 3. Smooth endoplasmic reticulum. 4. Mitochondrion. 5. Lysosome. 6. Rough endoplasmic reticulum. 7. Peroxisome. 8. Cytoskeleton. 9. Intermediate filament. 10. Microtubule. 11. Microfilament. 12. Nuclear envelope. 13. Ribosomes. 14. Mitochondrion. 15. Smooth endoplasmic reticulum. 16. Cilia. 17. Free ribosomes. 18. Golgi apparatus. 19. Microvilli. 20. Vesicle. 21. Nucleolus. 22. Nucleus.

Page 444 **Major Components of a Cell**
1. Cell membrane. 2. Cytoplasm. 3. Nucleus. 4. Organelles.

Page 444 **The Cytoskeleton**
1. Intermediate filament. 2. Endoplasmic reticulum. 3. Ribosome. 4. Microtubule. 5. Mitochondrion. 6. Microfilament. 7. Plasma membrane.

Page 445 **The Cell Membrane**
1. External membrane surface. 2. Phospholipid bilayer. 3. Internal membrane surface. 4. Carbohydrate chains. 5. Glycolipid. 6. Polar region of phospholipid. 7. Nonpolar region of phospholipid. 8. Protein. 9. Glycoprotein. 10. Cholesterol. 11. Membrane channel protein.

Page 445 **The Endoplasmic Reticulum and Golgi Apparatus**
1. Ribosomes. 2. Proteins. 3. Vesicle. 4. Cytoplasm. 5. Endoplasmic reticulum. 6. Cisternae. 7. Golgi apparatus. 8. Plasma membrane. 9. Secretory vesicle. 10. Vesicle containing plasma membrane components.

Page 445 **Cross Section of a Mitochondrion**
1. Outer membrane. 2. Inner membrane. 3. Matrix. 4. Cristae.

Page 445 **Cross Section of the Nucleus**
1. Nucleolus. 2. Nuclear pores. 3. Chromatin. 4. Nucleoplasm. 5. Nuclear envelope.

Page 446 **Longitudinal Section of a Long Bone**
1. Proximal epiphysis. 2. Diaphysis. 3. Distal epiphysis. 4. Articular cartilage. 5. Spongy bone. 6. Epiphyseal plate. 7. Red marrow cavities. 8. Compact bone. 9. Medullary cavity. 10. Endosteum. 11. Yellow marrow. 12. Periosteum.

Page 446 **A. Section of a Flat Bone**
1. Compact bone. 2. Spongy bone.

Page 446 **B. Magnification of Spongy Bone Tissue**
1. Trabeculae.

Page 447 **Longitudinal Section of a Long Bone and Magnification of Compact Bone Tissue**
1. Osteonic canal. 2. Osteon. 3. Periosteum. 4. Blood vessels and nerve in osteonic canal. 5. Volkmann's canal. 6. Compact bone. 7. Spongy bone. 8. Nerve. 9. Blood vessel. 10. Canaliculus. 11. Osteocyte. 12. Nerve. 13. Blood vessel. 14. Endosteum. 15. Compact bone. 16. Osteon.

Page 448 **Structure of a Muscle**
1. Tendon. 2. Muscle (fibrous fascia). 3. Axon of motor neuron. 4. Fascicle. 5. Blood vessel. 6. Muscle fibers. 7. Muscle fiber. 8. Myofibrils. 9. Filaments. 10. Myofibril. 11. Sarcoplasmic reticulum. 12. Nucleus. 13. Sarcolemma. 14. Endomysium. 15. Perimysium. 16. Perimysium. 17. Epimysium. 18. Bone.

Page 449 **Structure of a Muscle Illustrating a Sarcomere**
1. Actin filaments. 2. Myosin filament. 3. Myosin head. 4. Z-line. 5. M-line. 6. H-band. 7. A-band. 8. I-band. 9. Striations of skeletal muscle tissue. 10. Nuclei. 11. Muscle fiber. 12. Z-line. 13. Sarcomere. 14. Myofibril. 15. M-line.

Page 449 **Sarcoplasmic Reticulum and T Tubules of a Muscle Fiber**
1. Motor neuron fiber. 2. T tubule. 3. Synapse. 4. T tubule. 5. Sarcoplasmic reticulum. 6. Neurotransmitters in synapse. 7. Motor endplate. 8. Myofibrils. 9. Nucleus. 10. Sarcolemma.

Page 450 **Myosin and Actin Filaments – Top**
1. Actin subunits. 2. Actin filament. 3. Actin molecules. 4. Troponin. 5. Tropomyosin.

Page 450 **Myosin and Actin Filaments – Bottom Left**
1. Titin. 2. Actin filament. 3. Myosin filament.

Page 450 **Myosin and Actin Filaments – Bottom Right**
1. Titin. 2. Actin filament. 3. Myosin filament.

Page 451 **Sliding Filament Action – Top**
1. Actin filaments. 2. Troponin. 3. Tropomyosin. 4. Myosin heads. 5. Myosin filament.

Page 451 **Neuromuscular Junction**
1. Motor neuron fiber. 2. Muscle fiber nucleus. 3. Myofibril of muscle fiber. 4. Mitochondria. 5. Synaptic vesicles. 6. Synapse (synaptic cleft). 7. Neurotransmitters. 8. Motor end plate.

Page 452 **Structure of a Neuron**
1. Dendrites. 2. Cell body. 3. Nucleus. 4. Axon hillock. 5. Node of Ranvier. 6. Myelin sheath. 7. Axon. 8. Synapses with another neuron. 9. Collateral branch. 10. Synapses with muscle fibers. 11. Nucleus of Schwann cell.

Page 452 **Types of Neuroglial Cells**
1. Capillary. 2. Astrocytes. 3. Microglial cell. 4. Cilia. 5. Ependymal cells. 6. Oligodendrocyte. 7. Nerve fiber. 8. Myelin sheath. 9. Schwann cell.

Page 453 **Central and Peripheral Nervous Systems**
1. Cerebrum. 2. Brainstem. 3. Cerebellum. 4. Medulla oblongata. 5. Spinal cord. 6. Nerve. 7. Dorsal root ganglion. 8. Afferent nerve. 9. Efferent nerve to muscle. 10. Action potential (impulse propagation). 11. Muscle fibers. 12. Muscle fiber. 13. Neurotransmitters.

Page 453 **Myelinated Axon of the Peripheral Nervous System**
1. Node of Ranvier. 2. Neurolemma (sheath of Schwann cell). 3. Nucleus of Schwann cell. 4. Myelin sheath. 5. Plasma membrane of axon. 6. Neurofibrils.

Page 453 **Convergence of Neurons**
1. Cell body of postsynaptic neuron. 2. Axon of postsynaptic neuron. 3. Axon of presynaptic neuron.

Page 453 **Divergence of Neurons**
1. Axon of presynaptic neuron. 2. Cell body of postsynaptic neuron. 3. Axon of postsynaptic neuron.

Page 454 **Three Types of Fibrous Joints**
1. Bone. 2. Fibrous tissue. 3. Radius. 4. Ulna. 5. Interosseus membrane. 6. Parietal bone. 7. Frontal bone. 8. Coronal suture. 9. Coronal suture. 10. Periodontal ligament. 11. Root (of tooth).

Page 454 **Two Types of Cartilaginous Joints**
1. Ribs. 2. Costal cartilages. 3. Sternum. 4. Sternocostal joint. 5. Growth plate. 6. Bone. 7. Symphysis pubis. 8. Intervertebral disc.

Page 455 Structure of a Typical Synovial Joint
1. Bone. 2. Periosteum. 3. Blood vessel. 4. Nerve. 5. Articular cartilage. 6. Joint cavity. 7. Fibrous joint capsule. 8. Articular cartilage. 9. Synovial membrane.

Page 455 Various Types of Synovial Joints
1. Pivot joint (uniaxial). 2. Hinge joint (uniaxial). 3. Condyloid joint (biaxial). 4. Saddle joint (biaxial). 5. Ball and socket joint (triaxial). 6. Gliding joint (nonaxial).

Page 456 Diagram of the Skin
1. Hair shaft. 2. Stratum corneum. 3. Stratum granulosum. 4. Stratum germinativum. 4a. Stratum spinosum. 4b. Stratum basale. 5. Dermal papilla. 6. Tactile (Meissner) corpuscle. 7. Sebaceous (oil) gland. 8. Hair follicle. 9. Papilla of hair. 10. Cutaneous nerve. 11. Openings of sweat ducts. 12. Epidermis. 13. Dermis. 14. Subcutaneous layer (hypodermis). 15. Sweat gland. 16. Artery. 17. Vein. 18. Arrector pili muscle. 19. Pacinian corpuscle (joint receptor).

Page 456 Glands of the Skin
1. Epidermis. 2. Dermis. 3. Subcutaneous layer (hypodermis). 4. Hair follicle. 5. Sebaceous (oil) gland. 6. Eccrine sweat gland (in subcutaneous tissue). 7. Apocrine sweat gland (in dermis).

Page 457 Hair Follicle
Left Illustration
1. Dermal root sheath. 2. External epithelial root sheath. 3. Internal epithelial root sheath. 4. Germinal matrix. 5. Papilla. 6. Artery. 7. Vein. 8. Hair shaft. 9. Medulla. 10. Cortex. 11. Cuticle. 12. Hair root. 13. Arrector pili muscle. 14. Sebaceous (oil) gland. 15. Hair bulb. 16. Fat.

Right Illustration
1. Germinal matrix (growth zone). 2. Papilla. 3. Hair follicle. 3a. Medulla. 3b. Cortex. 3c. Cuticle. 4. Hair follicle wall. 4a. Dermal root sheath. 4b. External epithelial root sheath. 4c. Internal epithelial root sheath. 5. Melanocyte. 6. Stratum basale. 7. Basement membrane.

Page 457 Structure of a Nail
1. Free edge. 2. Nail body. 3. Lunula. 4. Cuticle. 5. Nail root. 6. Stratum germinativum. 7. Stratum granulosum. 8. Stratum corneum. 9. Nail body. 10. Cuticle. 11. Nail root. 12. Nail matrix. 13. Nail bed.

Page 458 Anterior View of the Heart
1. Superior vena cava. 2. Pulmonary trunk. 3. Right pulmonary veins. 4. Auricle of right atrium. 5. Right coronary artery. 6. Right cardiac vein. 7. Right ventricle. 8. Aorta. 9. Auricle of left atrium. 10. Left pulmonary veins. 11. Great cardiac vein. 12. Anterior interventricular branch of left coronary artery. 13. Left ventricle. 14. Apex.

Page 458 Posterior View of the Heart
1. Left pulmonary artery. 2. Left pulmonary veins. 3. Auricle of left atrium. 4. Left atrium. 5. Great cardiac vein. 6. Posterior artery of left ventricle. 7. Left ventricle. 8. Apex. 9. Aorta. 10. Superior vena cava. 11. Right pulmonary artery. 12. Right pulmonary veins. 13. Right atrium. 14. Inferior vena cava. 15. Coronary sinus. 16. Posterior interventricular branch of right coronary artery. 17. Middle cardiac vein. 18. Right ventricle.

Page 459 Anterior View of the Interior Heart
1. Superior vena cava. 2. Right pulmonary arteries. 3. Pulmonic valve. 4. Right pulmonary veins. 5. Right atrium. 6. Tricuspid (AV) valve. 7. Right ventricle. 8. Inferior vena cava. 9. Trabeculae carneae. 10. Aorta (thoracic). 11. Aorta (arch). 12. Pulmonary trunk. 13. Left pulmonary arteries. 14. Cut edge of pericardium. 15. Left pulmonary veins. 16. Left atrium. 17. Aortic valve. 18. Mitral (left AV) valve. 19. Chordae tendineae. 20. Papillary muscle. 21. Left ventricle. 22. Interventricular septum.

Page 459 Systemic and Pulmonic Circulations of the Heart
1. Systemic capillaries. 2. Right lung. 3. Left lung. 4. Systemic capillaries. 5. Pulmonary capillaries. 6. Pulmonary capillaries.

Page 460 Major Veins of the Body
1. Right internal jugular. 2. Right external jugular. 3. Right brachiocephalic. 4. Axillary. 5. Cephalic. 6. Basilic. 7. Brachial. 8. Median cubital. 9. Ulnar. 10. Radial. 11. Popliteal. 12. Small saphenous. 13. Anterior tibial. 14. Fibular. 15. Posterior tibial. 16. Left external jugular. 17. Left internal jugular. 18. Vertebral. 19. Subclavian. 20. Left brachiocephalic. 21. Superior vena cava. 22. Inferior vena cava. 23. Hepatic. 24. Splenic. 25. Hepatic portal. 26. Renal. 27. Inferior mesenteric. 28. Superior mesenteric. 29. Gonadal. 30. Common iliac. 31. Internal iliac. 32. External iliac. 33. Femoral. 34. Great saphenous.

Page 461 Venous Drainage of the Brain
1. Straight sinus. 2. Transverse sinus. 3. Occipital sinus. 4. Sigmoid sinus. 5. Superior petrosal sinus. 6. Inferior petrosal sinus. 7. Internal jugular vein. 8. Superior sagittal sinus. 9. Inferior sagittal sinus. 10. Cavernous sinus. 11. Ophthalmic veins. 12. Facial vein.

Page 461 Creation of Venous Blood Flow From Capillaries
1. Artery. 2. Arterioles. 3. Capillaries. 4. Venules. 5. Vein.

Page 461 Unidirectional Venous Valves
1. Normal vein/normal (unidirectional) valve. 2. Varicose vein/incompetent (leaky) valve.

Page 462 Major Organs of the Lymphatic System
1. Right lymphatic duct draining into right subclavian vein. 2. Axillary nodes. 3. Cisterna chyli. 4. Inguinal nodes. 5. Palatine tonsils. 6. Cervical nodes. 7. Thoracic duct draining into left subclavian vein. 8. Thymus. 9. Thoracic duct. 10. Spleen. 11. Area drained by right lymphatic duct. 12. Area drained by thoracic duct.

Page 462 Role of Lymphatic Capillary in Draining Intercellular Fluid
1. Arteriole (from the heart). 2. Intercellular fluid. 3. Blood capillary. 4. Lymphatic capillary. 5. Venule (to the heart). 6. Tissue cells. 7. Lymph fluid (to veins).

Page 462 Lymphatic Capillary Structure
1. Overlapping endothelial cells. 2. Fluid entering lymphatic capillary. 3. Direction of flow. 4. Valve closed. 5. Valve open. 6. Anchoring fibers.

Page 463 Lymph Node Structure
1. Capsule. 2. Medullary cords. 3. Medullary sinus. 4. Hilus. 5. Afferent lymph vessels. 6. Lymph. 7. Sinuses. 8. Germinal center. 9. Cortical nodules. 10. Trabeculae. 11. Efferent lymph vessel. 12. Venules. 13. Arteriole.

Page 463 Role of a Lymph Node in a Skin Infection
1. Site of infection. 2. Afferent lymph vessel. 3. Lymph node. 4. Efferent lymph vessel. 5. Venule. 6. Arteriole.

Page 464 Structures of the Respiratory System
Upper tract
1. Nasal cavity. 2. Pharynx. 3. Larynx.

Lower tract
4. Trachea. 5. Primary bronchus. 6. Lung. 7. Bronchiole. 8. Pulmonary vein. 9. Pulmonary artery. 10. Alveolar duct. 11. Alveolus.

Page 465 Lobes of the Lungs
1. Right upper lobe. 2. Major (oblique) fissure. 3. Horizontal (minor) fissure. 4. Right middle lobe. 5. Right lower lobe. 6. Left upper lobe. 7. Lingula. 8. Oblique fissure. 9. Left lower lobe.

Page 465 Bronchi of the Lungs
1. Trachea. 2. Right primary bronchus. 3. Left primary bronchus. 4. Segmental bronchi. 5. Lobar bronchi.

Page 465 Bronchiole and Alveoli
1. Bronchiole. 2. Pleura. 3. Alveolus.

Page 466 Anterior View of the Structures of the Urinary System
1. Kidney. 2. Aorta. 3. Ureter. 4. Bladder. 5. Urethra. 6. Inferior vena cava.

Page 467 Right Lateral View of the Bladder and Urethra of a Male
1. Pubis. 2. Penile urethra. 3. Penis. 4. Bladder. 5. Prostate. 6. Prostatic urethra. 7. Membranous urethra. 8. Scrotum. 9. Navicular fossa.

Page 467 Section Through a Kidney
1. Cortical arteries and veins. 2. Interlobar arteries and veins. 3. Segmental arteries and veins. 4. Renal artery. 5. Renal vein. 6. Ureter. 7. Lobar arteries and veins. 8. Renal pyramid. 9. Arcuate arteries and veins.

Page 467 Structures of a Nephron
1. Efferent arteriole. 2. Distal convoluted tubule. 3. Collecting tubule. 4. Papilla of pyramid. 5. Afferent arteriole. 6. Proximal convoluted tubule. 7. Glomerulus. 8. Descending limb of loop of Henle. 9. Ascending limb of loop of Henle. 10. Loop of Henle.

Page 468 Structures of the Gastrointestinal System
1. Oral cavity. 2. Salivary glands. 3. Liver. 4. Gall bladder. 5. Duodenum (small intestine). 6. Hepatic flexure (large intestine). 7. Ascending colon (large intestine). 8. Ileum (small intestine). 9. Cecum (large intestine). 10. Appendix. 11. Palate. 12. Uvula. 13. Pharynx. 14. Tongue. 15. Esophagus. 16. Common bile duct. 17. Stomach. 18. Splenic flexure (large intestine). 19. Pancreas. 20. Transverse colon (large intestine). 21. Jejunum (small intestine). 22. Descending colon (large intestine). 23. Sigmoid colon (large intestine). 24. Rectum (large intestine). 25. Anus.

Page 469 Accessory Organs of the Gastrointestinal System
1. Corpus (body) of gall bladder. 2. Neck of gall bladder. 3. Cystic duct. 4. Liver. 5. Lesser duodenal papilla. 6. Greater duodenal papilla. 7. Duodenum. 8. Sphincter muscles. 9. Right and left hepatic ducts. 10. Common hepatic duct. 11. Common bile duct. 12. Pancreas. 13. Pancreatic duct. 14. Superior mesenteric vein. 15. Superior mesenteric artery.

Page 469 Divisions of the Large Intestine
1. Hepatic flexure. 2. Ascending colon. 3. Cecum. 4. Appendix. 5. Anal canal. 6. Transverse colon. 7. Splenic flexure. 8. Descending colon. 9. Terminal ileum. 10. Sigmoid colon. 11. Rectum.

Page 469 Section Through the Abdominopelvic Cavity
1. Diaphragm. 2. Liver. 3. Stomach. 4. Transverse colon. 5. Greater omentum. 6. Mesentery of small intestine. 7. Small intestine. 8. Uterus. 9. Urinary bladder. 10. Symphysis pubis. 11. Lesser omentum. 12. Pancreas. 13. Duodenum. 14. Retroperitoneal space. 15. Sigmoid colon. 16. Rectum.

Page 470 Organization of the Immune System

1. Bronchial-associated lymphoid tissues. 2. Thymus. 3. Spleen. 4. Liver. 5. Gut-associated lymphoid tissues. 6. Appendix. 7. Tonsils. 8. Lymph nodes (cervical, thoracic, and axillary). 9. Lymph nodes (inguinal).

Page 470 Creation of B Cells and T Cells by the Bone Marrow

1. T cell. 2. Red bone marrow. 3. Thymus. 4. Lymph node. 5. B cell. 6. T cell.

Page 470 Activation and Effects of T Cells

1. Antigen. 2. T cell activated. 3. Cytotoxic T cells. 4. T memory cells. 5. Target cell. 6. Cytotoxic T cell. 7. Lysis.

Page 471 Actions of Antibodies

1. Inactivates antigen. 2. Binds antigens together. 3. Facilitates phagocytosis. 4. Antigen. 5. Antibody. 6. Phagocytic body cell. 7. Mast cell. 8. Activates complement cascade. 9. Initiates release of inflammatory chemicals.

Page 471 Action of Antibody-Activated Complement and Death of Bacterial Cell

1. Complement. 2. Bacterial cell.

Page 471 Types of Antibodies (Immunoglobulins)

1. IgM. 2. IgG. 3. IgA. 4. IgE. 5. IgD.

Page 472 The Major Endocrine Glands of the Body

1. Pineal. 2. Parathyroids (on posterior surface of thyroid gland). 3. Testes (male). 4. Hypothalamus. 5. Pituitary. 6. Thyroid. 7. Thymus. 8. Adrenals. 9. Pancreas. 10. Ovaries (female).

Page 472 The Thyroid Gland

1. Thyroid cartilage. 2. Right lobe. 3. Isthmus. 4. Left lobe. 5. Trachea.

Page 472 The Adrenal Gland

1. Adrenal gland. 2. Kidney. 3. Adrenal cortex. 4. Adrenal medulla.

Page 473 The Hypothalamus and Pituitary Hormones

1. Hypothalamic nerve cell. 2. Bone. 3. Growth hormone (GH). 4. Anterior pituitary. 5. Adrenal cortex. 6. Adrenocorticotropic hormone (ACTH). 7. Thyroid gland. 8. Thyroid-stimulating hormone (TSH). 9. Gonadotropic hormones (FSH and LH). 10. Testis. 11. Ovary. 12. Prolactin (PRL). 13. Posterior pituitary. 14. Antidiuretic hormone (ADH). 15. Kidney tubules. 16. Oxytocin (OT). 17. Uterus smooth muscle. 18. Mammary glands. 19. Mammary glands.

Page 473 The Pancreas

1. Duodenum. 2. Common bile duct. 3. Head of pancreas. 4. Pancreatic duct. 5. Tail of pancreas.

Page 474 Somatic and Stretch Receptors

1. Free nerve endings. 2. Krause's end bulb. 3. Pacinian corpuscle. 4. Merkel endings (Merkel's disc). 5. Meissner's corpuscle. 6. Ruffini's corpuscle (Ruffini ending). 7. Tendon. 8. Muscle fibers (extrafusal fibers). 9. Muscle spindle fibers (intrafusal fibers). 9a. Nuclear bag fibers. 9b. Nuclear chain fibers. 10. Neuromuscular spindle. 11. Type Ib sensory fiber. 12. Golgi tendon organ. 13. Capsule. 14. Perimysium of muscle fasciculus. 15. Gamma motor neuron. 16. Connective tissue capsule. 17. Type II sensory ending. 18. Type IA sensory endings. 19. Type II sensory ending. 20. Alpha motor neuron.

Page 474 Superior View of a Horizontal Section of the Eye

1. Fovea centralis. 2. Optic nerve. 3. Optic disc. 4. Retina. 5. Choroid. 6. Sclera. 7. Ciliary body. 8. Suspensory ligament. 9. Cornea. 10. Lens. 11. Pupil. 12. Anterior cavity (filled with aqueous humor). 13. Iris. 14. Posterior cavity (filled with vitreous humor). 15. Conjuctiva. 16. Extraocular muscles.

Page 475 External, Middle, and Internal Ear

1. External ear. 2. Middle ear cavity. 3. Inner ear. 4. Auricle (pinna). 5. Temporal bone. 6. External auditory meatus. 7. Tympanic membrane. 8. Semicircular canals. 9. Auditory ossicles. 10. Malleus. 11. Incus. 12. Stapes. 13. Oval window. 14. Facial nerve (CN VII). 15. Acoustic nerve (vestibulocochlear nerve) (CN VIII). 16. Vestibular nerve (CN VIII). 17. Cochlear nerve (CN VIII). 18. Cochlea. 19. Vestibule. 20. Round window. 21. Auditory (Eustacian) tube.

Page 476 Lateral View of the Internal Nose

1. Olfactory tract. 2. Temporal lobe – Olfactory cortex. 3. Olfactory bulb. 4. Olfactory epithelium. 5. Nasal cavity. 6. Mucous layer. 7. Cilia of receptor cell. 8. Odor molecule. 9. Cell body of olfactory neuron. 10. Supporting cells. 11. Cribiform plate of ethmoid bone.

Page 476 Dorsal Surface of the Tongue, Cross Section Through a Papilla and a Taste Bud

1. Palatine tonsil. 2. Circumvallate papillae. 3. Lingual tonsil. 4. Taste buds. 5. Gustatory cell. 6. Oral epithelium. 7. Nerve fibers. 8. Supporting cell.

Page 477 Male Reproductive Organs

1. Rectum. 2. Seminal vesicle. 3. Levator ani muscle. 4. Ejaculatory duct. 5. Anus. 6. Bulbocavernosus muscle. 7. Urinary bladder. 8. Symphysis pubis. 9. Prostate gland. 10. Corpus cavernosum. 11. Corpus spongiosum. 12. Urethra. 13. Testis. 14. Glans penis.

Page 477 Male Perineum

1. Location of symphysis pubis. 2. Urogenital triangle. 3. Anal triangle. 4. Location of ischial tuberosity. 5. Anus. 6. Location of coccyx.

Page 477 Tubules of the Testis and Epididymis

1. Nerves and blood vessels (vas afferens) in the spermatic cord. 2. Ductus (vas) deferens. 3. Epididymis. 4. Efferent ductules. 5. Seminiferous tubules. 6. Testis. 7. Rete testis. 8. Tunica albuginea. 9. Lobule. 10. Septum.

Page 478 Female Reproductive Organs

1. Sacral promontory. 2. Fallopian (uterine) tube. 3. Ureter. 4. Sacrouterine ligament. 5. Posterior cul-de-sac (of Douglas). 6. Cervix. 7. Fornix of vagina. 8. Anus. 9. Vagina. 10. Ovarian ligament. 11. Body of uterus. 12. Fundus of uterus. 13. Round ligament. 14. Anterior cul-de-sac. 15. Parietal peritoneum. 16. Urinary bladder. 17. Symphysis pubis. 18. Uretha. 19. Clitoris. 20. Labium minora. 21. Labium majora.

Page 478 Female Perineum

1. Mons pubis (without pubic hair). 2. Prepuce. 3. Labia minora. 4. Hymen. 5. Vestibule. 6. Labia majora (without pubic hair). 7. Perineal body. 8. Anus. 9. Clitoris. 10. Orifice of urethra. 11. Orifice of vagina. 12. Opening of greater vestibular gland. 13. Urogenital triangle. 14. Anal triangle.

Page 478 Anterior View of Female Reproductive Organs

1. Fundus. 2. Corpus. 3. Fimbriae. 4. Ovary. 5. Uterus. 6. Bartholin's gland. 7. Fallopian (uterine) tube. 8. Ovum. 9. Graafian follicle. 10. Perimetrium. 11. Endometrium. 12. Myometrium. 13. Cervix. 14. Vagina.

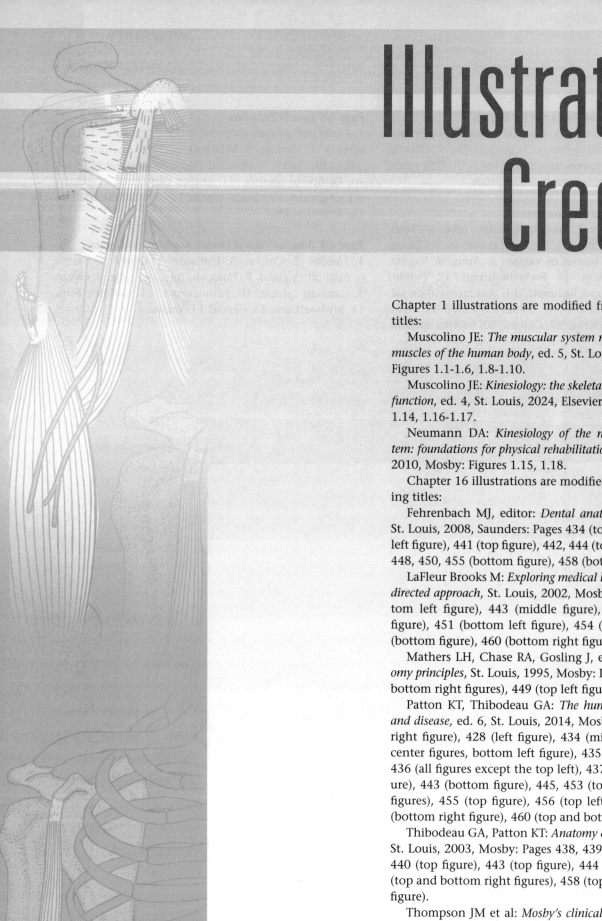

Illustration Credits

Chapter 1 illustrations are modified from the following titles:

Muscolino JE: *The muscular system manual: the skeletal muscles of the human body*, ed. 5, St. Louis, 2024, Elsevier: Figures 1.1-1.6, 1.8-1.10.

Muscolino JE: *Kinesiology: the skeletal system and muscle function*, ed. 4, St. Louis, 2024, Elsevier: Figures 1.7, 1.11-1.14, 1.16-1.17.

Neumann DA: *Kinesiology of the musculoskeletal system: foundations for physical rehabilitation*, ed. 2, St. Louis, 2010, Mosby: Figures 1.15, 1.18.

Chapter 16 illustrations are modified from the following titles:

Fehrenbach MJ, editor: *Dental anatomy coloring book*, St. Louis, 2008, Saunders: Pages 434 (top figure), 435 (top left figure), 441 (top figure), 442, 444 (top left figure), 446, 448, 450, 455 (bottom figure), 458 (bottom figure).

LaFleur Brooks M: *Exploring medical language: a student-directed approach*, St. Louis, 2002, Mosby: Pages 426 (bottom left figure), 443 (middle figure), 447 (bottom left figure), 451 (bottom left figure), 454 (right figures), 456 (bottom figure), 460 (bottom right figure).

Mathers LH, Chase RA, Gosling J, et al: *Clinical anatomy principles*, St. Louis, 1995, Mosby: Pages 447 (top and bottom right figures), 449 (top left figure).

Patton KT, Thibodeau GA: *The human body in health and disease,* ed. 6, St. Louis, 2014, Mosby: Pages 427 (top right figure), 428 (left figure), 434 (middle row left and center figures, bottom left figure), 435 (top right figure), 436 (all figures except the top left), 437, 439 (top left figure), 443 (bottom figure), 445, 453 (top and bottom left figures), 455 (top figure), 456 (top left figure), 457, 459 (bottom right figure), 460 (top and bottom left figures).

Thibodeau GA, Patton KT: *Anatomy & physiology*, ed. 5, St. Louis, 2003, Mosby: Pages 438, 439 (top right figure), 440 (top figure), 443 (top figure), 444 (right figure), 451 (top and bottom right figures), 458 (top figures), 459 (top figure).

Thompson JM et al: *Mosby's clinical nursing*, ed. 4, St. Louis, 1997, Mosby: Page 452 (top figure).